D0932279

DATE DUE

OCT 0 7 '04			
DC 08 '07			

617.89
F2295

DISCARD

Farley, Cynthia
Bridge to sound with a
'Bionic' ear

B.J. Harrison Library
Marshalltown Community College
Iowa Valley Community College District
Marshalltown, Iowa 50158

DEMCO

Bridge to Sound with a 'Bionic' Ear

By Cynthia Farley

IVCCD Libraries

MCC B.J. Harrison Library
Marshalltown, Iowa 50158

Published by Periscope Press

3030 Westwood Rd. Suite 102
Wayzata, MN 55391

Copyright © 2002 Cynthia Farley All rights reserved. No part of this publication may be reproduced, stored in a retrieval system, or transmitted in any form or by any means, electronic, mechanical, photocopying, recording, or otherwise without the prior written permission of the publisher.

For information on bulk purchases, corporate sales, or academic sales please contact the Special Sales Dept. at: Periscope Press 3030 Westwood Rd. Suite 102 Wayzata, MN 55391 (952) 471-3442

ISBN 0-9718546-0-2
LCCN 2002106538

   Farley, Cynthia.
      Bridge to sound with a 'bionic' ear / by Cynthia
   Farley.--1st ed.
   p. cm.
   Includes index.
   LCCN 2002106538
   ISBN 0-9718546-0-2
      1. Cochlear implants—Popular works. 2. Deaf-
   Rehabilitation. 3. Hearing impaired—Rehabilitation.
   I Title.
   RF305.F37 2002   617.8'9
                  QB102-200606

Printed and bound in the United States of America.

This book is intended to provide accurate information with regard to the subject matter covered. However the author and publisher accept no responsibility for inaccuracies or omissions, and the author and publisher specifically disclaim any liability, loss or risk, whether personal, financial, or otherwise, that is incurred directly or indirectly from the use and or application of any of the contents of this book. Readers are cautioned to consult with a physician should they have health concerns. No book can substitute for professional care or advice. The author and publisher are not engaged in rendering medical services.

I wish to dedicate this book to the 4,000 babies that are born deaf every year in America as well as the 12,000 babies who will leave the hospital with undetected hearing loss. Hearing loss is the #1 birth defect in America today. This tragedy could be eased and these childeren could have the opportunity for better hearing with assistive devices, if hearing screening programs were in place in all hospitals nationwide. There has been progress, however to date only 69% of all hospitals perform newborn hearing screening, causing far too many children to fall between the cracks with undetected hearing loss. For more information about hearing loss please visit: www.hearthisorg.com

Acknowledgements

While there are many people I wish to thank for their help, first and foremost, I want to thank those folks who took the time to share their stories. In doing so, they will make a difference in the lives of many people who read this book and will hopefully, be inspired by their experiences. The evolution of *Bridge to Sound* began when I was at crossroads about which path to take next in my life. I wanted to go in a new direction, one that had meaning, and would enable me to use my talents, energy, and experience to reach out to other people with hearing loss. Spreading the word about the wonderful benefits of cochlear implants is the path I've chosen!

I would like to thank the following individuals and organizations for their support and encouragement:

My physicians, Dr. Charles Luetje and Dr. Robert Schindler, who gave me a new lease on life via my cochlear implant, which in turn gave, me something to write about. You changed my life forever, as well as the lives of many others with your skills, and I honestly can't think of a better legacy than that.

Mardie Younglof for her friendship and mentoring as well as the excellent editing skills she brought to this project. She approached me in an email after reading a flyer about the book project and kindly offered her help. (Little did she know the work that it entailed or she might not have signed up so eagerly!)

The wonderful folks from Advanced Bionics, Cochlear Corporation and MedEl Corporation, who loved the idea for this book from the start and helped nurture it along. I will always be grateful for your encouragement and assistance.

All the organizations who so generously shared their press releases, studies, and news reports so that readers could have a one-stop-shopping experience in their desire to learn about the cochlear implant technology that enables the deaf to hear.

I also wish to thank my freelance graphic designers Heather Johnson and Katie Sonmor for their wonderful creativity. And I would be remiss if I didn't mention my teacher who helped me learn desktop publishing so I could put it all together; thanks, Nancy Wagner!

I also want to thank my husband Doug, as well as my parents Don and Velma for their love and support, as well as the endless hours spent reading and critiquing this book! I also want to give honorable mention to my wonderful son Zachary who is so patient and understanding with his mom's hearing loss. You are my sunshine, your good humor is so delightful, and you are the source of my inspiration.

INTRODUCTION

PERSONAL REFLECTIONS ON COCHLEAR IMPLANTS

R0BERT A. SCHINDLER, MD

SAN FRANCISCO, CALIFORNIA

Cochlear implants represent a classic example of a "scientific revolution." According to Kuhn, scientific disciplines undergo periods of "normal science" in which they obtain a high degree of precision and progress rapidly. Normal science is dependent on the adoption of a universally accepted paradigm that defines research problems for the scientist and provides the methods that should be applied to solve them. However, in the course of research, scientists inevitably stumble upon anomalies in the existing paradigm. Eventually, a competing theory proves relatively successful in explaining the anomaly, and the old paradigm is modified and replaced with a new paradigm. It is this process that defines "scientific revolution." Initially, the scientific community resists the replacement, but with time and successful application, the new paradigms gain enough support to win acceptance. In turn, the new paradigm creates new research questions, new methodologies, and new results.

To understand the nature of the scientific revolution that cochlear implants exemplify, we need to return to the early 1970s. In June 1973, a meeting was held at the University of California San Francisco (UCSF) entitled "First International Conference on Electrical Stimulation of the Acoustic Nerve as a treatment for Profound Sensorineural Deafness in Man." It was the first scientific gathering ever held to discuss cochlear implants. Prior to this conference, the public, the deaf community, and most physicians were largely unaware of these devices. Auditory physiologists and histopathologists dismissed them as misguided attempts by surgeons - who knew little or nothing about auditory neuroscience - to stimulate nerves that were already dead. Further, if they were not dead prior to inserting electrodes into the cochlea, they were certain to be dead after implantation. Ingrained in the scientific orthodoxy of the time was the belief that if cochlear hair cells died, then neurons also would necessarily degenerate.

Before the 1973 meeting, only one publication suggested that co-chlear implant systems could be built reliably for humans and provide useful sound sensations to deaf patients. By the time of the conference, House and Urban reported that their single-channel implant system was providing useful hearing to profoundly deaf subjects. Despite those reports, Merle Lawrence, PhD, then head of the Kresge Hearing Research Institute at the University of Michigan, summarized the prevailing attitudes of the scientific community when he stated that it would be impossible for a cochlear implant to replicate the complexities of the organ of Corti in order to produce speech understanding. "Regardless of the number of channels or electrode points, normal frequency specificity cannot be achieved. In other words, frequency-specific stimulation, regardless of the number of electrodes or their location within the cochlea, could never be accomplished. All that would be produced, he reasoned, would be noise, and even then, the dynamic range was liable to be extremely limited. Harold Schuknecht, MD, Professor and Chairman of the Department of Otolaryngology at Harvard and a noted cochlear histopathologist, was more direct when he stated, "I will admit that we need a new operation in otology, but I am afraid this is not it.

In spite of this prevailing attitude, cochlear implant research and development continued among small groups of investigators that were active at the time of the 1973 conference. They included Robin Michelson, Michael Merzenich, myself, and our associates at UCSF; William Home and Jack Urban at the House Ear Institute in Los Angeles; F Blair Simmons and Robert White at Stanford University; Donald Eddington at the University of Utah; Henri Chouard in France; and Graeme Clark in Australia. Other than these few physicians and scientists, the emerging cochlear implant technology was either ignored or dismissed as unlikely to produce a useful hearing device.

The dismissal of cochlear implants had its basis in historical events. Ever since 1800, when Volta reported that passing an electrical current through the ears caused an audible sound, scientists had hoped to use electricity to restore hearing. Little happened until 2 classic experiments were reported in the early part of this century. In 1925, radio engineers discovered the "electrophonic hearing" effect, noting that sound could be produced by electrically stimulating electrodes in the near vicinity of the ear. This report was followed in 1930 by one of the most exciting experiments in the history of auditory neuroscience. Wever and Bray accidentally discovered that researchers speaking near an anesthetized cat's ear could be distinctly heard on a loud-speaker in an adjoining room via an electrode surgically placed on the auditory nerve. They had discovered a phenomenon known as the "cochlear microphonic," an electrical potential arising from the cochlea as a result of acoustic stimulation. Their discovery gave rise to the hypothesis that the transmission of sound from the cochlea to the brain was analogous to a telephone, with the cochlear hair cells responsible for converting sound into an electrical analog that traveled along the auditory nerve to the brain.

Even though the hypothesis was eventually proven incorrect, Wever and Bray's findings suggested to some scientists that there was a possibility that hearing could be restored by stimulating the eighth nerve with an electrical analog of sound. Djourno and Eyries published the first data on direct stimulation of the auditory nerve in a totally deaf person in the mid1950s. During a reoperation for facial paralysis in a 50-year-old man who had undergone a radical mastoidectomy for cholesteatoma that had destroyed the cochlea, an inductively coupled electrode was placed into the stump of the remaining nerve and a current was delivered via a primitive speech processor. The patient heard sounds like "crickets" or a "roulette wheel." This research report attracted the attention of several surgeons in the United States and prompted them to investigate the feasibility of producing a device that would allow the profoundly deaf to hear. These surgeons included Drs James Doyle, William House, F. Blair Simmons, and Robin P. Michelson, each working in California at 3 independent facilities.

In 1961, William House and James Doyle designed a few implantable cochlear stimulating devices based on the work of the scientists at Massachusetts Institute of Technology and in the Soviet Union, and tested them in human patients. Due to limited understanding regarding the construction of an electronic implant, leakage and the toxic nature of some of the implant materials, they were forced to remove the devices after several weeks when the implant sites became inflamed. Nevertheless, House and Doyle's initial results indicated that patients could perceive the rhythm of speech and music and were aware of a variety of environmental sounds. Unfortunately, the technical difficulties they encountered reinforced the scientific belief that attempts to build a useful cochlear implant were doomed to fail.

The failure of the Doyle device was followed by an extensive assessment of the feasibility of cochlear implantation. At Stanford University, F. Blair Simmons placed an electrode into the modiolus of the cochlea of a terminally ill, congenitally deaf patient and demonstrated that the patient could perceive some sound when stimulated. Disappointed that the patient could not understand speech, Simmons stated that the chances were small that electrical stimulation of the auditory nerve could ever provide a useful means of communication. Negative opinions of cochlear implants were once again reinforced.

When Robin Michelson presented and published data on the first successful series of patients implanted with a single-channel cochlear implant, the prevailing negative views were dispelled and the scientific revolution truly was launched. Michelson obtained independent grant funding from the Department of Defense and brought his cochlear implant program to UCSF. He believed that a transcutaneous implanted receiver, with bipolar electrodes placed in the scala tympani close to the modiolus, would provide the best chance of delivering electrical signals to the auditory neurons. He tested preliminary devices in animals and became convinced that there was a real possibility of restoring hearing if the cochlear microphonic could be simulated. By the late 1960s, with the assistance of Arnold Beckman and Mel Bartz, he had constructed a device with biocompatible materials that could be implanted in human patients. Michelson's cochlear implant system consisted of a single-channel processor that converted speech into an electrical analog that was inductively coupled to an implanted passive receiver and bipolar scala tympani stimulating electrodes. The electrodes were covered in silicone and molded to fit into the basal scala tympani via a cochleostomy anterior to the round window. This system was implanted in 4 patients, and his report of their hearing results represents a watershed for clinically applicable cochlear implants.

The cochlear implant scientific revolution was launched with Robin Michelson's presentation entitled "The Results of Electrical Stimulation of the Cochlea in Human Sensory Deafness" to the American Otological Society, Inc, in May 1971. The discussion of this paper by distinguished members of the scientific establishment details their shock and complete disbelief in Michelson's results. His data were in direct conflict with existing concepts in auditory neuroscience and engendered extreme skepticism. Nonetheless, cochlear implant research and development expanded at UCSF. In 1971, Michael Merzenich and I joined Michelson in his work. Our objective was to understand what, why, and how patients heard with the Michelson implant and then to develop a strategy for building a multichannel system. The ultimate goal was the development of a device that could provide speech understanding to totally deaf patients. A series of animal studies and subsequent human investigations resulted in progressive improvements of a multichannel cochlear implant.

By June 1973, at the time of the First International Conference on Cochlear Implants in San Francisco, House had implanted 12 patients, Michelson and his colleagues had implanted 7 patients (1 still has a functioning unit as of this writing), and Simmons had implanted 2 patients. In spite of the modest initial success reported by each of these 3 groups, as well as by Chouard in France, the application of cochlear implants in deaf patients continued to meet with strong resistance in the scientific community. Scientists had 2 major ethical concerns about human implantation. First, they believed that safety and efficacy data could be obtained from animal experimentation. Second, they believed that the device itself could never work because of extensive and irreversible neural damage present in deaf individuals. In addition to these concerns, extravagant anecdotal. Claims began surfacing in public, including subjective patient testimonials about hearing birds again and enjoying music. This publicity further alienated the scientific community. Cochlear implant researchers were regarded as the pariahs of the academic community.

Undaunted by criticism, William House introduced the first widely applied clinical cochlear implant in 1973. This implant was a single-channel system that was later commercialized and manufactured by 3M and became known as the 3M, House implant. The device was implanted by many surgeons in hundreds of deaf adults and children throughout the world before 3M stopped production. Little progress in implantation would have been made without those pioneering efforts.

Much of the early cochlear implant work was supported by the National Institutes of Health (NIH), whose grants and contract programs facilitated implant development. This funding was encouraged especially by Terry Hambrecht of the then National Institute of Neurological and Communicative Disorders and Stroke, whose vision and belief propelled cochlear implant technology forward to the point at which implant recipients now hear and understand speech. In October 1974, the NIH sponsored a Cochlear Implant Workshop at UCSF to review the status of cochlear implants and to define the requirements for a multichannel device. The NIH not only sponsored basic research, but also was instrumental in developing clinical research programs. Notably, the NIH supported the first independent multicenter study of cochlear implant devices. Led by R. C. Bilger at the University of Pittsburgh, the study concluded that these devices were a definite aid in communication, particularly when combined with lipreading, and were also useful in voice modulation and recognition of environmental sounds. More important, the 1971, study provided substantial scientific evidence for the benefits of cochlear implantation and gave credibility to the emerging technology.

In 1981, 2 groups - Michelson and Schindler at UCSF and Clarke at the University of Melbourne - reported the first useful speech discrimination in cochlear implant patients. It is of note that each group used a different implant device to achieve their results.

In 1983, 10 years after the first conference on cochlear implants, a Tenth Anniversary Conference on Electrical Stimulation of the Ear was held at UCSF. Instead of the skepticism and controversy that permeated the first conference, optimism prevailed. Fourteen active research centers were represented, and over 1,000 devices had been implanted worldwide.

Research and development of cochlear implants has continued. To date, 3 devices have been released by the US Food and Drug Administration for commercial marketing in this country. The first was the 3M House single-channel cochlear implant (initially approved in 1984). The second was the Nucleus 22 channel cochlear implant, approved in 1985 for adults and in 1990 for children. The third was the Clarion Multi-Strategy Cochlear Implant, which was approved for adults in 1995 and for children in 1997. In addition, a fourth cochlear implant system, the Med-El Combi 40+, is undergoing clinical trials. These implant systems are far more sophisticated than those of a decade ago. They accommodate a variety of speech processing strategies and stimulation modes to address the individual needs of hearing-impaired patients.

For physicians interested in the benefits of implantation, the advent of competition in the industry is the most encouraging aspect in the history of cochlear implant development since its initial acceptance as a viable rehabilitative tool. As a co-developer of one of the first successful multichannel devices, I found that the inherent limitations of a university research facility in fabricating a sophisticated cochlear implant device became apparent. Although a university is ideal for testing ideas and developing prototypes, we must turn to industry for the manufacture of safe and reliable human implants. To further advance the fields these companies must have strong engineering expertise and a commitment to research and development. Given these requirements, it is no surprise that the 2 most successful cochlear implant manufacturers evolved from the cardiac pacemaker industry.

The university-based research team often finds it difficult to know when the time has come to give up control of their project, to talk to their office of technology transfer or parent office, and to request assistance in transferring core technology to an outside company. At UCSF in the mid-1980s, we had the assistance of the Storz Instrument Company in building the UCSF/Storz cochlear implant. That cooperative effort provided the opportunity to study multichannel stimulation in 16 patients implanted with that device between 1985 and early 1986. Speech recognition in these patients was very good, but design flaws related to the disconnect system led to direct current leakage in several patients, necessitating discontinuation of the device. It became apparent to both Storz and UCSF that significantly more engineering and financial resources than had been anticipated would be required to commercialize the multichannel system we envisioned.

In October 1985, at the NIH Neural Prosthesis Program meeting held annually in Bethesda, Maryland, UCSF presented data on the Storz patients. There we met Joseph Schulman of the Alfred E. Mann Foundation and explained our acute need for assistance to make the quantum leap from the Storz device to a small, hermetically seated 8-channel system that could handle both analog mid pulsatile stimulation in either bipolar or monopolar modes. Schulman suggested that we present our research to the leadership of a new research and development company, Minimed Technologies, that was headed by Alfred E. Mann, founder of Pacesetter Systems, the second largest cardiac pacemaker manufacturer in the world. Encouraged by his interest, I met with Al Mann and his team in spring 1986 in Sylmar, California, and presented the results achieved with the Storz device. When I showed a videotape of how well 3 of the patients heard with the device, and how they described their experiences, Al was moved to tears. He congratulated us on our work and inquired how much money would be needed to build and launch a new 8-channel system. I responded, "About $10 million." Al said, "Maybe, but I'll bet more." And then he said, "If you can get the university to take a reasonable royalty, I'll fund the project myself - my own money. That way I know it will get done." As I sat on the plane on my return to San Francisco, looking down at the rapidly shrinking San Fernando Valley, I felt my own tears. Finally - after all the struggles, all the failures, and all the false starts - there was someone who could make it happen. Today the Clarion cochlear implant is the result of Al Mann's commitment to his word, to the deaf, and to the dreams of the early cochlear implant pioneers. The papers that follow are a compilation of information and stories about the cochlear implant technology that has revolutionized hearing healthcare for those who are profoundly hearing impaired and unable to benefit from hearing aids. Hopefully, you will be inspired by patients stories as you read of their personal experiences as they gain the ability to hear and communicate.

ACKNOWLEDGMENTS - So many people have contributed to the development and success of cochlear implants it is impossible to mention them all. You know who you are, and the world owes you thanks. But it is Robin Michelson and his great contributions that I wish to acknowledge especially. He was my mentor, colleague, and dear friend for more than 27 years and he deserves credit for giving birth to the cochlear implant revolution that began in May 1971.

Reprinted Courtesy of Annals Publishing Company

Contents

Stories by Teenagers and Twenty-Somethings 167

Adults' Stories 215

Seniors' Stories 335

Resource Guide 427

Index 477

HEAR THIS

Hearing loss is America's invisible disability, affecting approximately 10% of the population—28 million people. Because of it's invisibility it has received little attention from researchers and little funding from public and privite funds. With the advent of the cochlear implant, more attention has been riveted on hearing loss and the terrible ramifications it has on these who are hearing impaired along with their families, friends, and associates. Numerous books have been written about deafness and a few have focused on cochlear implants. This book represents an effort to gather between it's pages information people should know about the cochlear implant technology. Readers will hopefully be encouraged to take action to address their hearing loss and inquire whether a cochlear implant would be the right approach to dealing with the degree of hearing they possess at that time.

Most people with hearing loss tend to wait seven years before seeking help for their hearing loss (source: Self Help for Hard of Hearing Persons, Bethesda, Maryland). They may be in denial or even unaware of technology that can help alleviate the problems caused by their inability to hear well. Information about hearing aids, cochlear implants, assistive listening devices such as flashing or viberating signalers for the home can be hard to obtain if one has no idea where to

1

begin looking for solutions and ways of coping. Internet search engines can bring countless websites to those who possess the necessary skills for scanning the Internet. Yet, not all the information on the Internet is accurate, and this is especially true in the case of cochlear implants, around which intense controversy swirled until the past several years. Reliable information about hearing loss and cochlear implants is now in your hands as you hold this book. We hope you will benefit from the cacophony of voices throughout it's pages.

Let's start with some facts about hearing loss:

- Over 4,000 babies are born deaf every year.
- Over 12,000 infants leave the hospital with undetected hearing loss annually.
- Almost 1/3 of all cases of hearing loss have been caused by loud noise.
- Noise induced hearing loss is the most common work related disability.

These facts do not take into account the human cost of deafness, which is immeasurable. As evident from the experiences recounted in this book, hearing loss affects every dimension of a person's life, as well as those around him or her. It affects marriages, parenting, friendships, dating, the ability to get and hold a job, the ability to aquire information (schools, colleges, classes, seminars, workshops, etc.), and the ability to function into the society which they were born and raised. People with hearing loss commonly experience a myriad of emotions such as depression, loneliness, irritation, frustration, and confusion. How do we add up the tremendous cost to society of hearing loss? How can we put a dollar sign on the impact of hearing loss?

Sensioneural hearing loss, the most common form of hearing loss and one of the most common disabling conditions in America today, can adversely affect one's physical, cognitive, behavioral, and social functioning. It is caused by a problem in the cochlea, the part of the inner ear that enables sound to reach the brain. People with sensorineural hearing loss have experienced a loss in the number of, and/or damage to, the cilia (hair cells) that line the cochlea in the inner ear. The cilia are then unable to properly send signals to the brain, where the signals are intrepreted as sound. For people with severe to profound hearing loss (70 dB to 90 dB), a cochlear implant may be the best means of intervention, often the only solution if they cannot benefit from the most powerful hearing aids.

While cochlear implant technology has been around since the 1970s, it's use took off in the past decade worldwide. Multichannel implants and concomitant improvements in thier design have enabled many implant users to understand speech and, in some cases, talk on the phone. Virtually all are able to discern various types of environmental sounds, such as gushing water, birds chirping, lawnmowers, and cars, etc. Below is an overview of what a cochlear implant is, the evalua-tion process, mapping, and auditory rehabilitation.

What is a cochlear implant?

A cochlear implant is a small electronic device that provides sound to those children and adults who have a severe to profound hearing loss (70db to 90db) who do not benefit from hearing aids. Cochlear im-plants enable sound to reach the brain by effectively bypassing the part of the ear that is damaged, to directly stimulate the hearing nerve electronically. A cochlear implant consists of three parts, of which only one is internal.

1) Receiver- The receiver is surgically implanted beneath the skin above the ear. A wire runs from the receiver, nestled in the mastoid bone, to the cochlea in the inner ear. The part of the wire that is threaded throughout the cochlea, a pea-sized organ that is curved like a snail, contains an array of electrodes. The operation last on average about three hours and is usually performed on an outpatient basis by an otolaryngologist

2) Microphone- Part of the "headpiece" that rests on the outer side of the skin that covers the receiver. The headpiece and receiver each have a magnet that enables each to cling to the other with the skin between them. The microphone then picks up sound in the environment and transmits it to the speech processor.

3) Speech processor- A microcomputer that can be worn behind the ear (it's appearance is similar to a hearing aid) or a body unit, which is worn on a belt or in a pocket. The microphone picks up the incoming sound and sends it via a small wire to the speech processor, which then transmits the signal to the receiver and electrodes, which then stimulate the auditory nerve fibers, which in turn transmit the signal to the brain where it is interpreted as sound. Thus the speech processor interfaces between sound in the environment and the internal implant electronics to send information to the hearing nerve. This process occurs in milliseconds enabling the listener to hear sound as it occurs.

The U.S. Food and Drug Administration (FDA) first approved cochlear implants for the treatment of profoundly deaf adults in 1985 and in 1990 for children. Today, over 70,000 people worldwide use a cochlear implant to hear. (Source: National Institute of Deafness and Communication Disorders January 2002)

You may be a candidate for a cochlear implant if:

Adults :
- Have a severe to profound loss in both ears. (70dB to 90dB or worse) hearing loss in both ears.
- Receive little or no benefit from a hearing aids.
- Have no medical problems that would preclude the procedure or limit it's effectiveness.
- Possess a strong desire to hear and understand speech.

Children 12 months and older may be a candidate if:
- Have a profound hearing loss in both ears. (90dB or more).
- Receive little or no benefit from hearing aids after a three to six month evaluation.
- Have no medical problems that would preclude the procedure or limit it's effectiveness.

Adult's who have lost their hearing later in life often benefit from a cochlear implant, because they have an "auditory memory" of what they were formerly able to hear. This allows them greater speech comprehension. As evident from their stories in this book, the vast majority report a better quality of life after receiving an implant. They also enjoy improved communication with their families, and friends, as well as with the world at large.

Young children may also benefit from implants. Cochlear implants can help them gain speech, language, developmental and social skills. Research is demonstrating that the earlier children are implanted, the more they tend to benefit from this technology.

How can someone learn if they are a candidate for an implant?

The first step is an evaluation at a cochlear implant center. The evaluation process, which is usually spread out over several weeks involves meetings with an audiologist and a otolaryngologist (an ear, nose, and throat specialist who performs cochlear implant surgery). The following steps are generally part of this process:

1) The initial consultation, during which the patient's history is taken.
2) Audiograms, with and without your hearing aid.
3) MRI and/or CT scan
4) Tests for balance/dizziness
5) Promontory stimulation test (done on ocacasion at some centers)

Sometimes a psychological evaluation is part of this process. It's purpose is to determine if a candidate has realistic expectations as to what the implant might do for him/her, and also to determine if there might be underlying emotional problems aside from those connected with hearing loss. Throughout this process candidates can and should ask any questions that come to mind, as well as perform their own research about the various brands of devices available at the center where they will have their surgery and subsequent mappings. Websites where you can begin your research are provided in the "Resource Guide" at the end of this book.

How much does the surgery cost and who pays for it?

As of 2002, the cochlear implant procedure costs on average about $60,000. This includes costs incurred during the evaluation process, all expenses associated with the surgery, the device, and the first year of mappings. Most insurance companies cover the costs and usually pay from 80% to 100% of expenses. Medicare, the Veterans Administration, and Medicaid also pay for the procedure in some states. Other services that may cover the implant are state Vocational Rehabilitation Services, and Children's Special Services.

The Surgery

Today cochlear implant surgery is usually performed on an outpatient basis and lasts about two to three hours. You will usually recover in a hospital room and be released within 24 hours. After the operation, you may be a little weak, nauseous, or have a headache. As with any surgery there are risks and you should discuss those with your cochlear implant surgeon. Side effects occasionally experienced included pain in the incision area and dizziness/veritgo. The dizziness can last from a couple of hours to several weeks.

After the surgery you will follow up with your surgeon, who will check for signs of infection and remove your staples, unless glue or soluable stitches were used. Once the incision is healed, in about four weeks, you will return to the implant center for your big day, the "hook-up".

The Mapping

On the day of "hook-up" (also referred to as "turn on" or "activation"), you will be given the external components of your cochlear implant system by the audiologist who will be working with you. She or he will then begin the process of activation of the device. You will hear a series of beeps at various frequencies and loudness. You will be told to tell the audiologist when you first hear the sound and when it becomes "loud but comfortable" to hear. (A different protocal is used with young children, who are not able to participate in this manner). After the programming session is complete, the audiologist will activate the switch that turns on your processor, and you will hear your first sounds with your new device. This is the good part, where you will suddenly be "on the air".

At first the sounds may sound strange. This is normal and you should expect this. After all, you have probably not heard for some time and your brain needs time and re-mappings to learn to adjust to your new hearing capability. People sometimes describe the initial sound of voices as "quacky," or "Donald Duck-like". Your perception of sounds should quickly improve over the next several months. Some of the sounds you hear initially may sound loud, such as gushing water from a faucet, the rattling of paper or plastic bags, vacuum cleaners, and other noisy machines. Keep notes on what you are hearing and how things sound, what you think you should be hearing but are not, and what sounds good or bad, and bring these notes with you to your next mapping session. Your audiologist will find them invaluable as s/he adjusts your maps to suit your changing auditory pathways. You will have several mapping sessions during the first month after "hook up." After that the frequency of mappings gradually decrease over time to the point that you will need just one or two per year.

Auditory Rehabilitation in Brief

You may want to practice your new listening skills in order to hone your speech discrimination. There are various ways to accomplish this, and you should experiment to see what works well for your particular situation, auditory history, and lifestyle. Many new users listen to children's books on tape reading the book as they listen. They then progress to adolescent materials and then on to adult-level books. Some people say nonfiction tapes are easier to listen to than fiction. There are also English-as-a-second-language tapes you can investigate at your local library. Many CI centers provide rehabilitation for adults, and most children receive auditory training. A good website for "listening practice" is www.esl-lab.com

Telephone use is a goal of many CI users, and an excellent way to achieve this goal is to dail 800 numbers. Job lines, weather/time reports, medical topics provided by insurance companies, and government topics are just a few of the ways you can get phone "therapy." You will also want to practice talking with friends and family in brief conversations. Generally speaking, the more someone practices with the phone, the easier it becomes. In time you will also want to experiment with different telephones to see which ones work well for you.

Music is an area that is highly individual, as you will infer from the stories that follow. The cochlear implant was developed as an aid to speech understanding, but naturally CI users want to enjoy the music they were once familair with. This can take time and remappings. You can also have a program developed specifcally for music enjoyment. You should communicate to your audiologist your thoughts about and perceptions of the music you are listening to, and s/he may be able to help make it a better, more "normal" experience for you. You may discover different types of music and different instruments sound better with your CI than when you had hearing. Be flexible when it comes to listening to music and give yourself time to adjust to hearing with your implant.

In the pages that follow you will find a treasure-trove of ideas and advice from other people who have "been there and done that." Their personal stories, reflecting the experiences of people from all walks of life, will hopefully be a source of inspiration for you and your family. Included also are reprints of various medical reports and news articles pertaining to cochlear implant technology. A resource section appears at the end of the book for those seeking further information which includes a list of cochlear implant centers by state as well as other helpful information. It is my sincere hope that you will gain valuable insight as you undertake your quest for knowledge about this technology that provides new hope and oppurtunities for people with profound hearing loss.

Graphic of Clarion CII Bionic Ear Cochlear Implant System

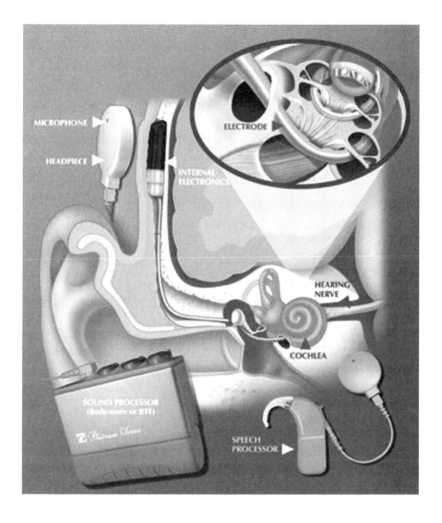

Photo courtesy of Advanced Bionics Corporation

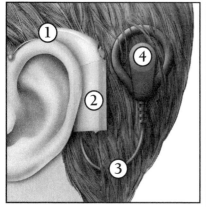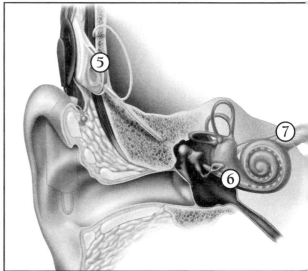

Pictures courtesy of Cochlear Ltd.

The Nucleus® cochlear implant system works in the following manner:

1. Sounds are picked up by the small, directional microphone located in the ear level processor.

2. The speech processor filters, analyzes and digitizes the sound into coded signals.

3. The coded signals are sent from the speech processor to the transmitting coil.

4. The transmitting coil sends the coded signals as FM radio signals to the cochlear implant under the skin.

5. The cochlear implant delivers the appropriate electrical energy to the array of electrodes which has been inserted into the cochlea.

6. The electrodes along the array stimulate the remaining auditory nerve fibers in the cochlea.

7. The resulting electrical sound information is sent through the auditory system to the brain for interpretation.

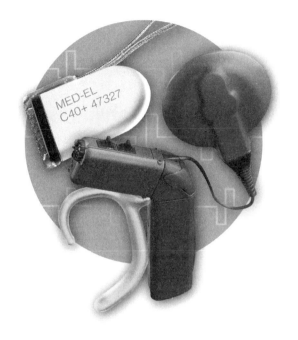

**Graphic of Med-El Cochlear Implant System
provided courtesy of Med-El Corporation**

Supporting Evidence Section

PRESS RELEASE: 29 APRIL 1999
Cochlear Implant Increases Access To
Mainstream Education

Reduces Need For Special Education Support After Two Years

Researchers at Johns Hopkins report that profoundly deaf children receiving a cochlear implant are more apt to be fully mainstreamed in school and use fewer school support services than similarly deaf children without an implant.

Results of the Hopkins-funded study, believed to be the first in the United States to examine the use of special education aids such as speech therapy, interpreters and tutoring in students with a cochlear implant, is published in the May 1 issue of *Archives of Otolaryngology—Head and Neck Surgery.* Specifically, the study showed children who received the implant plus one year of intense auditory and language development training were fully mainstreamed faster, at younger ages and at higher rates than a comparison group without implants. They also were less dependent on special education services after an average of two years. The study additionally placed the cost savings of educating a child receiving an implant at age three at $30,000 to $100,000 over the course of primary and secondary school education.

"The cochlear implant also appears to give children a significant educational advantage," says Howard W. Francis, M.D., assistant professor of otolaryngology—head and neck surgery at Hopkins and lead author of the study. "It offers the possibility for the development of verbal language, which increases the chance of English literacy, and better educational and vocational opportunities."

Francis and his colleagues reviewed the progress of 35 school-age (K-8) children with profound hearing loss. Prior to implantation, 22 attended special education classes full-time in public schools, five attended the Maryland School for the Deaf and eight were in special preschool classes. All received a multi-channel cochlear implant at the Listening Center at Hopkins and underwent one year of comprehensive auditory training and speech rehabilitation.

Following implantation and rehabilitative therapy, the Hopkins team found that during the first two years there was very little change in the children's education status. After two years there was a significant trend toward full-time mainstream placement; after four years, 75 percent of the children were in mainstream classes full-time, relying on an average of only one hour of special education support.

Francis says he'll now focus on how a child's age at the time of diagnosis of hearing loss and age of intervention impact his or her development and educational independence. Other studies will compare the type of intervention (lipreading vs. sign language) used.

"Our first priority is the development of verbal language regardless of the type of intervention," he says. "It appears that the cochlear implant enhances the achievement of this goal."

Francis cautions that their results may not be duplicated everywhere. "These results depend on the kind of rehabilitative training the child receives," he says. "The children in this study have undergone intense, comprehensive rehabilitation here. Many programs differ in their approach to rehab."

The cochlear implant is an electronic assistive listening device surgically implanted within the inner ear to stimulate hearing. Candidates for the cochlear implant have a severe to profound hearing loss (cannot discriminate sound in words and language) and do not benefit from high-powered hearing aids. Cochlear implants have been found to be among the most cost-effective medical procedures, ranking above other medical interventions like coronary artery bypass surgery and cardiac transplantation.

The study's other authors were Mary E. Koch, M.A.; J. Robert Wyatt, M.D., M.B.A.; and John K. Niparko, M.D., all of the Listening Center at Johns Hopkins.

Reprinted Courtesy of John Hopkins Medical Center

Study Finds Cochlear Implants Cost-Effective in Children
August 16, 2000
Technology improves quality of life and saves $50,000+ over child's life.

Researchers at Johns Hopkins report that cochlear implants, electronic devices surgically implanted behind the ear to bring sound to profoundly deaf people, not only improve children's quality of life, but also are highly cost-effective, with an expected lifetime savings of $53,198.

The study, published in the Aug. 16 issue of the *Journal of the American Medical Association* (JAMA), is the first to evaluate the cost of quality-of-life improvements in pediatric cochlear implant patients using U.S. cost data, the authors say.

According to Neil R. Powe, M.D., M.P.H., M.B.A., professor of medicine, epidemiology and health policy and management at Hopkins and one of the study's co-authors, the findings linking quality of life and cost-savings are unusual. "Most new interventions in medical care that improve health also raise the cost. In this case, we've found that when you include all the associated costs and consequences, the implant actually saves society money in the long term," he says. The cost-benefit comes in the form of fewer demands on special education and greater wage-earning opportunities of implant recipients.

Powe and his colleagues conducted a cost-utility analysis, measuring a cochlear implant's effect on quality of life against the costs of the device. They surveyed parents of children with implants, all patients at The Listening Center at Johns Hopkins. The children averaged 7.4 years of age with 1.9 years of implant use. Parents rated their children's health "now," "immediately before" and "one-year before" the implant, through a standard series of methods. The team also estimated the costs directly associated with the implant (device, surgery, rehabilitation, maintenance, etc.) and those indirectly affected by the device (time off work, travel, and change in educational costs, etc.), as well as cost savings.

In 1992, cochlear implants were approved for use in profoundly deaf children who fail to benefit from conventional hearing aids. Since its entrance to the market, cochlear implant technology has been one of

16

many new devices questioned by health insurers for reimbursement.

"Providing an option to profound deafness is neither easy nor cheap, and for many years we've ignored the financial aspects of this treatment, thinking that for young children, cost should not be an issue," says senior author John K. Niparko, M.D., professor of otolaryngology- head and neck surgery and director of The Listening Center. "However, rising health care costs have led to pressures that discourage technologies such as the cochlear implant, and many health care plans cite 'no timely cost-effectiveness data' as a barrier to reimbursement for the device. This study, by weighing costs of both the device and the benefit provided to a large group of children, provides the beginning of evidence that, from a societal perspective, cochlear implantation in children is highly cost-effective." Niparko hopes that these findings will encourage similar research on a national level.

Earlier research had shown the device was cost-effective in adults, and it was speculated that children, because of their prolonged use of the device, stood to reap a greater cost-benefit over a longer period of time. Previous pediatric cochlear implant studies either considered quality-of-life benefits in a hypothetical way or used data from adults and were performed in England or Australia.

Setting aside the special education and greater wage-earning opportunities of implant recipients, the cost-utility of pediatric cochlear implantation ($9,029 per quality adjusted life year [QALY]) compares favorably (less dollars paid for the benefit) to many other implantable technologies, including the implantable defibrillator ($34,846 per QALY), knee replacement ($59,292 per QALY), and adult cochlear implantation ($11,125 per QALY).

The principal investigator of the study is Andre Cheng, M.D., Ph.D. In addition to Powe and Niparko, co-investigators include: Haya Rubin, M.D., Ph.D., Nancy Mellon, M.S., and Howard Francis, M.D. Their work was supported in part by a training grant from the National Institute on Deafness and Other Communication Disorders, National Institutes of Health, and grants from the Deafness Research Foundation, the Advisory Board Foundation and the Sidgmore Family Foundation.

Reprinted courtesy of John Hopkins Medical Center

Deaf Children Who Get Cochlear Implants Early in Life Get the Biggest Language Boost, Concludes Largest-Ever Study

ANN ARBOR, Michigan. - The younger deaf and hearing-impaired children are when a cochlear implant awakens their hearing, the better they will do on speech recognition tests later in life, according to the new results of the largest and most carefully designed study of its kind.

In fact, University of Michigan Health System researchers report, the positive effect of early implantation is evident even in comparisons of younger and older children who have had their implants for the same length of time, despite the older children's maturity advantage.

The new evidence, published in the January issue of the *Journal of Otology and Neurotology* (formerly the *American Journal of Otology*), adds to the growing proof that eligible hearing-impaired children should receive cochlear implants as early as possible if they cannot benefit from hearing aids.

"We found a significant difference in speech recognition between those who got their implants between the ages of two and four years, during the critical language development period, and those who received them later," says Paul Kileny, Ph.D., lead author and professor and head of audiology at UMIHS. "We also found that the longer children had had their implants, the better they did, though the effect was still largest in those who were implanted earliest."

The study looked at test results from 101 children who received the same model of cochlear implant at UMIHS between the ages of 2 and 14 years. The group's size and the identical management of the patients make the study's results more relevant than those of past studies of the implanted electronic hearing devices. The children represent one-third of all pediatric patients ever treated in the UMIHS program, one of the oldest and largest in the country.

The children were divided roughly in half, to allow for two analyses that could help isolate the effect of age at implantation on speech percep-

18

tion. One group of 48 children had their speech-recognition skills tested when they turned 7, regardless of when they got their implants. The other group of 53 children of various ages was tested at three years after implantation, to isolate the effects of age at implantation. All children took a battery of six standard tests to measure their ability to recognize sounds, words and sentences. Overall, the results showed a strong combined effect of age at implantation and the length of time the children had had their implants.

Cochlear implants are electronic devices that transform speech and other sounds into electrical impulses that stimulate auditory nerves in the inner ear. They can restore hearing and improve communication for children and adults with severe to profound sensorineural hearing loss in both ears who get little or no benefit from hearing aids.

Kileny and his co-authors, audiologists Teresa Zwolan, Ph.D., and Carissa Ashbaugh, M.A., collected the data over several years from routine tests taken by UMHS cochlear implant recipients at regular intervals. The children were between ages 5 1/2 and 17 3/4 when evaluated.

The researchers grouped the children in each arm of the study into four subgroups. Children tested at three years post-implant were divided according to age at implantation, and those tested at age 7 were grouped according to time since implantation.

The differences between the groups were clearest - and most statistically significant - in the 7-year-olds who had had their implant for four or more years, and the children whose three years of implantation had begun between the ages of 2 and 4. But even those 7-year-olds who had only had their implants three years scored significantly better than those who had had them one or two years. And children who first heard between the ages of 5 and 7 did better than those who got their implants between the ages of 10 and 13.

Not all speech-perception tests produced results that showed clear differences among the groups. But Kileny notes that some tests required sophisticated linguistic and vocabulary skills, which the youngest patients may not have developed no matter what their implant age.
This effect of better speech perception performance with longer and

earlier use of an implant is probably linked to the effect that cochlear implants have on the developing auditory nervous system, Kileny explains. Basic research has shown that the nerve cells involved in the auditory system require early and constant stimulation in order to develop important connections and patterns of activation necessary for speech perception. And other clinical studies have shown that both children and adults keep improving their speech perception with time, though adults tend to plateau after a while and children continue to improve over a period of years.

Thus, according to Kileny, the "wait and see" approach in the case of newly diagnosed young children may be detrimental in the long run. "I have seen several youngsters whose parents have opted to wait for new technological developments, in some cases for two to four years. These patients, though they began with great potential, ended up deriving minimal benefit from their cochlear implant, having missed crucial speech and language development milestones."

This "plasticity," or ability to keep learning new things, adds still more fuel to the argument that children with hearing problems who do not benefit from amplification with hearing aids should get cochlear implants as early in life as possible. Researchers in childhood development have consistently found that toddlers and young children reach crucial milestones in speech and language development early in life. The new study's result may clearly point to the risk of missing or delaying those milestones because of hearing impairment.

The team is still looking at the long-term effects of cochlear implantation before the age of 2. The U.S. Food and Drug Administration has approved implants for use in children as young as a year, and clinical trials in 12- to 24-month-olds are now under way at UMHS and elsewhere. Initial data on these youngest patients are already showing a difference from those who got their implants later in life, Kileny says, but it will take time to accumulate a large number of patients with several years' experience to allow the type of analysis done in the current study.

Reprinted Courtesy of the University of Michigan

Cochlear Implants May Improve Quality of Life in Elderly

Description: The risk and cost associated with three hours of general anesthesia have caused many to question whether cochlear implantation is viable for the elderly hearing impaired, but researchers from the University of Minnesota Hospital and Clinics has found that elderly patients who have undergone implantation receive, with minimal risk, the same physical and quality-of-life benefits incurred by younger adults with minimal risk. 9/26/1999 Contact: Ken Satterfield

For the Elderly Who Have Profound Hearing Loss, Cochlear Implants May Improve Audiologic Function and Quality of Life. University of Minnesota researchers find that cochlear implantation may be a viable option for the elderly hearing whose hearing aids have failed.

New Orleans — The risk associated with three hours of general anesthesia and its high cost have caused many to question whether cochlear implantation is a viable medical option for the elderly hearing impaired. For many over 60, hearing aids have proved to be ineffective. Now, a team of researchers from the University of Minnesota Hospital and Clinics has completed research that reveals that elderly patients who have undergone implantation receive, with minimal risk, the same physical and quality-of-life benefits incurred by younger adults with minimal risk.

The results of the study, "Cochlear Implantation in the Elderly: Results and Quality of Life Assessment," were presented before the *American Academy of Otolaryngology—Head and Neck Surgery Foundation Annual Meeting and Expo* being held September 26-29, at the Ernest N. Morial Convention Center-in New Orleans, LA. At the gathering, the Academy's 13,000 members will have the opportunity to hear the latest research in the diagnosis and treatment of disorders of the ear, nose, throat, and related structures of the head and neck.

The authors of the study are Hamid R. Djalilian, MD, Timothy A. King, MD, Samuel C. Levine, MD, FACS, and Sharon S. Smith, all from the Department of Otolaryngology, University of Minnesota Hospital and Clinics, Minneapolis, Minnesota.

Study Methodology:

The study's objective was to determine if elderly patients (60 or older) received the same benefits from cochlear implantation as younger adults.

Accordingly, the research team identified the 130 patients who had undergone cochlear implantation at the University of Minnesota Hospital and Clinic in the past 13 years. Of that group, 94 were post-lingual, profoundly hearing impaired adults. Sixty-one of the cochlear implant recipients were between the ages of 18 and 59; 33 were older than age 60.

Each of the adults underwent extensive preoperative medical, audiological, and psychological testing to assess their candidacy for the procedure. Additionally, a 22-item questionnaire was mailed to all 94 adults to assess pre-implant history and post-implant use, communication, and quality of life.

As a means of comparing the two adult groups, the medical and surgical complications were classified as major or minor. Major complications were defined as those necessitating re-hospilitization for medical management, explantation of the device, surgical re-exploration, or any degree of facial paralysis. Analysis comparing pre-operative and post-operative results was performed using paired t-test, Chi-squared test, and when appropriate Fisher's Exact Test.

Results:

The findings revealed the following about the elderly in this study who received cochlear implantation in the following categories:

Audiology:

Prior to the implantation, the average pure-tone average among the elderly subjects was 100 dB. After the implantation, that average increased by 37 dB. Statistically significant improvement occurred in four choice spondee (bi-syllabic word with generally equivalent stress on each of the two syllables, used in hearing tests), vowel, medial consonant, NU-6 words, CID sentences, monosyllabic, and lip reading. There were no statistically significant differences in improvement between adults younger than 60 and those 60 and older. Postoperative puretone averages were 37 for the elderly, 36 for those below 60. Additionally, scores for the two groups on the Beck Depression Inventory revealed no statistical difference.

Quality of Life:

When compared to younger adult patients, there was no difference in hours per day of implant usage, ability to discriminate environmental sounds from human voices, or ability to communicate via the telephone.

The majority of elderly patients reported improved social life, confidence, and overall quality of life after implantation.

Complications:

The percentage of major surgical or medical complications in elderly cochlear implant recipients in this study was 6 percent, a value similar to that reported for all adult cochlear implant patients. Overall, the implantation surgery in the elderly was well tolerated, and complication rates did not differ from those of younger patients.

Conclusion:

For the elderly, the combination of central and peripheral degenerative changes in the auditory system explains why simple amplification with hearing aids fails as the hearing impairment progresses. Accordingly, the cochlear implant, which bypasses the cochlea, offers significant benefits to those over 60 with profound hearing loss.

Reprinted with permission of The American Academy of Otolaryngology Head and Neck Surgery

PROJECT HOPE CENTER FOR HEALTH AFFAIRS
Policy Analysis Brief   April 2000

Penny E. Mohr, M.A., Jacob J. Feldman, Ph.D., Jennifer L. Dunbar, M. H. S.

OVERVIEW

Severe to profound hearing impairment affects one-half to three-quarters of a million Americans. To function in a hearing society, hearing-impaired persons with this level of loss require specialized education, social services, and other resources. The *Project HOPE Center for Health Affairs* conducted a study to provide a comprehensive, national, and recent estimate of the economic burden of hearing impairment. Based on the findings of this study, severe to profound hearing loss is expected to cost society an average of $297,000 over the lifetime of an individual. Lifetime costs for those with pre-lingual onset of deafness exceed $1 million. The particularly high costs associated with pre-lingual onset suggest interventions aimed at children, such as early identification and/or medical intervention may have a substantial payback.

APPROACH

To estimate the lifetime costs of severe to profound hearing impairment, Project HOPE staff constructed a cohort-survival model. This model attaches resource utilization and costs to an age cohort in a given year. The population is then aged over their lifetime using standard survival curves. The severely to profoundly hearing impaired population was divided into five age cohorts, each representing life stages associated with the use of different types of economic resources. These five cohorts were pre-lingual (0-2), prevocational (3-17), early working age (18-44), later working age (45-64) and retirement age (65 and older).

Costs include both direct medical and non-medical costs and indirect productivity losses associated with hearing loss. Direct medical costs for the hearing impaired include the costs of diagnosis, periodic medical visits to assess the physical status of the ear as well as audiological evaluation of hearing and fitting of hearing aids, costs associated with other assistive devices, and visits to a medical doctor for concomitant middle ear problems. All costs are inflated to 1998 dollars using the Urban Consumer Price Index. Future costs are discounted at a rate of 3%.

Direct non-medical costs include those associated with special education and rehabilitation (including services of speech and language pathologists, educational audiologists, and vocational rehabilitationists).

24

Finally, we include reduced lifetime earnings due to the effects of severe to profound hearing loss on productivity.

To estimate costs for lost productivity due to premature mortality and disability, we used a human capital approach. This approach values foregone productivity at mean market earnings for a specific age and gender group. Transfer payments such as Social Security Insurance and Disabled Workers Insurance, are excluded. These transfer payments, which according to the Social Security Administration amounted to $600 million for deaf persons in 1998, are intended to offset losses in income or increased medical or educational costs associated with the disability. Including them would result in double counting economic losses.

Data for the model were derived principally from the analyses of secondary data sources, including the National Health Interview Survey Hearing Loss and Disability Supplements (1990-91 and 1994-95), the Department of Education's National Longitudinal Transition Study (1987), and Gallaudet University's Annual Survey of Deaf and Hard of Hearing Youth (1997-98).

Data on school placement by type of setting (e.g., residential, self-contained classroom, resource room, or regular education) were obtained from the Department of Education's Office of Special Education and Rehabilitation Services (OSERS) *Annual Report to Congress on the Implementation of Individuals with Disabilities Education Act, 1997.* Annual educational costs by setting were derived by updating previous estimates to the 1997-98 school year.

Hearing impairment has been variously assessed in secondary data sources, ranging from the outcomes of audiometric tests to self-reported hearing loss Using audiometric results, severe to profound hearing loss is commonly considered the inability to detect a sound at 70 decibels or greater (averaged across the frequencies of 500, 1,000 and 2,000 Hertz) in the better ear. Because audiometric results were not available on the NHIS, persons with severe to profound hearing loss were identified using responses to several questions on self-reported hearing loss. While the Gallaudet survey gathers information on audiometric test results, most other databases do not use this objective measure and simply use the term "deaf" to describe this level of hearing impairment.

RESULTS
The results of this study indicate that an additional $4.6 billion will be

spent over the lifetimes of the estimated 15,400 persons who acquired their hearing impairment in 1998. On average, an individual with severe to profound hearing loss is expected to cost society $297,000 over their life with this disability. Most of these losses (67%) are due to reduced work productivity and opportunity, although the use of special education resources among children contributes an additional 21%. Persons who experience severe to profound hearing loss before retirement are expected to earn only 50-70 percent of their non-hearing impaired peers and lose between $220,000 and $440,000 in earnings over their working life, depending on when their hearing loss occurs. About 60% of the special educational costs are for educating children in more intensive instructional settings, such as self-contained classrooms, with the remainder for supplemental services provided to students not in residential or day schools, such as speech/language therapy or sign language interpreters. Unlike many clinical conditions, severe to profound hearing loss largely impacts the social welfare system rather than the medical care system.

The magnitude of loss is directly related to age of onset, with persons experiencing severe to profound hearing loss in childhood incurring the largest expected costs. The expected lifetime cost of deafness for a child with prelingual onset, for example, exceeds $1 million. By contrast, societal losses for persons who acquire their hearing loss late in life are expected to average $43,000. Notably, our approach to cost estimation, known as the human capital approach, places a heavy emphasis on earnings potential and does not value intangible losses, such as the social isolation and psychological stress imposed by the condition. Among the elderly, who represent nearly 40% of new cases, costs will be especially undervalued by this approach.

CONCLUSIONS

Severe to profound hearing loss imposes a substantial social cost. Although its incidence is relatively low when compared with other conditions, per case losses are large, amounting to more than a million dollars for a prelingually-deafened child.

Early identification of hearing loss in children can significantly improve language development and possibly other developmental outcomes.' While the cost per infant identified with significant hearing loss varies with prevalence estimates, these costs pale by comparison to expected lifetime expenditures for severely to profoundly hearing-impaired children. A cost per infant hearing screening of $25 and a prevalence rate of 3.2/1000, which has been found in the Colorado screening program, would cost $7,800 per identified case.' If early identification can shift just an additional ten percent of pre-lingual deaf children into mainstream classrooms, the return on investment would more than double even when not including possible effects on earnings.

Cochlear implantation offers a medical approach to reducing the level of hearing impairment and improving function. Several studies have shown cochlear implantation can make a significant and positive impact on quality of life. Also, cochlear implantation has been found to improve earnings among adults.' In another study, profoundly deaf children who had more than two years experience with a cochlear implant were able to move out of special education into a mainstream setting at twice the rate of their age-matched peers without a cochlear implant.'

The costs of cochlear implantation and associated rehabilitative services reported in the literature range from $29,000 to $63,000. Studies conducted to date have consistently found cochlear implantation to be cost effective among appropriately selected candidates. Regrettably, the benefits of this medical intervention are not realized by health insurance plans, and, thus, payment often has not adequately covered the costs of surgery and rehabilitation, resulting in a strong disincentive for hospitals to provide cochlear implantation.' Regardless of the approach taken, this study shows aggressive and early intervention to reduce the level of hearing impairment may produce savings to society.

References

Chaikind, S., Danielson, L.C., Brauen, M.L. What do we know about the costs of special education: A selected review. *Journal of Special Education,* 1993, 26(4), 344-370.

Moore, M.T., Strang, E.W., Schwartz, M., Braddock, M. *Patterns in special education service delivery and cost.* Washington, DC: Decision Resources Corporation, 1988.

Yoshinaga-Itano, C., Sedey, A.L., Coulter, D.K., et al. Language of early- and late-identified children with hearing loss. *Pediatrics,* 1998, 102(5), 1161-1171.

Downs, M.P. Universal newborn hearing screening: The Colorado story. *International Journal of Pediatric Otorhinolaryngology,* 1995, 32, 257-259.

Harris, J.P., Anderson, J.P., Novak, P. An outcomes study of cochlear implants in deaf patients. *Archives of Otolaryngology and Head*

IVCCD Libraries

MCC B.J. Harrison Library
Marshalltown, Iowa 50158

and Neck Surgery, 1995, 121, 398-404.

Francis, H.W., Koch, M.A., Wyatt, J.R., Niparko, J.K. Trends in educational placement and cost-benefit considerations in children with cochlear implants. *Archives of Otolaryngology and Head and Neck Surgery,* 1999, 125, 499-505.

Kane, N.M., Manoukian, P.D. The effect of Medicare prospective payment on the adoption of new technology: The case of cochlear implants. *New England Journal of Medicine,* 1989, 321, 1378-1383.

Reprinted courtesy of Project Hope Center for Health Affairs

Interview with Dr Samuel Levine, Neurotologist 9/16/2002

HH/Beck: Good Morning Dr. Levine. Thanks for your time this morning.

Levine: Thanks Dr. Beck. I am happy to meet with you.

HH/Beck: Before we get into issues related to cochlear implants, let's talk a little about your professional history. Can you please tell me where you went to school?

Levine: Sure. I went to Northwestern University for undergraduate work, and my bachelor's was actually in engineering, and I earned that in 1976. Then from 1976 to 1980 I was at the Hannemann Medical College, and earned my MD there. I did my otolaryngology residency at the Cleveland Clinic from 1980 to 1985, and then I did my neurotology fellowship under Michael Glasscock, in 1985 and 1986, and since then I've been here at the University of Minnesota.

HH/Beck: Very good. Please tell me about your current practice?

Levine: The university practice is quite large. We have 12 otolaryngologists on staff here, and we service 4 separate hospitals. We also have 7 audiologists, who do pretty much everything, and so the group is large and very busy.

HH/Beck: Dr. Levine, how long have you been a cochlear implant surgeon?

Levine: Since 1986. I started a year or two after the FDA approved cochlear implants.

HH/Beck: Can you recall, back in 1986, when you discussed cochlear implants with patients, what was it that you felt comfortable telling patients? In other words, what were the expectations that you had, and what were the expectations you felt comfortable telling your cochlear implant candidates in 1986?

Levine: I used to tell patients that if they got sound awareness - that would be a wonderful and amazing thing. In 1986, I told them they could count on the fact that they would not be able to hear normally, in fact, we tried to disassociate cochlear implants from the actual sense of hearing at that time. I used to tell cochlear implant candidates they would get an awareness of sound, or a perception of sound, and that was about it. The expectations were cochlear implants would be useful to help people read lips, but again, we didn't want to have the patients think of it as "hearing" back in 1986, because it was too crude, and not really what any of us considered true hearing - back then.

HH/Beck: And how would that contrast to what you tell patients at this time?

Levine: Well, I primarily use the Advanced Bionics Clarion, and of course there are others available too. But I tell patients that 98 percent of the cochlear implant recipients like the implant, they use it on a regular basis, and the cochlear implant is useful for many different sounds and situations. I feel very comfortable telling them about 3/4's of the current cochlear implant users are able to use the telephone, and they can expect to understand about half of what is being said without visual cues, and that in real sentences such as day-to-day situations, they can expect almost 100 percent comprehension. But I also warn them that we cannot accurately predict outcomes for any individual ahead of time, and that in fact, each patient is different.

HH/Beck: Dr. Levine, sometimes I get email from cochlear implant candidates who write me and ask about "failure rates." In other words, I believe they are asking, what percentage of patients who receive cochlear implants, are not able to use it because it simply doesn't work? My answer is that in working with cochlear implant patients for almost 20 years, I have only seen two patients that didn't "stimulate," and they were both in the 1980s. What do you tell patients with regard to this issue?

Levine: I tell them about the same. The success rate, if it is defined as "successful electrical stimulation" or as "perceiving sound through the cochlear implant" is probably just about 100 percent. I cannot recall the last time someone didn't stimulate, and that is based on our doing about 50 implants per year, or maybe a little more.

HH/Beck: What do you tell patients regarding their aural rehabilitation and the time it will take to learn to effectively, efficiently and maximally use their cochlear implant?

Levine: Like most good surgeons, I refer them to the audiologist! Sharon Smith is our lead cochlear implant audiologist and she addresses this topic with the patients. I think the bottom line is that aural rehabilitation (AR) is necessary and the AR treatment course varies based on the patient and their needs, and we know that the more they work on it and the more they attend to the issues, the better their eventual outcome will be. So it really is driven by the patients. Those that do the best are usually those that work at it the hardest. We know that simply turning on the implant is not enough, and we know that the audiologist working with the patient is the most important factor post-op, in determining their final outcome.

HH/Beck: Can you tell me, when did we actually "turn the corner" on cochlear implants? When did we go from an awareness of sound, to actually hearing?

Levine: Great question. I'm not sure that there was a singular moment, but we did go through a series of tests that helped lead to the Advanced Bionics CII cochlear implant, and I remember realizing at that time that something had changed dramatically. I like to tell the story that sometimes between the Wright Brothers and the 747, air travel got a lot safer and a lot cheaper, and it's the same with cochlear implants. Somewhere between 1990 and 2002 we've made a few quantum leaps. Not only are the devices significantly better, but the complication rates have fallen way down, and the results are typically excellent.

HH/Beck: What are the surgical and post-op complications you discuss with patients?

Levine: I tell my patients that the biggest complication issue is the wound itself. Sometimes the wound can break down, and sometimes the wound will need medical or surgical attention. Of course that is extremely rare, but it is possible. Once you have a foreign body implanted, there is always a risk that it might need further attention. Again, those are rare issues, but these are the issues I discuss with my patients.

HH/Beck: What was the single most impressive advancement you've witnessed in the last 2 or 3 years with regards to cochlear implants?

Levine: The modular hugging electrode array has been evolving for the last few years, and in the last year this has really improved dramatically. So I think that would probably be the most important new development in cochlear implants. Of course the hardware and the software have both improved dramatically over time, and the improvements have been significant.

HH/Beck: Dr. Levine, it has been a pleasure speaking with you. Thanks for your thoughts and insight on this topic.

Levine: Thanks for inviting me Doug. It's been a pleasure for me too.

**Reprinted with the permission of Dr. Douglas Beck,
Dr. Samuel Levine and Healthy Hearing
please visit www.healthyhearing.com**

Interview with Sharon Smith M.S., CCC-A, Clinical Audiologist,University of Minnesota at Minneapolis. 9/23/2002

HH/Beck: Hi Sharon, thanks for joining me today.

Smith: Hi Doug, thanks for the invitation.

HH/Beck: Sharon, before we get to the topic of the day, which is cochlear implants, can you please tell me where you went to school?

Smith: I did my undergraduate work at the University of Wisconsin- Eau Claire and I received my Master's in Audiology at Syracuse University in upstate New York.

HH/Beck: Sharon, I know you have lots of experience with cochlear implants, and in particular with adults. Can you tell me a little about the cochlear implant program?

Smith: Sure. The University of Minnesota Cochlear Implant Program began as a tiny program around 1984. Since that time, we have evolved from a program from one cochlear implant recipient in 1984 to a program with more than 300 patients. In the mid-80's we had an average of about 9 adult recipients per year; this year we will have over 60 adults and children receive cochlear implants at our facility. And, we have evolved from a one-audiologist and one surgeon program to a team consisting of 4 audiologists, two health psychologists, a speech/language pathologist, a behavioral pediatrician and 2 surgeons.

HH/Beck: How many children receive cochlear implants at the university each year?

Smith: Children began receiving cochlear implants at our facility in 1990, the same year the FDA approved pediatric implantation. That year we implanted three children; the number of pediatric recipients has been rising steadily ever year since then. Last year 30 children received cochlear implants at the University of Minnesota.

HH/Beck: What is the age of the youngest child that has been implanted?

Smith: At our facility the youngest recipient was 2 months old, although I believe that worldwide the youngest was 5 months of age. Next month we will have a six-month old undergo the procedure.

HH/Back: Can you describe the differences between the children implanted in 2002, as compared to the kids implanted ten years ago?

Smith: Absolutely. There are many differences. First, the implant technology today is far more advanced than the technology from 10 years ago. Better technology has yielded better speech and language outcomes when combined with appropriate aural rehabilitation. For instance, speech and language milestones which used to take a year to reach are now achieved in months.

Another difference is that children are getting implanted at younger ages than they were 10 years ago. With the FDA lowering the age criteria, in combination with today's infant and newborn hearing screening programs, we are now identifying, amplifying and implanting children at younger ages than we were 10 years ago. This in turn, with appropriate intervention, has allowed for earlier and earlier acquisition of receptive and expressive spoken language than we were seeing 10 years ago.

Education and aural rehabilitation are other areas which have expanded over the past 10 years. Our school systems have become accustomed to addressing the needs of cochlear implant children, and we have become wiser about the amount of rehab children need, and we have see the emergence of oral schools for the deaf across the nation.

HH/Beck: So you are indeed implanting children at an earlier age, and you are seeing clinical outcomes that demonstrate improved results?

Smith: Yes. Ten years ago, kids were implanted later, for instance, 24 months or older, and it usually took a year for a child to respond to his or her name or to begin to produce speech. Today we have children implanted at 12 months of age, responding to their names two weeks after hook-up and reaching near age-appropriate milestones by the age of 24 months, following appropriate aural rehabilitation.

HH/Beck: Can you tell me a little about post-implant aural rehabilitation for children?

Smith: Aural rehabilitation is a must for all pediatric cochlear implant recipients. It includes at a minimum; speech and language services provided by the child's school system, and individualized auxiliary rehab through our speech pathologist on the team or a practitioner in the community. Having private rehabilitation allows additional needed therapy and helps distribute the responsibility of the therapy from just the school, to another professional and allows another professional to be looking at the child in a one-to-one setting. Many of the parents of our pediatric recipients have opted to enroll their children in the Moog Oral School here in town, to enable them to receive intensive speech and language therapy all day long in an oral educational environment.

Parents are a key component to a child's aural rehab program. Cochlear implantation requires a high level of commitment from parents-both for getting the child to their rehab and programming appointments, as well as being able to continuously provide the child with auditory input. The cooperation among the clinical and educational audiologists, the speech language pathologists, the parents, the school administration and the educators is essential. They each provide a building block toward the child's ultimate success with a cochlear implant.

HH/Beck: What about your adult cochlear implant program?

Smith: Our adult program is currently larger than our pediatric program. We have more than 190 adults whom we follow, and probably 100 of those come in every year for reprogramming, or to check on their units, or just to have an annual follow-up.

HH/Beck: What is the typical entry point for adults into your cochlear implant program?

Smith: There is a bit of variation there. Sometimes they are referred by their family or friends, have seen an article somewhere and come self-referred, but most often they are referred by their doctors or their audiologists.

HH/Beck: And then once they come in to see you?

Smith: We put them through pretty much the same diagnostic work-up that most cochlear implant centers do. Our pre-implant evaluation requires a current hearing test, and a trial period with appropriate hearing aids. With today's digital technology and the benefits realized with it, it is important that the patient is offered every opportunity to try out all amplification options before settling on a cochlear implant.

When the patient comes in for a cochlear implant evaluation, their aided open-set word and sentence recognition is tested, with the criteria being set at 30% or worse on open set word recognition (CNC test) and 50% or worse on sentence recognition (HINT scored for percentage of words correct). If the patient meets these criteria, we spend over an hour discussing how implants work, what they look like, the surgical procedure and its associated risks, and the bulk of the time spent discussing appropriate expectations. Following the appointment with the audiologist, the physicians go through the medical history and their diagnostic work-up too, to make sure that the patient is a candidate from a medical and surgical viewpoint. Patients are required to undergo a CT scan, and at this facility, they also undergo a consultation with a Health Psychologist.

HH/Beck: What is the largest diagnosis code, or etiology, of the adult implant candidates you see? In other words, what is the cause of their hearing loss?

Smith: Interestingly, for adults, it is cause undetermined. In other words, we really don't know why some of these people lost their hearing. Probably the second largest category is otosclerosis, and then after that, perhaps Meniere's disease.

HH/Beck: One question I get lots of email on, usually from adult cochlear implant candidates is what percentage of patients can expect to use a telephone after they receive their cochlear implant?

Smith: That's a question we get too. I usually tell people that there are two important parts to the answer. The first is nobody can guarantee any results with a cochlear implant! The second is, of my patients, and with the current cochlear implant technology, about 70 percent of the post-lingual cochlear implant patients will be able to use the telephone.

HH/Beck: That's quite a bit better than the results from ten year ago too!

Smith: Yes, it really is. Ten years ago, it was the exceptional patient that could use the phone, and now it's the exceptional one that cannot. It's the same with music too. I'd guess that probably some 70 percent of the patients are able to appreciate music while using their cochlear implants too.

HH/Beck: Very good. Thank you so much for the information and for your time today.

Smith: It's been my pleasure, thank you for the opportunity.

Reprinted with the permission of Healthy Hearing

Interview with Nathan Schepker, MED-EL, Patient Support Manager and Cochlear Implant Recipient
10/21/2002

HH/Beck: Hi Nathan, thanks for taking the time to speak with me today.

Schepker: Hi Doug, nice to finally get together!

HH/Beck: Nathan, please tell me a little about your education, and how you came to be an employee of MED-EL?

Schepker: I graduated from college in 2000 with a degree in International Business from Mary Washington College in Virginia. I started working for MED-EL between my junior and senior years, and I basically served as an intern at MED-EL for that summer. I went around the country to different trade shows, state meetings and exhibitions addressing cochlear implant issues and speaking with people about my implant experience. I really started to enjoy the work and the information exchange and so when I finished college, I came back to work here full-fime.

HH/Beck: Nathan, I am not quite sure what you do as the Patient Support Manager, can you please tell me about that?

Schepker: Sure. My position is such that the goal is to provide programs for cochlear implant candidates, and for MED-EL users to help provide a support network for people entering the cochlear implant arena, and for those who are already into it, but need more information and direction. In other words, I correspond with, and coordinate information flow between MEDEL, the candidates and the patients. I try to help people understand what an implant is, what it's all about, what they can expect and whatever else they need. Sometimes I help put candidates and their families together with cochlear implant users, and this is very gratifying. We also have the Hearing Companions program, which is a network of volunteer MED-EL users, and they are available to help people get through the process and to share their stories. We sometimes are able to match up people who are actually quite local to each other. These are really important services.

HH/Beck: Do you also help coordinate cochlear implant candidates and implant centers?

Schepker: Yes, I do. Sometimes people are looking for local audiologists or surgeons, and I can help direct them to the appropriate professionals. Sometimes there are small support groups of cochlear implant patients that just like to get together and talk about their experiences, problems and solutions, and I try to help as best I can in bringing these people together. I also help individuals both candidates and implantees locate community resources that might be available for them in there area, such as these support groups or organizations.

HH/Beck: Nathan, I know that you too, are a cochlear implant patient. Can you tell us a little about your personal cochlear implant?

Schepker: Sure. I was actually born with hearing loss and they suspect it was probably moderate-to-severe at birth. My hearing loss wasn't detected until I was almost two years old, because there was a question as to my speech development, which is why they started to investigate my hearing! Anyway, by the time my hearing loss was detected, it was a profound hearing loss. I was fitted with hearing aids right away and I wore hearing aids throughout my education. I went to a preschool and kindergarten for the deaf and I learned to sign there. I was mainstreamed in the first grade with an oral interpreter and I stayed mainstreamed throughout college. By the time I graduated I had had oral interpreters, note-takers, FM systems and a lot of support from speech therapy too.

HH/Beck: Nathan, how old were you when you received your cochlear implant?

Schepker: I was 20 years old when I was implanted. It was between my sophomore and junior years of college. My implant was in 1998.

HH/Beck: I probably should point out to the readers that you are in North Carolina and I am in Texas, and we're communicating over the telephone, virtually without repeats or problems while wearing your implant.

Schepker: Yes, I use the phone all the time - every day! In fact, using the telephone is one of the best things for me, regarding using a cochlear implant. The fact that I can use the phone is amazing - it really opens up the world to me.

HH/Beck: What has been the biggest surprise for you regarding your implant. In other words, was there any one thing that just really went way above and beyond your expectations with the cochlear implant?

Schepker: That's really a difficult question ... if I had to pick one thing, I would just say "sound" in general. Now what I define as a sound is clear and easy to listen to. But, when I was first hooked-up, I wasn't really able to identify sound as sound. Early on, it was just a sensation in my head. I knew what sound was - or at least I thought I did, and that sensation through the cochlear implant wasn't sound. I had a 110 dB loss, which is way past profoundly deaf, so maybe the sounds I was used to weren't quite right either. Anyway, as a week or two became three and four weeks, the sound started to make sense, very slowly at first. But eventually my brain started to recognize the sensations the cochlear implant was providing as sound, and it was amazing to start identifying sounds as related to a certain object or event. I never heard high frequencies until I got my cochlear implant, and at first, the high frequencies kind of overrode all of the sounds I was hearing, everything sounded high pitched and it was very hard to listen to the sound easily. It was pretty confusing. In fact, it was almost like I was hearing two versions of each sound at the same time- the high pitched and the low pitched. But eventually, the high-frequencies and the low frequencies began to blend together into a whole and complete sound that began to make sense.

HH/Beck: What was the approximate time frame from the time your cochlear implant was activated, until sounds started to make sense?

Schepker: Actually associating sounds with basic sound sources took about 3 to 4 weeks, but it took longer for speech sounds to make sense and to be clearly understood. It was probably about three months before I could understand speech without lip-reading. Music took a while too. I love music and I used to listen to it with my hearing aids, but with the cochlear implant I am better able to get the harmonics and sometimes I get the melody too. I just started playing guitar a few months ago, and I can now tune the guitar and play a few chords by ear while wearing my cochlear implant. So it gets better all the time, and I always work on my listening skills to become a better listener.

HH/Beck: Nathan, what can you tell me about the aural rehabilitation process, as someone who has gone through it?

Schepker: The most important thing is to have reasonable expectations. Some people expect that as soon as they get their cochlear implant activated, everything will be great. That happens sometimes, though rarely, and more often, it takes time and practice. If the expectations are too high, that sets up the individual for failure. Everyone reacts differently to a cochlear implant and no two experiences are alike. It's best not to compare your experience with others, but to compare to how you were performing before you got the implant. That's a better indication of how you, personally, are doing. It is also important not to set a time frame for certain achievements, such as, "I want to hear on the phone in 6 months." You can't be rushed or timed in this manner, because that's simply not how the brain adapts.

HH/Beck: Supposing someone wants to get in touch with you, what's the best way to do that?

Schepker: They can write to me at my email address: nschepker@medelus.com, and I'll be happy to get in touch with them.

HH/Beck: Thanks Nathan. I appreciate your time.

Schepker: Thank you too, Doug. It's been fun.

**Reprinted with the permission of Healthy Hearing
please visit at www.healthyhearing.com**

Transcript of NIDCD interview with Director Dr. Battey
By Mardie Younglof

As we wrote in the previous issue of *CONTACT* (First Quarter 1999), *CONTACT* Associate Editor Mardie Younglof (MCY) and CICI Executive Director Peg Williams, Ph.D. (PW), spoke with Dr. Battey in December at his office on the NIH campus of Bethesda, Maryland. Dr. Battey is the Director of the National Institute on Deafness and Other Communication Disorders (NIDCD). This is the concluding part of the interview.

PW: I want to tell you how much I appreciate the work of the NIDCD Clearinghouse and how helpful its cochlear implant information packet has been to CICI's efforts to respond to consumer requests for information. In the future, CICI would be very interested in conducting a co-sponsored educational symposium with NIDCD to provide and share information about research findings and consumer needs. Would this be of interest to you in your work at NIDCD?
NIDCD would be very interested in a conference whose focus would be to help people understand much better exactly what the cochlear implant does, why it works, and the good outcomes that can happen when individuals are implanted at an early age. NIDCD would be quite anxious to make that information available to the public so they are aware of the progress that has been made in this area, because it is really quite significant. It would also be important for them to know what the limitations are and to understand what the compelling research questions are for the future.

PW: While we focus a lot on what the cochlear implant has done for children, it also has had a remarkable impact on the lives of adults. Many have told me that, when they lost their hearing, they also lost jobs, marriages, family relationships, and friends. After receiving a cochlear implant, they have been able to regain some of this loss and move back into social and work settings. It seems society also benefits when implanted people can get their lives back. Ultimately there is an economic return to society for the funding provided to support cochlear implant research.
I completely agree. Certainly in the adult population, there is a remarkable role for the cochlear implant, particularly in an individual who undergoes sudden and profound loss of hearing. By performing the implant surgery in a timely manner, you can keep the areas of the brain

43

needed for speech and language perception actively stimulated, thereby optimizing language and communication skills. So, you are absolutely right, there is an important role there and, in fact, it is in that arena that we are asking the question, "Is 88 decibels of hearing loss the right number to consider for implantation, or would individuals with 60-65 decibels who may get benefit from hearing aids, but not a lot of benefit, be better off with an implant?" That is a very important question we need to answer. The number of individuals who are candidates for implants will expand. NIDCD will continue to support research whose goal is to use the implant as an auditory prosthesis in a greater number of individuals with hearing impairment as we learn more about the best ways to use the device.

PW: A lot of calls that I get, perhaps one-third, are from parents who are concerned because their child had meningitis and experienced damage to the inner ear. Are there any plans or thoughts about studying the differences in this kind of disorder versus one that is genetically based?

Clearly, the biological bases are very different from hearing loss due to infection as compared to hearing loss due to a genetic cause, which presumably will interfere with either the development or survival of critical cellular elements within the inner ear that are necessary for hearing. By understanding the mechanisms whereby mutated genes cause hearing impairment and comparing that with what we see mechanistically and anatomically in the scenario of an infectious cause for hearing impairment, I think we will gain a great deal of insight as to what aspects of the biology are the same and what are different when hearing impairment is caused by these two very different etiologies.

MCY: How many genes for deafness have been mapped? Is it currently feasible for the average person to be tested for the presence of these genes?

That is an interesting question. If you include hereditary hearing loss that is syndromic, which means hearing impairment in connection with other clinical problems, with non-syndromic hearing loss, there are literally over 100 genes involved in hearing impairment. If you talk about just the non-syndromic hereditary hearing impairment - hearing impairment without any other clinical symptoms - a little over 40 genes have been mapped, and roughly 10 of those genes have been cloned. Much of that activity has taken place within the last year and a half. Now, in terms of whether or not it is feasible to test for the presence of these genes, that is also a complicated question, because we are only now learning the basics of the genetic epidemiology of hearing impairment. What I mean by that is to say that some genes cause hereditary hearing impairment more often than others. For example, there is a gene called Connexin 26, in which a single base or nucleotide is dropped, and this relatively common mutation is the cause of perhaps as much as 40% of the hereditary hearing impairment among some groups of Americans. This would be a very straightforward mutation to identify, using either polymerase chain reaction or direct sequencing of the gene itself. But for the remaining 60% of those with hereditary hearing loss, we don't yet know how much the contribution is from other genes besides Connexin 26. This is a very active area of research, both among our extramural grantees and in our intramural laboratories here in Bethesda.

PW: I was reading the article, "A New Era in the Genetics of Deafness," in a recent issue of *The New England Journal of Medicine*. It mentioned research results showing genetically based hearing loss that doesn't really appear until adulthood. We tend to think of genetic testing only as it relates to children. It was eye-opening to me that a genetic factor responsible for hearing loss may not be apparent until hearing loss appears in adulthood, even late adulthood. Is it your impression that this kind of information is new, obtained from recent genetic research, and that it gives us an explanation for many types of progressive hearing loss that, till now, we have not attributed to genetics?

This is absolutely true. There is hearing impairment that runs in families that is not early onset, but shows up in the second, third, or fourth decade of life. Some forms of hereditary hearing impairment affect the low frequencies more than the high frequencies, and there are forms that affect the high frequencies more than the low frequencies. The same mutation, such as the Connexin 26 mutation, in some individuals causes a profound early-onset hearing impairment and in others a less profound onset. A different mutation in Connexin 26 might give you a dominant disorder, and another would give you a recessive disorder. Then there is the equally interesting possibility that, for a given gene, two copies of the mutated gene cause early-onset profound hearing impairment, but a single copy of the mutated gene contributes to hearing loss that accompanies aging, or noise-induced hearing loss. Now that we know the genes and the mutations, we can do systematic studies to determine the importance of all these factors for hearing impairment both early and late in life.

PW: I find this exciting. When I worked with clients clinically, in taking a history, they always said, "No, there is no history of hearing loss in my family. Oh, maybe a relative had hearing loss as they got older." And we always attributed the clients' hearing loss, just as you said, to noise pollution or the aging process. It never occurred to me back then that it could be genetic.

This is the really exciting area of human genetics, not just for hearing impairment, but for all sorts of other disorders where, by identifying the genes that underlie susceptibility to various disorders, the medicine of the next millennium will take advantage of that information, helping individuals to make the right choices, to minimize their risk of developing problems for which they are perhaps more susceptible than others. One simple example would be that, if you knew you were more susceptible to noise-induced hearing loss, you probably would not operate a jackhammer for a living. Instead, you would make a career choice that minimized the risk to your hearing.

MCY: Victor McKusick, who is considered the father of modern genetics, has said that numerous genes, not just one, may be responsible for most genetic syndromes. In light of this, can you tell us how many causes of deafness are likely to be from multiple genes? Has progress been made to "turn off" any of these genes?

Hearing impairment is a good example of a human genetic disorder where many genes can cause hearing impairment. But within a given family, it is usually just one gene, or predominantly one gene, that is causing the hearing impairment. We inherit hearing in Mendelian fashion. Dominant inheritance occurs when just one copy of the mutated gene causes the hearing loss; when the inheritance of a copy from each parent is required for the hearing loss to show up, that is recessive hearing impairment. For many other common afflictions, such as diabetes or hypertension, there isn't a single gene involved, but it is the effect of multiple genes working in concert that cause the hypertension or the diabetes. So hearing impairment is different in that regard. As for turning off any of the genes, we first need to understand what they do and how they are regulated before we can even imagine that we can intercede with a genetic medicine approach of actually modifying the way the genes work. So we are a ways off, I think, from being able to intervene at the genetic level in the arena of hereditary hearing impairment.

MCY: Would people who once had normal hearing be better

prospects for hair cell regeneration than those who are congenitally deaf?

I wish I understood the molecular mechanisms that regulate hair cell regeneration, since much of hearing loss is a consequence of the death of these wonderful sound transducing cells in the inner ear. We have a whole collection of basic and translational scientists who are studying very carefully what prevents a hair cell from regenerating in the inner ear. In fact, some significant progress has been made within the last year in that area, and I'm hopeful that we will ultimately be able to send molecular signals into the inner ear that stimulate hair cell regeneration after they have been lost through some sort of disease or environmental process. We know that it is possible, because in other species, such as birds, for example, or some reptiles, hair cell regeneration happens. And if it can happen in birds, I'd like to think that if the scientific community is clever enough we can figure out how to make it happen in mammals and in humans.

MCY: How can CICI support funding for NIDCD programs on cochlear implants?

I think your organization is doing among the best things you could possibly do. Help get out the word that the cochlear implant is a wonderful device, that the device has enormous utility, and that the utility is expanding. We are learning that more individuals are potential candidates for cochlear implants, the technology is improving, the speech processing algorithms are improving, and we are becoming much more knowledgeable about how to use the implants. There is too little public awareness among average people about the cochlear implant and, in fact, about hearing impairment in general and what a devastating disorder it is. It is one of the most debilitating problems that an individual can have in modern society. If I can borrow an idea from my colleague Bob Rubin up in New York for a minute, he makes the point that in the early 1900s most people made their living by lifting things or pushing things, with physical skills. In that era, communication skills were probably not as big a factor in having and keeping a good job as they are today. Now, virtually all jobs, or good jobs, involve having good communication skills. Individuals who are hearing impaired, without the benefit of a cochlear implant or the right assistive devices and the right rehabilitation, can be at a tremendous disadvantage in this employment arena. So, if that message can be made known to the public and if they could appreciate the number of individuals we are talking about - estimates are as high as 28 million Americans who have hearing impairment-then

I think the public will realize that the answer to this problem is better understanding, more research, and translating those research findings into better ways to help individuals with hearing impairment. In general, I feel the American public is tremendously supportive of biomedical research, and we are enormously grateful for their support. We would just like them to know that we are making great progress and that that progress, we hope, will rapidly translate from the laboratory to patients so that the public that is supporting the work becomes the beneficiary of the research that has been done.

MCY: How can CICI work together with NIDCD and what support can NIDCD offer to CICI?

I think by developing good information pieces for the public, both for older people and school-age children, that will get out the word on what a problem hearing impairment is and how more research will bring about benefit to hearing-impaired individuals, and that giving hearing-impaired individuals the best communication skills possible will actually be an economic benefit to the United States because these individuals will be able to be more productive with better communication skills. Getting all those messages out is something that NIDCD would very much like to do with CICI, whether it is in developing written material or working together with you on conferences. I think there is a lot we can do together to make that happen, and I look forward to the opportunity to work with you on those important areas.

PW: Our respective organizations are both engaged in disseminating and exchanging information for diverse populations. We serve not only English speakers but also those who speak other languages. We also need to meet the needs of those who cannot afford services and who may not know of available assistance or even the existence of the cochlear implant In addition, the different professions, schools, employers, and the community at large also need information on new research findings. Communication and joint efforts are vitally necessary. And, of course, it is communication that is often lost for the hearing impaired consumer. We appreciate the research efforts underway at NIDCD that explore ways to restore this lost ability to communicate and to help any hearing impaired person, not just those with cochlear implants, to communicate with the world at large.

The NIDCD remains very much committed to helping individuals with hearing impairment, with the primary focus being on optimizing their communication skills, because that is one of the many things one loses

48

when hearing is lost. Losing the ability to communicate is a devastating blow, in that people become isolated and have difficulty taking full advantage of all the great opportunities that exist in America today. The cochlear implant is one very important tool for optimizing communication skills. But I think it is important to keep in mind that there is no one size that fits all. While the implant has proven to be a wonderful tool for many individuals, there are individuals for whom other intervention strategies are a better route to go. NIDCD is committed to exploring all avenues to improve the communication skills of individuals who have hearing impairment.

PW: Thank you, Dr. Battey, for the generosity of your time, and we also thank you on behalf of CICI for all that NIDCD does to support cochlear implant research. A great many people, including our membership, have benefited from your Institute's findings.

It's really my pleasure, and we hope to work together with organizations such as yours in getting the message out that there are important things to do, we're doing some of these things, and we want to do more in the future. But it is only with the help and support of organizations like yours and the generous support of the American public that we can do all that we do to further this important area of research. We would very much appreciate any thoughts or ideas that you might collect about areas in which we could move our research to continue to make a difference to people with hearing impairment.

Reprinted courtesy of Marjorie C. Younglof

The Cochlear Implant : A Parent's Perspective
By Melody James Parton

This article is the text of a statement made by Melody James Parton before the Ear, Nose and Throat Devices Panel of the Food and Drug Administration on May 21, 1997, in Washington, D.C. Ms. Parton's testimony was part of the, fact-gathering process to determine whether FDA approval should be granted to the Clarion, a new cochlear implant device for children. This speech was reprinted in the League for the Hard of Hearing Rehabilitation Quarterly, Vol. 22 #2, 1997.

I would like to thank this FDA Advisory Panel for the opportunity to testify regarding the cochlear implant. My name is Melody James Parton, and I am the parent of an implant child. I am also the Director of Public Education for the League for the Hard of Hearing in New York, a member of the Executive Board of the Parent Section of the Alexander Graham Bell Association for the Deaf, a member of the Board of Directors of the New York Chapter of this organization, and a member of the Cochlear Implant Club International.

I am also here to represent the hundreds of cochlear implant families we have met, shared concerns with, as well as achievements and joys, over the last ten years. Strangers at the beginning, we parents quickly find our common ground: our children are deaf. We wrestle with the implant decision. Once made, we continue to face challenges regarding services, school options, and their well being each step of the way.

The network of implant families is now extensive. We meet at conferences, through cyberspace, print, and phone. All of the families I know and speak with regularly would tell you the implant works for their child, that it is an effective tool helping their child. It does not solve, fix, or end the challenges of raising one of our children.

Our daughter Caitlin contracted meningitis at the age of 22 months. She emerged with a profound hearing loss. We chose for Caitlin to receive the Nucleus 22 channel cochlear implant eight months later. At the time of her operation in January 1988, the implant was still under 'investigative status' for children with the Food and Drug Administration. Caitlin was one of the first toddlers in the world to pioneer the device. We are glad to have this opportunity to thank you for allowing the implant option years ago. Some of her abilities are a result of being implanted so young. For our child, our family, and the others we know, the implant has made a world of difference. Each external upgrade has brought improvements, and Caitlin's ability to use this tool keeps getting better. Those who propagandize that parents like us make this choice cavalierly, or for our own convenience, quite simply *just don't know us*. If as a parent, you look forward to sharing life with your child, and you believe that your child will benefit from who you are, your vision and experiences, and you will mutually benefit from this close bond, then you need to share a common language. "A different language is a different vision of life." For us, it was common sense to try our native language first. If it hadn't worked, we would have moved to a different option.

Another significant point leading us to an oral/aural approach and then to the implant is the low test scores in reading and language skills of deaf students educated in non-oral programs, where ASL is the mode of communication. The norm for these deaf high school graduates is to read on a fourth grade level. American Sign Language is beautiful but its syntax is very different from that of English, and it is without a written form. These facts present obstacles to becoming fluent in English. Education is the great equalizer in a society, and the most important gift to give a child. In our country, English is the language of the majority. Reading, writing and speaking it well mean access to information and possibilities; access to more fulfilling jobs, and a positive self-image that is based on accomplishments. The abilities to maneuver and feel comfortable in the dominant culture and excellent communication skills if possible are extremely helpful in one's life. We wanted these opportunities for our child. We believed to not try to teach Caitlin English first, to wait till "later," was to risk sentencing her to functional illiteracy. It is well recognized that the window of opportunity to develop any language is the first five years of a child's life.

Caitlin is happy, tenacious, and enjoys life. She has friends, both hearing and deaf, and is fully mainstreamed in an academically challenging school. She gets support services funded through the Board of Education. Her language and reading skills are three years above the norm for her age level. She studies piano, flute, French, and sings in the school chorus. Caitlin is a member of the National Dance Institute and last weekend performed with over a thousand kids in Central Park. She knows how to fingerspell and some ASL. Let me assure you: Caitlin is in there participating, learning, and exploring many different ideas and ways to express herself.

We have a close, extended family. We discuss, argue and laugh together. Caitlin has the ability to form her own opinions and speak her mind. She can disagree with her parents and sometimes does. So far we have the tools to navigate our differences. The implant, our shared language, and our love form the bridge. For us, deafness threatened something we value: freedom. If you do your job well as parents, your child grows up to be a happy adult, free and capable of choosing for herself from the broadest possible spectrum of life's adventures. Love, self-esteem, education, curiosity, community, independence, openness to other people, cultures, and the world - possessing a passion for life - were the dreams we discovered we valued and wanted for our child.

Most of us parents, the 90% who are hearing, face awesome questions in the initial days: Where do we start? What world will my child feel part of, comfortable and at home in? "What can I do to give my child the best chance at a happy, productive life?" Whatever our choices, there are no guarantees. But making our child "just like us" was never the issue.

Some of the best advice we got came from an oral-deaf otolaryngologist, Dr. Paul Hammerschlag. "Deafness is something that happens to a family, not just the child." Deafness affects communication, which is integral to healthy family life. The family is recognized as the initial place, the fragile equilibrium system that gets our new little people on firm foundation. Some don't get this foundation; they are injured and play "catch up" their entire lives. We know deaf children have the same needs as all children: to love and be loved; to be cherished, supported, responsibly cared for, well educated; and to learn to respect themselves and others. Implant families don't see our children as deprived of cultural identity. Those who argue hearing parents can't and shouldn't parent their deaf children because they can't be proper role models, baffle us. We know they have not spent time with our children.

We believe the implant was our responsibility and our decision to make as Caitlin's parents. We will answer to her. No one was going to represent Caitlin's individual needs, abilities, and interests the way we would. Our course has been to nurture and help her become all she can be. The extraordinary professional and community support we receive from the League for the Hard of Hearing's rehabilitation program with its high expectations, careful monitoring, guidance, and family-centered philosophy - as well as the A.G. Bell Association with its education, advocacy, and scholarship aid programs and also the Cochlear Implant Club International's adult role models and generous advice - has been essential to our family's well being. These organizations, the implant center at New York University Medical Center, her school, and her family form Caitlin's team. Caitlin is an example of what a "village" can do for a child when we work together.

Caitlin has been labeled an "anomaly" by the implant opposition. Her accomplishments and the *truth of her* have been marginalized. I am here today to lasso her back from that ostracized place. Shame on those who label and dismiss our implant children and families who bravely stand up to dialogue and speak about this tool. Our kids are not "solo stars that pro-implant people trot out to mislead and recklessly give false hope to other parents." Why would I do that to another parent? To another child? It would be cruel. Caitlin is special, all kids are, and she's mine, but she is not an anomaly. Labeling people and suppressing information has never been good strategy! This spreading of false information serves a political agenda, not the children. It was never our desire to have our child rejected by the deaf community because she uses an implant. But parents-like us aren't imagining what these implant kids are doing. We see it, hear it, and live it. I can tell you from my work at the League and international conferences, hearing impaired kids play, laugh, and have friends. They are doing amazing things: jabbering away, talking non-stop, playing musical instruments, boasting about their undefeated baseball team, winning spelling bees, performing on or above grade level, participating in the life of their school, community and family. The children benefiting from an aural/oral program are doing particularly well.

Deaf children cannot be caught in the middle of this ideological debate. We all need to create a climate that recognizes there is no one answer or correct way This means accurate information, quality options, improved technology, and parent advocacy training. Programs to help children maximize the use of this tool must be ensured. Funding and policies that respect and enable choices to work must be put in place everywhere.

Caitlin and the children like her have a miraculous tool to use. My daughter can turn her implant off and be in a silent world. She can learn sign language as well as hearing interpreters can. She already has a remarkable command of English. Caitlin has choices. She can go anywhere in the world and speak for herself.

Reprinted courtesy of Melody James Parton as previously published in League Rehabilitation Quarterly

With Implant, She Doesn't Miss a Beat
New York Times Sunday, August 1, 1999
by Leslie Feller

CAITLIN PARTON, a 14-year-old honor student at Westport's Coleytown Middle School, is deaf, but she can hear. In 1987, bacterial meningitis left her profoundly deaf at age 2. At 2 1/2, she was the youngest child in the country, and one of the first in the world, to receive a cochlear implant, a prosthesis that provides useful sound information by directly stimulating auditory nerve fibers in the inner ear, or cochlea.

More than a decade later, thanks to modern technology and much hard work, the eighth grader leads a remarkably normal life in a world filled with sound. She talks on the phone with friends, loves to watch MTV, listens to "everything but country on her radio and studies classical piano.

Soon after her implant surgery, the little girl and her parents, Melody James and Steve Parton, became the focus of controversy. In 1990, the National Association of the Deaf, representing what is called "the deaf culture," published a position paper opposing the cochlear implant particularly for children. "At the time, Caitlin was making wonderful progress," Ms. James said. "We felt we needed to let other parents know there was a choice." The Partons said they were shocked at what they felt was "very slanted" coverage in the deaf press. "Still, here we were just trying to do the best for our daughter who had almost died and, in addition to speech and hearing, had also lost her sense of balance," Mr. Parton said. When she returned from the hospital, the formerly active toddler could no longer hold her head straight, sit up, walk or talk. "Suddenly we were being vilified as these hearing parents who were ignorant, trying to fix their deaf kid instead of loving her just as she was," Ms. James said. "They said we had no right to decide to use artificial technology to deprive Caitlin of her deafness."

The Nucleus Spectra 22 Cochlear Implant System made by the Cochlear Corporation consists of a tiny receiver/stimulator implanted in the bone behind the ear. It is connected to 22 electrodes inserted into the cochlea, or inner ear. A small external microphone worn behind the ear is wired to a speech processor contained in a box the size of a deck of cards that can attach to a belt or fit in a pocket. Sounds are relayed to the processor which, powered by one AA battery, changes them into electrical impulses. These are transmitted to the nerve fibers of the cochlea, which send signals to the brain that are interpreted as sound.

54

Dr. Noel Cohen, the surgeon who did Caitlin's implant at New York University Medical Center, said her success is no longer unusual. With proper follow-up therapy, he said, the procedure has a 75-80 percent success rate and is an option for those whose deficit might be less severe, but who want access to a greater range of sounds. Success is considered the ability to understand a reasonable amount of speech without lipreading. Dr. Cohen said that 25,000 successful implants have been done worldwide, about 20,000 of them in the United States, where the operation, priced around $40,000, is considered minor surgery and is covered by most insurance companies as well as Medicaid and Medicare. The essential auditory and speech therapy require additional funding, which may not be covered by insurance.

"One cannot look at patients who have had cochlear implants in 1999 and say they that they don't work, because they do work," said Dr. John Kveton, a professor of otolaryngology at Yale School of Medicine. "It's critical to understand that the success rate will vary significantly depending on the individual's history." Dr. Kveton added that the goal is to push the operation "closer and closer to birth."

In November 1992, when Caitlin was 6, CBS news magazine *60 Minutes* broadcast a segment on her progress. It included comments from the author of the National Association of the Deaf position paper, Harlan Lane, a Ph.D. in psychology. During the *60 Minutes* telecast, Dr. Lane called surgeons, audiologists and speech therapists "the bigots of the world," accusing them of being motivated only by profit.

The associations president at the time, Roz Rosen, told Ed Bradley of *60 Minutes* through an interpreter that to be a part of the deaf culture, that approximately 2 million people learn to use American Sign Language, was a better alternative. "Instead of thinking of deafness as a disability," she said, "we think of it as an enhancement of vision."

Caitlin, who is an active spokeswoman for the device, disagrees. "I don't understand why these people are in denial," she said. She first testified before Congress when she was 5 and later at age 11. She recently appeared on the Nickelodeon channel's *Nick News* on a panel discussing disabilities with the journalist Linda Efferbee and the actor-director Christopher Reeve. "A person normally has five senses," she said. "If one is impaired, the others do enhance, but what's missing certainly constitutes a disability. At the very least, deafness is a difference that can isolate you and severely narrow your options." Caitlin adamantly supports her parents' decision about the implant. "They had to act for me because I was too young to act for myself," she said.

"There are people in the deaf culture who called my parents cruel and the implant a form of genocide, killing off deafness in the world. But I'm still deaf. Without the implant, I hear practically nothing. I'm part of their culture whether they want to accept me or not."

Caitlin and her parents emphasized that the implant was not a quick fix. "You don't pop it in and suddenly hear," Caitlin said. "It's a tool you have to learn to use, which takes years of intensive speech therapy and support from family members. It is a miracle device, but you have to put in the hard work to make the miracle happen."

Dr. Cohen cited research indicating that, with the right training, virtually all children who have the implant before the age of 5 can learn to use the device to understand speech and develop normal spoken language. Some recent recipients have been as young as 13 months. "The earlier, the better," he said, "because the most rapid development of speech and language takes place in the first two years of life."

Ms. James, now Director of Resources for the League for the Hard of Hearing in New York City, said that it is difficult for people who grow up as manual communicators to pick up oral language later on. "They don't develop the muscles that are used for speech," she said, "and when the auditory nerve has not been stimulated for many years, it atrophies." Ms. James is working to correct what she said was the distorted perception of the implant. "Television shows like *E.R.* and *Guiding Light*, watched by millions, often sacrifice accuracy for melodrama," she said. "They portray the implant as something perpetrated by incompetent money grubbing surgeons." The message of a movie like *Children of a Lesser God* is that it is traumatic for a deaf person to learn to speak, Ms. James said. "Once that may have been true," she said, "but not anymore." Positive support, backed by determination, has fueled Caitlin's accomplishments, including adjusting to the loss of balance that is a second consequence of meningitis.

Caitlin said she now hears "just like that," even first thing in the morning after sleeping all night minus her microphone and processor. "In less than a split second from hearing nothing to hearing everything," she said. She said, however, that functioning well as a deaf person in a hearing world required concentration and multiple strategies. Along with hearing skills, she relies on lipreading and intelligent guessing. She does not hesitate to ask friends to repeat things when necessary. "The effort can be exhausting," her father said, "especially in situations like car pools and going to uncaptioned movies. Caitlin's gotten so good at appearing normal, it's easy to forget she's a disabled person using a

56

prosthetic device." At school, a cacophony of background sound requires deciphering. "There are bells ringing, chairs scraping, pencils dropping, people whispering," Caitlin said. With Coleytown Middle School being renovated, construction noise has made the past year even more difficult. Along with her book bag, she must carry a personal sound system from class to class. "The teacher talks into a remote microphone," she said, "and I hear it directly from a small speaker that sits on my desk."

In French class, Caitlin looks just like any other student at first glance. A slight quaver in her voice, the tiny microphone and double wires snaking down behind her left ear are the only indications of difference. "There are times I wish I were like everybody else," she said. "But what's the point of that? In general, I like the way my life is turning out."

In 1998, the National Association for the Deaf withdrew its original position paper, saying that the issue of childhood cochlear implants was undergoing re-evaluation. Meanwhile, at Coleytown Middle School's year-end talent show, Caitlin will perform a piano solo. "I'll be playing Battle by Burgmufler," she said, adding that of all the sounds that fill her world, piano music is a particular pleasure.

"When she first got back from the hospital," her parents said, "Caitlin would go up to the stereo speaker and put her hands on it. That's how she would listen to the music. Shortly after the implant, Caitlin had to learn how to use the implant to recognize each note. "I don't have to analyze it anymore," she said. "I am just in the music."

Reprinted with permission by The New York Times

S.F. Woman Hears What She's Missed
By Zoe Mezin
The San Francisco Examiner
Published June 20, 2001

For the first time in more than four decades, Julie Stephens sat down to dinner with her husband and discovered sounds she had never heard before: the clinking of silverware slicing meat and vegetables, the din of dishes being thrown into bins by busboys, and the creaking of chairs as restaurant patrons hoisted themselves in and out of seats. At home, she heard her toilet flushing "like a big Niagara Falls" and the tip-tap-typing of her fingers on a computer keyboard. Her husband, itching to talk, no longer poked her to get attention. He simply spoke.

Stephens is the first patient fitted with the new "bionic ear" by a team of researchers at University of California San Francisco. In March, doctors, using cochlear implant technology, surgically imbedded a quarter size microprocessor in Stephens' skull and 16 electrodes in her inner ear. Behind her right ear, she wears a device that acts like a miniature radio station. It sends signals through her skin to the microprocessor that in turn activates the electrodes to stimulate nerves in the inner ear, thus creating the sense of sound.

This "bionic ear" not only helps her hear and understand conversation again, but it also gave her the chance to recognize sounds she never knew existed.

"There were so many little sounds I wasn't aware of," Stephens said in a phone conversation Monday. "I was amazed at what I was missing."

Totally deaf in her left ear and profoundly deaf in her right, Stephens is one of an estimated 28 million Americans who suffer from hearing loss. Though about 700,000 people in the United States are severely or profoundly deaf, only about 40,000 people worldwide currently use cochlear implant technology. Many simply wear external hearing aids.

Stephens has relied on hearing aids since age 4, when an infection took away her ability to hear. But in the past few years, the hearing aids, which amplified sounds, no longer seemed to work. She could no longer hear the two or three words she long relied on to piece the puzzles of a sentence together. She stopped calling friends and shied away from group conversations.

Last year, her audiologist asked her if she knew about cochlear implants. She said yes.

Shortly after graduating from college in the early 1980s, her parents took her to UCSF to be fitted for one of the first-generation cochlear implants. They were bigger and heavier in those days, Stephens said, and not as technologically advanced. She decided to pass on the implant and wait for the next big technological leap.

This leap, the third of its kind in the field, didn't come until early this year, when the FDA approved the Clarion CII Bionic Ear implant.

The technology was developed in the early 1970s and gave patients only a general awareness of sound. The pea-sized inner ear cochlea looks like a snail shell and is filled with fluid. Sound waves agitate the fluid, making it move like the waves in an ocean. About 40,000 microscopic hair cells, also located in the inner ear, sway and bend like sea algae caught in a tidal thrust, providing the electrical stimulation that's ultimately transmitted to the nervous system.

Understanding speech remained elusive until the mid-1980s, when two research teams in San Francisco and Australia -started inserting multiple electrodes in the ear. These electrodes could transmit 20,000 to 40,000 pulses per second of information to nerve endings, helping severely to profoundly deaf people distinguish the wail of a siren from the cry of a baby.

"It's all about resolution," said Doug Lynch, communications director for Advanced Bionics Corporation, the makers of the bionic ear. "The more sound information delivered to the inner ear, the better the person hears."

The new bionic ear can act as a regular cochlear implant, sending 64,000 pulses of sound information per second to nerve endings. It also can be revved up to 1 million pulses per second when switched to bionic mode. UCSF researchers are prepared to test the effectiveness of this new wave of cochlear implants and are seeking six more volunteers to participate in the nationwide study.

The surgery, implant and one-year post-operative visits costs from $45,000 to $50,000. Unlike hearing aids, it is covered by most public and private health insurances.

Jan Larky, coordinator and lead audiologist at the Douglas Grant Cochlear Implant Center, encourages everyone to come in and be evaluated, even if they don't want the implant.

"They can choose not to be implanted," she said, adding that she wants them to at least have the opportunity to experience hearing again. Said Larky of the results: "They're pretty immediate. First, they're not hearing, and then they're hearing. And that happens in a day. It's pretty exciting."

Reprinted with permission from the San Francisco Examiner

The Richest Man in Town
By William E. Saracino

December 18, 2001 Source: *California Political Review Online*
The small, everyday things make a wonderful life. William E. Saracino
is a member of *California Political Review's* editorial board.

A whim of my esteemed editor some months ago determined that my
column appears on Tuesday. A whim of an esteemed calendar-maker
centuries ago determined that this year Christmas and New Years fall
on Tuesday. Hence, this will be my last offering for the year. That
being so, I hereby invoke a point of personal privilege, opting out of my
usual political ponderings to offer thoughts more apropos of the season.

You don't have to know me very well to discover that I think *It's A
Wonderful Life* is perhaps the finest movie ever made. Oh not judging
on technical standards, though the movie is quite well done. *It's A
Wonderful Life* is a great movie - perhaps the greatest - because of the
messages that are imparted in it. And though it is ubiquitous on television this time of year, do yourself a favor and buy the video cassette, or
better yet the DVD, to avoid the editing done for the tube. Avoid the
colorized version like you would a letter from Osama Bin Laden with
powder on it.

It is a rare person who is not familiar with the scene at the end of the
movie, where all of George Bailey's (Jimmy Stewart) friends and family have gathered round him to help him through a tough spot. That
scene, to me, is the essence of a successful life, of a wonderful life -
having those you love and who love you surround you with comfort
when you need it most.

I know from whence I speak. In September of 1998 I went completely
deaf in the space of three hours one morning. I recovered my "hearing" in April of 1999 after successful cochlear implant surgery. During
the seven months of my 'Simon and Garfunkel' period, from September
to April, (think sounds of silence ... ahem) and for the first few months
after surgery while adjusting to the cochlear implant, I discovered how
George Bailey must have felt. I could not possibly have made it through
that very rough time without the support and love of my family and
friends delivered on a daily basis.

One of the messages of *Wonderful Life* I find most compelling is how George got into the position of having all those friends willing to rally around him. The answer lies in the way he lived his life. He was constantly looking out for other people, always willing to help out, eager to do the right thing. He was always happy to engage in kindnesses that, while they might appear trivial on the surface, meant a great deal to the people on the receiving end of them. It was the small things, the every day things that made the difference. George Bailey didn't change the world. But he did make it a much better place, one person at a time.

I learned the importance of "small kindnesses" when I went through my great (non) hearing adventure. During my seven months of deafness, there were times I would get down, dispirited, or stressed. Every time that happened and I mean this quite literally—one of my family or friends would call, write, stop by, send an e-mail, or do some small thing that picked me up. It may have taken them 30 seconds and might have involved the most trivial of things—but it made my day, many times. Many good things have come out of that time in my life. Among the foremost is my understanding now that the little things can mean a lot to people in day-to-day living.

Let me make clear I'm not talking about the moronic "random acts of kindness" mantra that the Cumbaya crowd prescribes as a cure for the world's ills. What I'm talking about is specifically not random. Spur of the moment perhaps, but not random. I'm talking about premeditated acts of charity and love for those we know are in need of succor. Or even for those we only suspect are in need of it. I'm talking about appreciating the importance of taking time in our busy lives to do the small things—acts of friendship, for lack of a better description—that which is so easy to put off until "tomorrow."

Don't do that. Tomorrow is promised to none of us, and the spirit of somebody you know may well need a lift today. At 9 a.m. on September 18, 1998, I could hear just fine. At noon I was stone, cold deaf. Tomorrow may not bring you the opportunity to help someone that today carries. While we are busy trying to do the big things in our lives, let's not forget what George Bailey teaches us - that often we do the most important work of living just by being a friend - one person at a time.

Mother Theresa put it this way: "Only rarely in our lives are we called upon to do great things. But every day of our lives we are called upon to do little things with great love." I expect that sounds hokey and maudlin, yet I know the truth of it. During my challenging times I was, of course, cheered by the big things done and grand gestures made on my behalf. But it was the small, day-to-day kindness and thoughtfulness really got me through.

Doing 'little things with great love' can be a challenge, as it requires a humility that isn't necessarily natural to us. We, after all, grow up dreaming of big things, especially those of us in politics or the public eye. Most of us, myself included, define a successful life in financial terms way too frequently. Following Mother Theresa's road may make the world better, but it's unlikely to make us rich or famous. It probably won't even get you noticed - except of course by the recipient of your thoughtfulness.

But there are other rewards. Standing before the Almighty on judgment day, would you rather be able to say you helped elect presidents, senators, and governors, or that you helped mend someone's spirit when that spirit was tattered? That you drove only the finest cars, or that you took the five minutes necessary to brighten an estranged friend's heart? That all your sweaters were cashmere or that you comforted all you met with love and laughter? All these things aren't mutually exclusive certainly, but far too many of us do not have them prioritized properly.

As we approach December 25, let us contemplate the message of the child born in Bethlehem. And as we do so, let us keep in mind the admonition of Mother Theresa, who is doubtless one of his saints. Let us, by all means, do the 'great things' that life brings to us, if that is our lot. But let us every day remember to do the little things with great love. By doing so we can impact the world enormously, just as George Bailey did, one person at a time. It's the secret to a wonderful life.

Reprinted with permission of William E. Saracino who serves as the CFO of the Parents Television Council

Now Hear This!

People Weekly, **August 1999**
Deaf since childhood, a TV actress celebrates the gift of hearing.

You'd almost think Amy Ecklund is a contestant on a game show called 'Guess That Sound.' "That's a glass!" she proudly exclaims as she hears a clinking noise in the New Haven pub where she's having lunch. "Silverware!" she cries at the clang of a fork. When a hammer bangs, Ecklund gets really excited. "Wow!" she says, "that is loud!"

Life's everyday clatter is a symphony to Ecklund, 29, who for four years has played deaf hospital administrator Abigail Bauer on the CBS soap *Guiding Light*. Hearing-impaired since age 6 (doctors never determined the cause) Eckland no longer has to read lips to do scenes. Last January she had a Nucleus 24 cochlear implant put in her right ear, thus becoming one of the 2,000 people in the U.S. to have benefited from the revolutionary hearing device.

The two-part implant - an internal receiver and electrodes that stimulates hair cells in the cochlea (the canal in the inner ear where the auditory nerves originate), paired with an external sound processor hidden behind the ear - has allowed Ecklund to hear nearly normally, dramatically changing her life. "It's like watching a child being born," says Michael O'Leary, who plays her husband, Dr. Rick Bauer, on *Guiding Light*- which Ecklund's character also received a cochlear implant in May. But trying to understand thousands of sounds - dishwasher, her dogs flapping their ears - has been disorienting for the Nevada-born daughter of an attorney father and artist mother. Married to Jon Ecklund, 29, a Yale School of Drama graduate, and living in New Haven, Ecklund met with correspondent Cynthia Wang to explain what it's like to hear again after so many years.

I started losing my hearing when I was 3 or 4, and every year it got harder to hear voices or talk on the phone. But between my hearing aid and reading lips I was able to get along socially and at work. Last year, though, things got so bad that at the grocery store, people would poke me in the back and say, "Would you get out of the way. I've been asking you to move for five minutes!"

Every once in a while I would ask my audiologist, Amy Popp, about hearing-enabling devices, but for years I just wasn't ready to get one. Then, last November, Amy showed me the Nucleus 24 implant, which you can't even tell someone has on. That kind of did it for me. I decided to just jump off and do it. I know there is a controversy about the implant. Many people in the deaf community believe that being deaf is not a defect, and that's a valid viewpoint. But because of the career and the life that I choose, I am really in the thick of the hearing community. I'm an adult, and I made the choice that's right for me, and all of my deaf friends are very supportive of my decision.

The operation happened on Jan. 13, and it lasted an hour and 40 minutes. I had to wait about a month for my head to heal, and there was more pain than I thought there would be. When they first turned on the implant in February, things all sounded the same, like a high, Mickey Mousey sound. The first thing I heard was my audiologist's voice, and I made her stop talking and start whispering. Even fingernails tapping on a table were too loud. For two days after that my husband and I had to whisper because everything was so loud.

My audiologist adjusted the implant and then made me go walk around the street for five minutes, and that was really weird. I was aware of people staring at me because I was walking like a zombie. I think I might have even been drooling. Then I had to start learning and identifying all these new sounds, and that was tiring. I knew what some noises were because I could see what was happening. But on the first day, I heard a noise in the kitchen that sounded like a slide whistle, and I asked Jon, "What's that?" He said, "That's the dog drinking out of the bowl." And I thought about it and all of a sudden the sound changed, like from Chinese characters to English, and I heard the dog drinking.

The thing that I was really excited about was using the telephone, and for my first call I dialed my mom. But she wasn't home, and I got my brother Nick, who's 18, then I said, "Hi, it's Amy," and he said, "Oh, hi." He didn't realize I could hear him. So I said, "Nick, do you realize this is my first phone conversation in 18 years?" And he goes, "Oh, my God, you can hear me?" And we both just started crying.

After that, I think I called everybody - even my ex-boyfriend from college! I'm learning phone etiquette, about not cutting in and who talks first. I tried listening to music in the first week, and it wasn't so good. But by the third week I was on the floor sobbing - going, "It's the Doobie Brothers!" I also went to see *Saving Private Ryan*, and I was in shock. I could tell the difference between the machine guns and the rifles, which was great. I giggled through the whole movie, which I know was inappropriate.

Everything changed. I used to flood the kitchen a lot because I'd turn on the water and go do something else. Not anymore. My two miniature pinschers, Eloise and Marcella, were always aware I couldn't hear. Someone would be at the door, and they would come and get me. Now they notice I tell them to be quiet a lot more. Even hearing myself pee was a real revelation. Now I can tell when I'm finished!

On *Guiding Light*, I used to memorize every actor's lines to do a scene. Now I can just take in what they're saying. I can close my eyes and still talk to the makeup artist, for the first time! Michael O'Leary, my costar, has been belching in front of me a lot. He does this impression of William Shatner and belches, which really cracks me up. But there was a downside to this: I would get depressed - I'm not sure why. I had to deal with other people's happy emotions, with them wanting to know how I feel. But lots of times, I don't know how I feel. It's an enormous experience, and it's not all clear to me. I don't think I would have been able to go through this without Jon's support.

Still, I wouldn't change this experience for anything. I connect with people better now because I'm so much more able to be myself rather than putting up a shield to hide my fears. My whole place in the world has changed, just from understanding more of what is going on. Before, I didn't even realize some of the things I was missing, but that's okay. Every day is different now. Every day is a miracle.

Reprinted with permission from People Weekly

Hear US
FOR IMMEDIATE RELEASE August 17, 2000

NOISE-INDUCED HEARING LOSS IS LEADING OCCUPATIONAL DISEASE IN TODAY'S WORKFORCE. Working Americans Reminded to Care for their Hearing Health this Labor Day

Washington, D.C.- Noise-induced hearing loss is one of the top occupational hazards in the modern workforce. This Labor Day, the National Campaign for Hearing Health urges all Americans to take care of their hearing, and is offering free earplugs in order to ensure hearing safety while on the job.

According to a recent Harris poll, nearly half (48%) of all Americans have not had their hearing checked in the past five years despite the daily bombardment of toxic noise, the medically approved phrase the National Campaign for Hearing Health uses to describe noises that can damage and destroy hearing. And, the majority of Americans (68%) have let three years go by without a hearing check-up. Yet, over one-third of those polled report having some degree of hearing loss. To keep in good hearing health, the National Campaign for Hearing Health recommends making hearing exams a part of every routine medical examination.

Approximately 30 million workers are exposed to workplace toxic noise. Symptoms of exposure to toxic noise include ringing or pain in ears, muffled sounds, difficulty hearing quiet sounds, a feeling of fullness in ears, or awareness of transient hearing loss. An additional nine million are at risk for hearing loss from other agents such as solvents and metals, according to the National Institute for Occupational Safety and Health (NIOSH). In addition to being the most common occupational disease, noise-induced hearing loss is the second most self-reported occupational illness or injury.

"Workplace toxic noise causes one-third of all hearing loss in the U.S.," said Elizabeth Foster, director of the National Campaign for Hearing Health. "In a workplace where state-of-the-art technology, equipment and communications devices are commonplace, we want to ensure that the basic provisions — such as protective equipment and quiet work areas — are made available to everyone."

To promote hearing health work environments, the Campaign is offering free earplugs through their Web site (www.hearinghealth.net)

or by calling 1-800-829-5934.

According to NIOSH, those most at risk for hearing loss are workers in the agriculture, mining, construction, manufacturing, utilities, transportation and military industries. Any sound produced at or above 85 decibels (dB) threatens to damage the ear. Normal conversation measures at approximately 60 decibels and the average phone rings at 80 decibels, but many sounds we commonly encounter register at a much higher level - from 90 to well over 100 decibels. Elements within those high-risk toxic noise environments include tractors (95-100dB), hand drills (95-100dB), ambulance sirens (120dB), and airplane engine noise in cabins (90-110 dB). However, without proper protection from toxic noise everyone is at risk of hearing loss, whether in the office, at the job site, or while working at home.

Noise-induced hearing loss is a preventable occupational disease. The National Campaign for Hearing Health recommends following these simple steps to guard against hearing damage in the workplace:

Keep it quiet - Encourage your employer to select quieter equipment when purchasing new items; affordable sound meters are available for measuring dangerous areas or pieces of equipment.
Keep it short - Minimize duration of exposure to loud noises; take regular breaks from particularly loud jobs/assignments.
Keep it covered - Use earplugs, earmuffs or other protection when working around loud equipment or in loud areas.
Keep it monitored - Have your hearing tested every year; it is an easy, inexpensive and non-invasive way to ensure healthy hearing, to prevent further deterioration if possible and to get appropriate remedies or treatments before it's too late; contact the National Campaign for Hearing Health for information on health care facilities that conduct hearing tests in your area (1-800-829-5934).

The National Campaign for Hearing Health was launched in March 1999 by the Deafness Research Foundation, the nation's largest voluntary health organization devoted to research and public education related to hearing loss and hearing health.

Reprinted with permission of the Deafness Research Foundation

NATIONAL CHILDREN'S HEALTH CRISIS LOOMS AS INFANT HEARING SCREENING RATES STAGNATE FOR AMERICA'S NUMBER ONE BIRTH DEFECT: HEARING LOSS

National Campaign for Hearing Health Releases Data Showing a Marginal Increase In Newborn Screenings From 65% to 69%

Washington, D.C. - On Tuesday, May 21, the National Campaign for Hearing Health (NCHH), in partnership with the American Academy of Pediatrics, Members of Congress, hearing health experts, pediatricians and daytime drama stars who have dealt with this issue, will hold a National Update on Infant Hearing Screening from 10:00 am to 11:30 am in SR-485 Russell Senate Office Building on Capitol Hill. Preliminary data released by NCHH indicates a minor increase in newborn hearing screenings since the release of the Campaign's last annual report card in May 2001. In November 1999, the Campaign released data that indicated only 25% of U.S. newborns were screened for hearing loss. Since that time there has been steady and substantial progress — until recently. In April 2000 - the number had risen to 46% and in May 2001 65% of infants were screened. One year later, that number has only made a marginal rise to 69% of babies born in the U.S., an increase that is worrisome -especially since funding for infant hearing screening programs was eliminated from the President's FY 2003 Budget.

"Considering that hearing loss is our nation's number one birth defect and a reliable hearing test costs as little as $20, it is unbelievable that all infants are not automatically screened at birth," said Elizabeth Thorp, Director of the National Campaign for Hearing Health.

"As a pediatrician, I cannot overstate the importance of early detection," said Dr. Louis Cooper, President of the American Academy of Pediatrics, "Hearing loss is the most common birth defect and, if undetected can impede speech, language, and cognitive development."

Held during Congressionally recognized Better Hearing and Speech Month, the event on Capitol Hill will unveil the most recent data on newborn screenings and increase awareness for the importance of early detection of hearing loss. The panel will include:

- Kassie & Jim DePaiva, *One Life to Live* actors and parents of a child with hearing loss
- Louis Z. Cooper, M.D., President of the American Academy of Pediatrics
- Karl White, Ph.D., Director of National Center for Hearing Assessment and Management
- Elizabeth E. Thorp, Director of the National Campaign for Hearing Health
- Representative Jim Walsh (R-NY), Congressional Hearing Health Caucus Co-Chair
- Representative Jim Ryun (R-KS), Congressional Hearing Health Caucus Co-Chair
- Representative Rosa L. DeLauro (D-CT)
- Elvir Causevic, D.Sc., and Mike Scholin, MS, CCC-A, GSI Infant Hearing Screening Demo

Approximately 33 babies with significant permanent hearing loss are born each day and experts have stressed the importance of screening all babies at birth in order to prevent these children from leaving the hospital with undetected hearing loss. Yet, almost one-third of newborns are still going home undetected. Although hearing health and pediatric experts have emphasized how critically important it is to have universal newborn hearing screening, currently only 37 U.S. states and the District of Columbia have laws mandating hearing screenings at birth.

According to Dr. Karl White, director of the National Center for Hearing Assessment and Management at Utah State, "Newborn hearing screening is a simple and inexpensive procedure that results in dramatic benefits for babies and their families. It is a tragedy that nearly a third of all newborns in the United States still leave the hospital without anyone knowing whether they can hear."

The Campaign will release its third annual State-by-State Report Card that analyzes the current status of infant screening. Preliminary findings indicate the following:

- **15 Excellent** states-Almost all babies are screened (95%+), and a statewide system for coordination, training, quality assurance, and follow up has been established.

- **22 Good states-**At least 75% of babies are screened, and a statewide system for coordination, training, quality assurance, and follow up has been established.
- **7 Fair** states-At least 45% of babies are being screened, and a statewide system for coordination, training, quality assurance, and follow up is being developed.
- **6 Unsatisfactory** states-Less than 44% of babies are being screened.

The state-by-state report card and state map can be seen on the Web at www.hearinghealth.net.

"As the mother of a child with hearing loss," said actress Kassie DePaiva, "It is so important for parents - even those with no family history of hearing loss - to take an active role in their child's hearing health. Without newborn hearing screening, parents have no idea whether they are really communicating with their baby!"

The National Campaign for Hearing Health, launched in March, 1999 by the Deafness Research Foundation, is working to put hearing health on the national agenda by promoting awareness, advocacy, education and legislation of the number one birth defect in the United States — hearing loss.

Reprinted courtesy of the Deafness Research Foundation

Educating a Child Who Has a Cochlear Implant
By Peg Williams Ph.D. of Cochlear Implant Assoc. Int.

As the parent of a child with a cochlear implant (CI), you need to become familiar with the Federal and state services that are available to provide your child with a free and appropriate education designed specifically to meet his or her needs. You should be aware of and take an active role in obtaining these services, which are available to your child either until he or she graduates from high school or reaches age 21, whichever comes first.

Background

The Federal law that supports special education and related services programming for children and youth with disabilities is called the individuals with Disabilities Education Act (IDEA). Under this law, which was originally enacted in 1975, all eligible school-age children and youth with disabilities are entitled to receive a free and appropriate public education (FAPE) in the least restrictive environment. The least restrictive environment entitles most children to be educated with non-disabled children, to the maximum extent possible, where they can benefit from the stimulation and social contact and where appropriate supplementary assistance is provided. In addition to this law, amendments were passed in 1986 that include:

> · Provisions to help states develop early intervention programs for infants and toddlers with disabilities, and special funding incentives for states that make a free appropriate public education available for all eligible preschool children with dis abilities ages three through five.

It is important for you to become familiar with your state special education law. The IDEA is a Federal law and as such, provides minimum requirements that states must meet to receive Federal Funds to assist in providing special education and related services. Your state law and regulations may go beyond the Federal requirements, and it is important to know their specifics. You may want to contact your State Department of Education, Division of Special Education, in your state capital, and ask for a parent handbook on special education.

Obtaining Special Education Services for Your School-Age Child

The first step in obtaining special education services for your school-age child is to arrange for your child to receive an evaluation by the district's Committee on Special Education (CSE). This evaluation process gathers and uses information to determine whether a child has a disability and the nature and extent of the special education and related services that the child needs. The public schools are required to conduct this evaluation of your child at no cost to you.

The evaluation process should look at the "whole child" and include information about your child's total environment. Performed by a multidisciplinary team (including appropriate specialists, such as a school psychologist, speech-language pathologist, occupational therapist, physical therapist, medical specialist, educational diagnostician, classroom teacher, and others), the evaluation process includes observations by professionals who have worked with your child, your child's medical history, and information and observations from the family. There are at least three ways for your child to receive an evaluation: You can request an evaluation; the school may ask permission to evaluate your child; or a teacher or doctor may suggest that your child be evaluated.

Following the evaluation, if your child is found to be eligible, the evaluation results will form the basis for developing your child's Individualized Education Program (IEP) This is a written statement of the educational program designed to meet a child's special needs. It is designed to: (1) establish the learning goals for your child; and (2) state the services that the school district will provide for your child. It is developed by a multidisciplinary team that must include one teacher or other specialist who is knowledgeable about hearing impairment, along with the child's teacher(s), a representative of the school system, the parents, and the child (when appropriate).

A child's IEP should include statements of the child's strengths and weaknesses and describe the instructional program developed specifically for him or her. This plan shows the child's current educational level, short and long-term goals, and adaptive listening devices that may be required to achieve these goals. It should be provided at the district's expense, not yours. It also includes transportation and any related services your child will require. It is very important for parents to be entirely satisfied with the IEP prior to signing, as this document will direct the services your child will receive. Remember, however, that the IEP can be changed. You may request a review or revision of the IEP at any time. If the school system is reluctant to provide the proper training for your child, you need to be assertive and persistent. The rehabilitation team at the implant center may be able to assist you in working with the school to develop an appropriate program for your child.

Under the Federal and state special education regulations, a variety of services must be made available if needed by your child. These related services can include but are not limited to the following: physical therapy, occupational therapy, speech/language therapy, adaptive physical Education, vocational placement services, counseling, transportation, assistive technology and Training necessary for professionals to use/teach with the device rehabilitation counseling Orientation and mobility services.

If you are unable to reach agreement with the school on the placement of your child, a specific procedure, called Due Process, is available, but you must ask for it. Due Process also is available if a disagreement arises concerning identification, assessment, or placement of a child. You should be notified of this process in writing when the school advises you about the recommended placement of your child.

Tips for Parents

There are a number of things you can do to ease your child's transition into the classroom. Meet with your child's teachers to explain the cochlear implant and/or provide pamphlets and brochures about cochlear implants. Some cochlear implant centers provide in-service training for teachers who will be working with cochlear implant children. This will be especially helpful if the child is mainstreamed in a hearing class where the teacher may not be familiar with cochlear implants.

Emphasize that the benefits gained by the child's participation in a regular school program. Provide a telephone number should an emergency arise. Ask the teacher to explain to the other children about why your child has a cochlear implant. Explain to the teachers that it is best for your child to be treated the same as the other students, equally and without special favor or attention. After your child turns 14, the IEP must include a statement of transition needs. Transition services are defined by the IDEA as a coordinated set of activities for a student that promotes movement from school to post-secondary activities, including education, vocational training, adult services, and independent living.

College

In most cases, the only deterrent facing a student with a cochlear implant in choosing a college is optimum accessibility of the facilities. Many colleges and universities have support services to assist in the accommodation of students with hearing impairment. Personnel providing these services can often be helpful in providing information to help prospective students determine whether the college will meet their needs. A visit to any college being considered is imperative to judge the degree of accessibility.

Reference: Some of the information included in this fact sheet was abstracted from:

Estes, J.M. (1997). Advocating for your child's education. Atlanta: The Georgia Advocacy Office.

Additional Readings:

Anderson, W., Chitwood, S., & Hayden, D. (1997). Negotiating the special education maze: A Guide for Parents and Teachers (3rd ed.). Bethesda, MD: Woodbine.

Apicella, R. (1993, Summer). Special Education Meetings. In *CONTACT*, Washington, DC: Cochlear Implant Association, Inc., p.35.

Nevins, M.E., and Chute, P.M. (1996). Children with cochlear implants in educational settings. Florence, KY: Thompson Learning.

Reprinted Courtesy of Cochlear Implant Association International

GETTING THE MOST OUT OF YOUR PROGRAMMING SESSION

Presented by Advanced Bionics in conjunction with the Cochlear Implant International Convention 1999

Don't just tell your audiologist that you are not hearing well. You need to give him or her more detail. <u>What</u> are you not hearing well, and <u>when</u> are you not hearing well? Keep a journal. Write down which situations are working well for you, and which ones are not. For example, you might be having problems at work when certain machinery is in use, or you could not hear well at a family gathering or when a TV was playing in the background. Perhaps you are having difficulty with men's voices on the telephone, but women's voices and children's voices are fine. Write that in your journal and take it along to your mapping session so your audiologist can help you with those circumstances. You might want to have a map just for those circumstances, or maybe one of your maps needs adjustment for it. Do write them down so you can remember them when you get to the audiologist. You will both find this very helpful.

When to go for a new program:
-Changes in your voice have occurred (people will tell you)
-Changes in clarity of speech (either your speech or the speech of others)
-Changes in listening at a distance (used to be able to hear at that distance, and now you can't)
-Frequent asking for repetitions (huh, what?) -Some sounds are uncomfortable
-Need a program for a particular listening situation
-Missing sounds, consonants, or parts of words

What should you bring?
-Journal of listening experiences
-Rating of your processor in different listening situations (example: one-on-one conversations (good), listening to the radio (fair), hearing the minister at church (poor)
-Report of whether volume or sensitivity button is used more
-Description of needs or problems
-Special media that you would like to use such as a telephone adaptor,

walkman with patch cord, etc.

What makes it easier?
-Establish a vocabulary with your audiologist that describes sounds
(see below for some suggestions)
-Practice loudness comparisons at home
-Practice pitch comparisons
-Practice speech listening activities (have someone read the same
article, for example)
-Practice listening at different distances

Before you leave your appointment:
-Listen to multiple speakers with your new program
(both men and women)
-Listen to your program through your processor
-Listen in quiet and in noise (try going out in the waiting room or down
to the cafeteria for a few minutes and then come back)
-Try to re-create special media needs in the audiologist's office by bringing along your telephone adaptor or walkman so you can try a new
program before you leave.

Some people take a tape of their favorite type of music and have their
spouse read a newspaper article aloud. If both things sound good with
the new map, they know the map will work for them.

Be sure you ask for enough time when you go in for a map. Even
though you may be done with your mapping in 30 minutes, you want
time to be able to go out and test it, and then come back if necessary.
Even if your audiologist sounds good, that is just one voice in perfect
quiet. Try other voices in other listening situations if you can before you
leave for home.

A great website for honing your listening skills is: www.esl-lab.com

Reprinted Courtesy of Advanced Bionics Corporation

Children's Stories

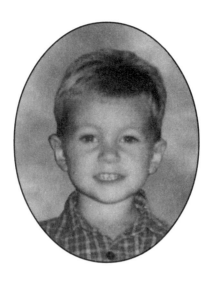

A Mother's Story of Doubt…By Stacy Thurman

Do you have doubts or concerns about your child's health? Get them checked out. Shortly after my son was born, I started having concerns about his hearing. These concerns increased as time went on. I would try my own hearing tests like setting off the smoke alarm or banging on pots and pans. I was always sure I had seen some reaction from him. I was in denial. When I did bring myself to mention the idea to others, most would try to ease my worries by reassuring me "newborns could sleep through most anything." Still I knew something wasn't right. When I questioned Eli's pediatrician, I was told I was imagining things. I was put off time and time again. I tried to make an appointment with a specialist. I needed my pediatrician's referral. At this point I went to Eli's pediatrician and demanded my son's hearing be checked.

When my son was 4 ½ months old, all my fears were confirmed. I was told my son had profound hearing loss in both ears. He was deaf. What I felt was indescribable, I was devastated…I had never been more confused or scared in my entire life. How were my husband and I going to provide Eli with the life we had always dreamed of giving him? Immediately I had all these thoughts going through my mind. Would Eli need to go to a deaf school or could he attend a public school? Would we need to relocate? How would I communicate with my son?

Would I ever hear Eli say, "Mom, I love you," or could he ever hear me say I love him? So many "Whys?" How could this happen? While pregnant with Eli I didn't drink or smoke; what did I do wrong?

Right away Eli was fitted with two of the most powerful hearing aids made. After months of wear he received minimal benefit. Although Eli's communication was progressing wonderfully using sign language, our hopes for better hearing and speech were being discouraged. In the meantime, we began using sign language with Eli. I am so glad we chose to sign with Eli as it is such a beautiful language. It was amazing how quickly he picked up signs. Eli did learn to communicate to me. He was signing, "Mom, I love you," and he understood that I loved him as well.

At last, another option appeared for Eli that might provide him with better hearing and the tools to learn speech. We learned that Eli was a candidate for a cochlear implant. But it was hard to make decisions for someone that you know will affect the rest of their life. All along, my husband and I had tried to keep an open mind and explore all our options. In our minds, we needed to know as much as we could about Eli's loss in order to make the best possible decision. We finally felt we had reached that point. We wanted to give our child every opportunity we could to hear and speak. The decision to have Eli receive a cochlear implant was not made quickly, nor easily. We read piles of literature and spoke with a number of individuals who had dealt with the same decision.

Once again I went to Eli's pediatrician. I told him that we were considering cochlear implantation. He told me that cochlear implants "were something that you hear about on *60 Minutes*" and really "were not a good alternative." We pursued cochlear implants anyway. The decision came down to what was in our hearts.

Prior to implantation, we met with Eli's ear doctor (Dr. Scott Estrem) for several counseling sessions. At one point he told us that this was his favorite surgery. This statement caught me by surprise. But he continued, "that it wasn't the surgery itself, but because I get to see the wonderful results." At last the day of the surgery arrived. I don't think my husband or I slept a wink the night before. I'm pretty sure we were not alone. The waiting room was filled with family and friends. A lot of people love our special little boy. Those who weren't there were putting up prayers. But Eli came out of surgery with flying colors! Those are four hours of my life I do not want to relive. Now it was time for waiting.

We waited an entire month before Eli could be hooked up. A month filled with high hopes and trying to keep realistic expectations. On August 3rd, 2000, the day we had been waiting for, our son could hear! Our prayers had been answered. We knew choosing the implant would require lots of work, intensive therapy, and many follow-up visits with the audiologist for programming and mapping. We have kept up with this hectic schedule and it has paid off. It is all worth it when I hear him say, "I love you." After only three months of implant use, he spoke 10 words! Ten words that *others could understand.* Wow! This was so much more than we ever would have dreamed possible. And now after one year of implant use, he is a chatterbox. He listens without lip-reading or sign language and understands most things. Every day we get to see the look on his face when he hears a new sound or recognizes a sound that puts a smile on his face. The large vocabulary he had in signing has made the transition to speech and language a much easier bridge to cross.

I have no regrets in the choices we have made. Even though I was frustrated that I got nothing done until Eli was 4 ½ months old, all the professionals say that actually that is early, so we are very lucky. We have a loving and supportive family that have always stood behind our every decision. We thank everyone for their support and prayers. We have no doubt that we did the right thing.

An Audiologist Without A Doubt…By Lisa Geier

As an audiologist who has been in the implant field for 13 years, I have no doubts that cochlear implants are effective. They change lives in a positive way. When I began working with implant patients, it changed my life. I found a field of work where you could observe miracles every day.

I was lucky enough to work with Dr. Luetje at the Midwest Ear Institute for five years. When my husband and I moved to a smaller city, I was disappointed that there were no clinical cochlear implant jobs in the area. But the next thing I knew, I was working for a cochlear implant company (Advanced Bionics Corporation) as a clinical specialist. I traveled around the world helping other audiologists work with *their* patients. I was working with some of the brightest people in the implant field. The implant industry was exciting and fast-paced. I loved it, except I really missed working directly with patients. In the spring of 2000 I heard that an experienced implant surgeon had moved to Springfield, Missouri, where I live. I was hoping that he would want to start a local, quality implant program. As I had counseled others, I tried not to have "inappropriate expectations," but I wanted that job! I started buying toys for the clinic before I was ever offered the job.

Dr. Scott Estrem hired me to direct the cochlear implant program here in Springfield, Missouri. His first patient in Springfield was one of the most beautiful children I have ever seen. This is remarkable, since it seems that all children with cochlear implants are gorgeous. But this kid was *really* cute. He was a spunky little "tow-head" with the smile of an angel and the mischievous grin of the devil. He was two years old, smart and very expressive. His name was Eli and he had these parents that were wise beyond their years. Eli's first experience with sound through the implant was an event no one will forget. The room was packed with family and audiologists. All eyes were on Eli as the stimulation level was slowly raised. His first reaction was one of calm awareness. He simply tapped his ear and then looked straight at his mom as if to say, "Mom, did you have any doubt I'd hear this?"

Since that time, Eli has made huge gains in his use of hearing and speech. He is able to understand the speech of others, and his own speech has made impressive gains. I knew all these things would occur. I have seen it with more than a hundred patients, yet when we conducted his first "cochlear implant-aided" hearing tests, I was still in awe of the miracle. Here was this little kid that didn't hear a jet plane engine with his hearing aids, yet was now perceiving very soft sounds with his implant. He is now repeating words I say, virtually verbatim. They pay me to watch miracles happen. Needless to say, I have no doubt that I am back where I am supposed to be, in clinical work, with implant patients.

Lisa Geier, Ph.D., CCC-A, Audiologist
Director, Cochlear Implant Program
Regional Ear, Nose & Throat
St. John's Hospital and Clinics
1965 South Fremont, Suite 1950
Springfield, MO 65804
Voice/TTY: 417-887-9828

84

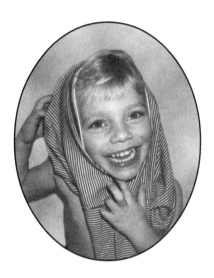

William's Story…By Cindy Wallace

The pale blue beautiful eyes of a man will one day grace these pages as they read and try to comprehend what pain and anguish his parents went through so many years ago. I wonder? What will he be thinking as he reads? Will he understand the debt of sorrow that filled his parents hearts? Will he have realized by now that his unborn sister lay sleeping safely in his mother's womb the day he almost died? Will he ever know the debt of torment his parents went through as they watched the emergency crew running down the corridors with their baby boy? Echoes of a voice that will haunt them for the rest of their lives, "Mr. and Mrs. Wallace if it were my son lying on that table I would want no one other than Dr. Peterson caring for him. If anyone can save him, he can!"

September 27th, 1999 will forever be engraved on my heart as "The day the walls of my sheltered life came crashing down." Gone are the days of "it can't happen to me."

One in 200,000 my son William was that one percent. I will NEVER view life the same again. I live in the world of reality now. I appreciate every moment and have learned the painful lesson well, it can happen to you. I was seven and a half months pregnant at the time and had been on bed rest for nearly five months with a fragile pregnancy. I had naively thought the hardest part was behind us. My mother-in-law was

85

kind enough to take us in temporarily. This worked out well because she ran a small day care out of her home. My son William was 20 months at the time and would play all day long in her house and about every 15 minutes would run down the hall to hug and kiss me. The nightmare began when William's cold turned into a sinus infection. I didn't think anything of it at first, but then slowly I noticed his fevers were getting worse jumping up and down sporadically, only temporarily lowered by Tylenol and Motrin. If only he could tell me what was wrong or what was hurting, it would have been so much easier. I started keeping a journal of his temps and symptoms, calling nurses around the clock. Everyone told me the same thing, "Ma'am, we understand that you're concerned, your son simply has the flu." There I was again alone with my thoughts in the middle of the night with this unbelievably nagging feeling that something was very wrong. We took him to the pediatrician the next morning (of course our favorite doctor was out of town). He said he had a bad case of the flu, then we left. Later that evening it appeared that William was getting better, as he was actually moving around and playing a little. We all took a big sigh of relief.

Late into the night things took a turn for the worst. When everyone was asleep I lay there awake holding him, afraid to fall asleep. I could tell he wasn't breathing peacefully and seemed agitated. This was one of the scariest moments of my life, instinctively knowing something was terribly wrong and all I could do was wait for it to happen. The next morning I got up to use the restroom (as we pregnant ladies do) and William started to follow me. He seemed rather lethargic and sort of slumping over. I called Nurse Connection again and got the same response, except this time they were not as friendly as before. I set up another appointment with the doctor anyway. An hour later not wanting to take my eyes off him, I called for William to follow me again, except this time when he got up it was as if time 'STOPPED'. I can remember turning toward him in slow motion and thinking, "Oh, dear God, he's dying". This time he was slumped a little lower to the floor, a difference that was almost undetectable. I could feel the hairs on the back of my neck stand up, an anguished sob stuck in the back of my throat. I dropped to my knees and prayed to God for direction. "Dear God tell me what is happening?" I heard the softest sound of a whisper say, "Watch him walk".

As I did the Lord helped me see that he was slightly lower to the ground than just one hour before. I knew then what was happening! I began to scream for help as I picked him up in my arms and started running for the car.

They call it "The Baby Killer." The symptoms mimic the flu and by the time you realize it's something worse, your small window of opportunity to save him is up. When my sister-in-law, Julianne, and I arrived at Children's Hospital, he was almost unconscious and barely alive.

William had contracted bacterial meningitis. He had only a few hours left to live. The next couple of days and nights were the worst of our lives. They couldn't be sure if the pneumococcal meningitis he had contracted was contagious or not and if the baby I was carrying was infected as well. I was at risk of losing not one but both babies! The question of whether or not William had brain damage was yet to be determined. This was inconceivable; to this day I won't even entertain the thought.

The infectious disease specialists kept asking me, "How did you know it wasn't the flu? How did you know to get him here in time, before it was too late?" My answer was one that I'm sure they'll ponder over and over throughout their career. I said, "Jesus told me to "watch him walk" and when I did I was able to notice a slight change from one hour before; this was my warning sign.

Eleven long days and nights we stayed at that hospital, each day, longer then the last. Waiting for anything, some sign that showed he was responding to the "cocktails of antibiotics" they were giving him to kill the infection. They had determined that it wasn't contagious. Three spinal taps, two CT scans, and two MRI's all led up to the conclusion that our son was going to pull through with no brain damage! PRAISE GOD!

In those dark hours my husband, Dave, and I both found our own way to deal with the immense pain we were experiencing. He somehow knew all along that William had lost his hearing. In a numb hazy memory I can recall him saying over and over, "William, can you hear Daddy, can you hear me?" I suppose I knew that something was terribly wrong but the truth was I couldn't go there. I had to stay focused, my contractions were already too close together, and I knew any negative thinking would send me straight to triage! William needed me. This is one of the greatest lessons we learn as parents, that 'it's not about you anymore'. I desperately wanted my son to live and I was holding onto that prayer very tight. When I was certain he was out of harm's way then I could focus on the road ahead.

The morning we were to be discharged, the hospital sent for a coordinator from Speech and Hearing to run the BER test. I was still in denial, only wanting to believe that he was fine. She took the test and said, "Your son has a profound hearing loss." (You have to understand if you have lived in a world void of any sort of disability, the word "profound" simply meant "mysterious or intellectual." The description of what she was suggesting didn't compute.) I had to ask her to clarify; she seemed somewhat put out at this notion and said a little louder, "Your son has a profound hearing loss, and he is completely DEAF." I got it that time. As the tears of disbelief and shock over came me, I asked her, begged her "Is there ANYTHING we could do to restore my baby's hearing?" She looked me in the eyes and said, "No, I will connect you with an ASL liaison. She will help you to get started in a sign language program for your son."

You have never seen a more pitiful couple, heads lowered in defeat as my husband pushed his crying, pregnant wife in a wheelchair down a dimly lit corridor toward the cafeteria. Just then we could hear the distant sound of an angel, my husband's brother Jim saying, "Wait!! Wait, it's going to be o.k.!! Have you every heard of a cochlear implant?"

From that moment forward we had HOPE! I can't tell you how devastated we were. First we almost lost William, thinking we made it through the fire, only to have a coordinator for Speech and Hearing who in fact was working for the same hospital that put the implant in tell us that there were NO OPTIONS OTHER THAN SIGN LANGUAGE! I really don't have to say much more about this particular issue. I believe those of us who have had to "fight the battle" for the implant understand all too well what we're up against with the majority of the Deaf community. Not to mention a select few working in related fields who have their own "personal agenda," one that clearly DOES NOT look out for the "best interest" of the patient. What a sad day it is when the victim is a defenseless child who tragically lost his hearing and for the parents who had the misfortune of hearing the shocking news first through a biased employee!

On William's 2nd birthday, January 5th, 2000, my "Warrior Son" was about to be reunited with the hearing world. I say "Warrior" because his full name is William Tecumseh Wallace, named after two famous warriors. William survived a pre-term delivery and a near-death battle with a deadly disease; I would say he's living up to his legendary name! The day of his "hook up" we all sat holding our breaths. It had been three months since he had last heard and needless to say, we were all a little giddy with anticipation. Well, I wish could say something really dynamic, but the truth is, besides letting out a scream upon hook up the whole thing was anticlimactic. Two weeks later, however, it all came back to our little man who worked so hard to gain his strength and walk again. The kids and I were in the kitchen. I was washing the dishes and said over my shoulder, "William, are you all done?" He replied, "Yes, mama." I thought I was going to fly through the roof! I ran to him and made him repeat it over and over until he finally took off running all through the house laughing in delight as I chased him. This is truly a miracle. Where there was silence now there is sound! Praise God!

Lessons learned, lives changed. We all have changed tremendously due to this tragedy. Because of our son, my husband became a humble man looking to "Christ first" for guidance over decisions that need to be made.

Unfortunately, sometimes it takes a tidal wave in some cases to get a person's attention. This was our tidal wave. My entire family has drawn closer to God in search of their own need for peace and understanding. I have discovered that the answers are not found in daily routine. For me to begin to make "peace" with this life-altering tragedy I had to first seek out "compassion." I found myself consumed with "what if" and in order to put this in perspective and behind me I started helping others, trying to be a kinder person. Showing compassion in areas that were 'uncomfortable' for me before William's illness. As I did this, my anger, bitterness, and guilt seemed to dissipate I could feel God's presence in me working to restore my faith. I began the healing process in the starting of a CIAI support group (Cochlear Implant Association Incorporated) for San Diego, California. I also found healing in the starting of an Internet support group called "Parents-of-CI-Kids." My family joined a new church and has found comfort there. My husband has taken on 'pro bono' work at his law firm helping children in need receive a cochlear implant; I help the struggling parents and their need to understand the system. There have been many blessings along the way if you choose to see them; the problem is the blessings are not what we think they should be, therefore we miss them if we don't humble ourselves before the Lord and ask for "his perspective." We are a success story! The cochlear implant has given back to my son what was rightfully his!

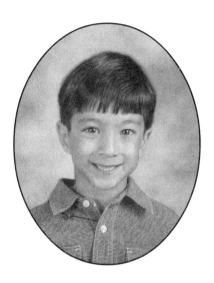

It's a Miracle! – One Mother's perspective…By Mary Olsen

Discovering the hearing loss:

Mitch, our first child, was born eight weeks premature on July 18, 1993. Our first few months with Mitch were spent trying to save his life and bring him home from the hospital. Looking back, we were told, Mitch had several risk factors for a hearing loss (extended ventilation, high bilirubin counts, low birth weight, extended use of oxygen, and cycles of gentamycin to fight infection). We discovered Mitch was deaf at eleven weeks of age. We were all sitting around with Mitch on my lap, when a very loud balloon popped. I noticed that Mitch was the only one who did not seem to get startled. I spent the next couple of days making every loud noise behind him (from clapping hands to banging pots and pans), with no reaction. If he didn't have a hearing loss, we probably gave him one! Luckily, since he was born premature, his pediatrician took my concerns seriously and scheduled us to obtain a hearing test. The test showed that Mitch suffered from a profound bilateral hearing loss. Our immediate response was, of course, shock, grief, and then self-pity. We could not imagine what hardship's he would face, not being able to hear.

Dealing with the hearing loss, the early months

Once we accepted Mitch's hearing loss, we were appreciative that he was otherwise fairly healthy after his rocky beginning. We set out to figure how to deal with it. We were guided to our local Special Education Center and enrolled Mitch in the 0-3 program. Within six months Mitch was fitted with hearing aids and we started using sign language with him. The center we were going to never even mentioned using a cochlear implant. We discovered later that the district we were in did not really believe in the cochlear implant, but instead relied strictly on a total communication approach. I learned about cochlear implants from Northwestern University where I started taking Mitch for supplemental speech therapy. I saw videos of children implanted at various ages and hearing loss and the progress they made over the next few years. I was amazed by what I saw, but was still a bit skeptical that this was a common result from the implant. I asked the Special Education Center about the implant, and they told me that the implants were all hype and the results I saw were not typical. By now Mitch was a very active 18-month toddler, able to communicate with sign language, but was seeing no result from the hearing aid use or speech therapy. After attending a seminar on cochlear implants, we decided to work with Children's Memorial Hospital in Chicago to determine if Mitch was a candidate. I had came to the decision that if they said he was a candidate, I was going to let him have it, even if at a minimum he would be able to hear environmental noises or at least react to my voice. I cannot tell you how many times I was given the scare of my life and had to run after Mitch in a parking lost, walking down a street or in a mall (he loved those escalators!).

Implantation and immediate results, right?

Once Children's Hospital was able to confirm Mitch as a candidate (through physical exams, hearing tests, physiology tests), we had to choose which brand of implant we wanted. We were immediately attracted to the Clarion model based on the simple design of the headpiece (Mitch hated having the hearing aid mold in his ear) and the advanced technology of the processor at the time. We decided that we would have Mitch participate in the FDA children's trial of the Clarion implant. The requirements were the severity of loss (for which he qualified), hearing aid use for at least 12 months, and a minimum age of at least 24 months. We had a few more months to wait, and we concentrated on working with Mitch on auditory response training (so he could be tested and mapped for his implant).

Finally, Mitch was implanted at 27 months of age and was "turned on" four weeks later. Mitch's first reaction to the implant was immediate; he heard the noise and grabbed his blanket and jumped onto my lap. We were in awe, especially after spending months almost screaming to get him to even turn his head to a noise with his hearing aids. During the first couple of weeks we were planning on gradually having Mitch wear it a couple of hours a day, but to our amazement, he would bring the processor to us and sign "listen." Mitch spent the first month becoming acquainted with general noises, the phone ringing, us calling his name, and his favorite game was an electronic drum that would play for about 20 seconds every time you pushed a button. He would push the button and then dance around until the noise stopped, and then repeat this. Meanwhile, we continued with auditory training and speech therapy at Northwestern, still using sign language along with our voice, but started investigating alternatives for Mitch's continued "training" for his implant. Just a couple of months after his implantation, we decided to use Auditory-Verbal therapy with Mitch and stop using sign language. We found that since Mitch had relied so much on sign language, he found it easier not to try and use his voice and would sign instead. We figured he was young enough and if it didn't work out, we could always sign with him again. The Special Education Center was not able to work with us when we made this decision, so we now were only seeing an Auditory-Verbal therapist.

Mitch loves learning how to hear and talk. I made a whole cabinet full of therapy games for him, so much that he would constantly drag me to it to give him his lessons at home. I would say during that first year after his implant, we averaged three hours of "therapy" time at home a day, in addition to seeing an Auditory-Verbal therapist two times a week. When we first started out, I used to be the teacher eliciting responses to my sounds and commands, and Mitch would respond, but I quickly learned the best way to get Mitch to use his voice was to have him be the teacher!

The pre-school years

When Mitch reached that key age of three, we went through the IEP process for his placement into school. We had decided that Mitch was doing so well with his implant that we would continue to pursue a verbal communication approach with him. Our school district did not agree and recommended the local Total Communication program. They had not really seen the progress we did (since he was no longer seeing them), and our battle began. We did not place him where they recommended, but instead found a wonderful new Oral Education school called Child's Voice. The school was over 50 miles from our house one way, but they knew how to work with children with implants. We eventually won our battle with the school district and Mitch attended the school for three years. We continued to work with Mitch at home to constantly improve his hearing and verbal skills. I also worked with our implant center regularly to maintain proper mapping for Mitch and to make sure we were getting the full use of his implant.

Mainstreamed!

After the second year at Child's Voice, we started actually believing Mitch would soon be ready for the regular school district. We decided to move to a school district that had a great reputation for its education system. During his third year at Child's Voice, we made sure we enrolled him in the local Park District programs so he would make some local friends and interact with normal hearing children. Since Mitch had a late summer birthday, we decided to start him in kindergarten after he turned six. He had started reading at age four, when he started kindergarten, he was reading fluently above age level in reading and language. He was able to adapt to his new school as well as any child starting kindergarten. He had speech therapy and a hearing itinerant along with a portable FM system. In addition to the school activities, Mitch has participated in many extra-curricula activities, including drama (he has been in two plays), basketball, soccer, karate, gymnastics, drawing classes, and baseball. His second year of school, 1st grade, was just as successful as his first year. He continued to progress in all subjects as his peers and stays ahead in reading. He is doing so well with his speech that we will be reducing his pull-out speech therapy during the upcoming year. Mitch will start second grade after this summer, and I expect him to continue to successfully progress. He may need additional help as subjects get harder, with note taking etc., but we know we can tackle all challenges ahead, thanks to his implant!

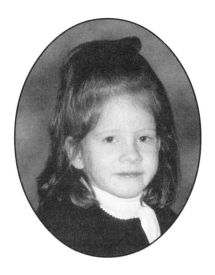

Erica's Story…By Erica King

My mom tells me I'm the prettiest little redhead girl and some day I want to be a dentist. Mom also tells me that I can out-talk any eight or nine year old from miles around. This is something I take pride in, since I'm not quite six and I was born with a profound hearing loss.

I was fitted with hearing aids at eleven months of age and received a cochlear implant when I was 3.5 years old. One of the first things I heard that I thought was really cool was the slurpy sound I could make while drinking my milk at the supper table. The whole family was so excited that we all took turns making slurpy sounds.

I love to talk to people about my cochlear implant. I'm not at all shy about my hearing loss. I've even met the President of the United States of America and told him about my implant. Once I got to fly to New York to meet Diane Sawyer and tell her about my implant. (This was an ABC flick.)

My sister now has an implant too. She's only two years old and can talk really well too! We both love to talk on the phone with Grandpa and Grandma. I love to listen to the birds and crickets! I love to sing too but Daddy says I sing like Mommy, so I'd better go to dental school.

If I didn't have a cochlear implant I don't think I'd be able to go to dental school because I wouldn't be able to talk to my patients or hear them tell me which tooth was hurting them.

I know a lot about Helen Keller. She was deaf too, but she lived a long time ago before they had cochlear implants. I'm glad I have a cochlear implant because the world is a beautiful place full of wonderful sounds and I can hear them all with my implant!

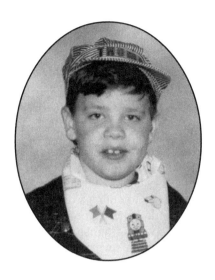

Our Family's Long Road...By Dan Heeb

Our son, Jacob, was born on March 1, 1994. Although we had suspicions about Jacob's lack of speech development and expressed concern to our pediatrician, it was not until he was 21 months old that an audiologist tested his hearing. Auditory Brainstem Response (ABR) testing in January 1996 confirmed his hearing loss, which was 90-100 dB bilaterally. Despite two trips to Boys Town National Research Hospital for genetic testing, and recent testing for the Connexin 26 gene, the cause of Jacob's hearing loss is unknown. Brenda was extremely careful during pregnancy, and there is no family history of hearing loss. The following story discusses the many challenges we've faced in trying to provide Jacob the best rehabilitative therapies and hearing technology. These challenges were compounded due to our living in a rural area that has few services.

Jacob was fitted immediately bilaterally with behind-the-ear hearing aids. The audiologist gave us a few references to get us started. I checked all these sources and searched the Internet for any information about deafness. We signed Jacob up to work with a speech/language pathologist (SLP) who used a Total Communication approach, as TC and ASL approaches to deaf education were all that were available in our rural area in Missouri. We also enrolled in a Signed Exact English course at the local vocational-tech school. Our IDEA Early Childhood caseworker was a staunch TC advocate. He wouldn't approve an oral school placement (we had to contact a top state official to get permission to send Jacob to an oral school later). When I called the state school for the deaf for information, and mentioned that the clinic where Jacob's ABR was done had said that Jacob might be a candidate for a cochlear implant, the outreach worker said that she could provide us with a lot of reasons not to have a cochlear implant. We weren't aware at that time about the battles between signing and oral deaf education approaches - this was our abrupt introduction to the controversy.

We continued with the TC approach for about seven months. During this time, we attended a "Family Fun & Learning Weekend," sponsored by the state school for the deaf. It turned out to be an intensive push for the use of ASL. Two weeks later I attended the A.G.Bell Convention in Snowbird (1996), primarily to gather information about cochlear implants, to see if Jacob could benefit from one. While there, I also saw deaf children who used spoken English for communication instead of sign language and talked with several of the oral school representatives. Shortly after Snowbird, we were invited for a visit by one of the new oral schools. We were impressed by how well the children there appeared to be doing, and the school personnel said they were impressed by Jacob's outgoing personality and that he just jumped right into the middle of things with the other children. They said he was the best candidate for an oral education that they had seem

Soon afterward we started driving 250 miles round-trip once a week to have Jacob work with the preschool teacher at this oral school. After about six months of this weekly commuting, we decided it was time to have Jacob attend the school full-time. He was, at 2 years 10 months old, their first preschool age student. We rented an apartment near the school and the entire family moved. I relocated my office to a bedroom of the apartment, and our other son, Alex, was enrolled in a new school.

We soon realized that this school was too structured for a two-year-old and that they were unwilling to adapt to Jacob's learning style. Jacob had been speaking several words when he started at the school, but had totally stopped verbal communication within two months. Seeing this regression, and also seeing his personality drastically changing to becoming very withdrawn, we saw no choice but to take him out of the school. As the other oral schools had no openings, we had no choice but to return to our rural home and resume TC therapy with our former SLP.

Jacob had used his hearing aids for a little over one year, and he wasn't getting much benefit from them. We started to seriously consider a cochlear implant for him. We visited three cochlear implant centers, including Boys Town National Research Hospital, even though it was too far from our home for us to actually consider using it. Dr. Lee Harker at BTNRH concurred that Jacob was an appropriate candidate for an implant.

During this period, we also visited a private TC preschool with an excellent reputation. We were told before visiting that we would see several children with cochlear implants and see how well they were speaking. However, all we saw at the school were children using sign language, without any use of speech. This gave us the impetus to reconsider what communication approach we wanted to use.

In September 1997 at age 3 1/2, Jacob was implanted at the Shea Clinic in Memphis, Tennessee. Dr. John J. Shea III reported that the surgery went well and that all electrodes were implanted and functioning. We were startled when we heard how hoarse Jacob sounded (an effect of the anesthesia and the tube inserted for breathing), and by the huge bandage dressing on his head. Surgery was on an outpatient basis and we spent the night in the hotel next to the clinic. It was a long, sleepless night, as Jacob threw up a couple of times and his head movements kept pushing the dressing out of place. We drove the 300-mile round-trip to Memphis about 25 times over the next two years for CI mapping and troubleshooting.

During the fall of 1997, Brenda took a couple of college courses in teaching speech and language to the deaf, which required her to commute twice a week 250 miles round-trip each time. I rearranged my schedule to working Saturday and Sunday so I could watch the boys on the days Brenda had classes.

We took two trips to Chicago in the spring of 1998. One was to a regional Auditory-Verbal International conference featuring Daniel Ling. As a result of hearing Ling and the other speakers at the conference, Brenda's eyes were opened to what the Auditory-Verbal Approach really involved. One big plus for her was how the speakers emphasized that parents were the primary participants in teaching their deaf child to talk, rather than passive observers while a teacher of the deaf or an SLP worked with their child. Brenda also attended a Network of Educators of Children with Cochlear Implants (NECCI) workshop in Chicago featuring Pat Chute, Ed.D., and Mary Ellen Nevins, Ed.D. As a result of the Ling conference, our interest in the Auditory-Verbal Approach was sparked, but there was no place locally that provided an A-V therapist or training. We had heard of the Helen Beebe Center in Fort Washington, Pennsylvania, near Philadelphia, and I asked about it on the CI Circle parents listserv. It received glowing recommendations. So off we went in May 1998 to the Beebe Center in Philadelphia for an intensive one-week training.

June 1998 saw us at the A.G.Bell Convention in Little Rock, Arkansas. We attended many beneficial workshops - especially, for Brenda, the ones given by Judith Simser. As a result of attending this conference, we found a therapist who was familiar with the A-V Approach and who could work with us. This was Sister Arline Eveld, who was retired from St. Joseph Institute for the Deaf after working there almost 50 years. She had started and supervised their parent/infant program for many years. Sister Eveld began working with Brenda and Jacob once a week. Her vast experience gave Brenda the help she needed to proceed confidently as Jacob's primary teacher, speech teacher, and oral motor/myofunctional therapist (under the direction of SLP Sharon Wexler). We also were fortunate to be able to talk with Pat Chute at the convention about some of the problems Jacob was having with his implant.

In September 1998, I went to Portland, Oregon, to take a weeklong class at the Oregon Graduate Institute of Science and Technology to learn about the Center for Spoken Language Understanding's (CSLU) interactive learning tools for language training with profoundly deaf children. This CSLU Toolkit combines computer-based speech recognition, speech synthesis, an animated 3D face that produces speech, and face tracking and speech reading of the child by the computer, along with an ability by the parent or teacher to custom design language and speech lessons. These tools have been used at the Tucker-Maxon Oral School in Portland. More information about the CSLU Toolkit can be found at their website.

While we were fortunate in finding a therapist to work with us using the A-V approach, Jacob was having problems with his implant. The third medial electrode went out completely about four months after activation. Jacob's performance also was erratic - he would sometimes appear to be improving, but then would lose what he had gained. We were loaned a portable CI tester and used it to test impedance of the electrodes at home on a regular basis. We found that several other electrodes were also showing a high impedance, which would have compromised the speech processing strategies available to Jacob. Although the implant company kept insisting that Jacob's implant was functioning well enough, we knew from his performance and from the numerous electrode problems that something was wrong with it. By June 1999, we had started checking into implant centers experienced in reimplantation. Just in case his hearing wouldn't be adequate with the new implant, we decided to learn Cued Speech as a backup. We brought in Pam Beck to give a class on Cued Speech to everyone involved with Jacob. We were convinced that Cued Speech would provide a better path than SEE or ASL for English literacy if the implant by itself didn't provide adequate hearing.

In August 1999 Jacob was reimplanted at Lenox Hill Hospital in New York City by Dr. Simon Parisier and activated in September. While we were able to fly in for the surgery, we were advised against Jacob flying for at least a month following the operation. Consequently, we drove back to Missouri and then drove round-trip for the activation. We've been able to do subsequent mappings in St. Louis.

At Jacob's one-year evaluation for his new implant, he was shown to

100

have emerging Category Six open-set speech perception, which represents the highest level of open set comprehension. His improvement has been dramatic in the past year. He speaks in complete sentences and engages in conversations. We know that if we had listened to the first implant company and not opted for reimplantation, he would never have reached this level. Also, we're convinced that the intensive therapy and Brenda's one-on-one work with Jacob have given him the educational foundation and helped him to regain the confidence he needed to make this leap. He has also long since regained his outgoing personality. In addition to attending a regular child development center two afternoons a week, Jacob participates in 4-H, and he also picks up a lot of words from his ten-year old brother Alex.

As a result of a contact made with Melissa Chaikof on the CI Circle listserv, we also realized that Jacob may have some oral motor problems that were interfering with his speech. She referred us to an SLP who specializes in myofunctional/oral motor therapy, and who had worked with several children with implants. Jacob has progressed steadily with this therapy. Since the therapist, Sharon Wexler, is located in Atlanta, we've made several 1000-mile round-trip drives for this therapy. We have thus attempted to meet Jacob's needs by a combination of traveling elsewhere for services, bringing in therapists locally, and developing Brenda's skills in teaching a child who is deaf. Brenda has a master's in Education and had been a teacher. The local Oran, Missouri, school district has been very supportive of these efforts. However, seeing the need for improved services locally, we have also been active in trying to get more services for deaf children in the area. For the last two legislative sessions, I have contacted a local state senator to sponsor a bill that would require the state of Missouri, rather than the local school district, to cover all special education costs for deaf and hard-of-hearing children. I have also worked with a local Missouri House member to introduce a bill to establish regional schools and resource centers for deaf children from birth through grade six, with an oral education option offered. I also serve on the Missouri Newborn Hearing Screening Advisory Committee.

In conclusion, while it has been a long, almost five-year journey since finding out Jacob is deaf, he is now well on the way to having completely intelligible speech and excellent listening abilities. Additional language acquisition and refinement of speech are our target areas for the near future.

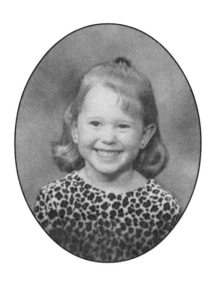

Kyann's Story...By Darlene Eslick

It was June 6th, 1999. We sat in the restaurant trying to enjoy my birthday dinner, but couldn't get our 2 1/2 year old, Kyann, to sit down. She ignored repeated requests to turn around and be seated. Lately, she had been very irritable. She had been a little bookworm, who sat spellbound when I read to her. Then one day while reading, she blurted out angrily, "Read the book! Read the book!" I watched in dismay as she stormed away in a rage. My husband, Courtney, and I definitely were aware that something was wrong with Kyann, but we did not recognize the symptoms for what they were! We couldn't understand why our sweet, compliant child had suddenly become so irritable and disobedient. Just days earlier she walked away at a picnic despite my telling her to come back. A friend there said, "Mom, you'd better get control of her! She seems very strong-willed." I felt so insulted! After all, my 7-year-old daughter, Paige, was proof that I knew what I was doing. Up until then, both girls had similar behaviors. Both girls respected adults, had nice manners, and were loving to others. Why then was Kyann suddenly so different?

Back at home, the cake cutting had just begun when Kyann tipped over her bar stool, slamming her chin against the edge of our island.

We rushed to the emergency room, Kyann sporting a deep gash and lots of blood. The doctor quizzed us about Kyann, and then began a lengthy struggle to stitch her chin. It was a frightening, painful ordeal for her, and we simply could not console her. Afterward the doctor said he wanted an MRI because he was suspicious that something just wasn't quite right with Kyann.

We brought home a pale, disoriented, weak child late that night and put her to bed. Her MRI results had been normal, but Kyann was suffering horribly. By morning she was limp and couldn't support any part of her body, not even her head. She was still displaying the night's symptoms, and was now dry-heaving. I was terrified she would die! And my attempts to reach the doctor were fruitless. He was "too busy" to call me back. At 5:00 p.m., I pleaded with another doctor who agreed to meet us at the emergency room. I buckled up my rag doll child, and drove to the gas station, with my husband on the way from the high school where he teaches. Waiting for the gas to fill, I knocked on the car window to smile at Kyann. She did not look. She did not blink. I knocked again. She did not react at all. A shocking dread washed over me... Kyann couldn't hear!

Two days, numerous doctors, and two towns later, we arrived in Kansas City at Children's Mercy Hospital. There Kyann was subjected to daily appointments that stretched out for weeks. Answers did not come immediately, but we knew for certain that Kyann couldn't hear. We spent many hours driving between Kansas City and Topeka (where we were staying with family), and in hospital waiting rooms and clinics. On top of our already difficult situation and all of the scheduled procedures, Kyann continuously seemed to be sick, and not in a way that was logically connected to her hearing loss. She developed a bad rash, then a fever. Her pediatrician did not know what was wrong with her. We started her on an antibiotic, but could not resume hospital appointments until her symptoms cleared up. Then late one Friday afternoon Kyann's eyes began to do bizarre things. They were askew and droopy. One eye wandered, then one became dilated. An intern examined her, but was limited in what he could do. He simply said he thought her vision was normal. We were sent back to Topeka with no answers, terrified Kyann might lose her vision too.

Finally, the weekend passed and we visited a pediatric optometrist who squeezed Kyann into a full schedule. He didn't find anything wrong. Over the next week her eyes slowly returned to normal. Our relief was enormous! However, at the same time, her neurologist thought Kyann had no nerve response or deep tendon reflexes. He said parts of Kyann's body seemed to be shutting down, area by area, and that he was suspicious of Dejerine-Sottas syndrome. He referred us to a clinic that tested Kyann's nerves. Needles were inserted into her body, legs and feet. She was given light shocks over and over as a computer picked up her brain responses. We literally felt sick with agony as we sat helplessly by, while Kyann struggled and cried, no doubt wondering why we didn't save her from these strangers who just kept hurting her. Most days, Kyann was subjected to the agony of no food or drink from midnight until noon because of repeated sedations for procedures, many of which were painful.

We soon learned that Kyann's hearing loss was profound. The news came like a nightmare, from which we couldn't wake. Even the most powerful hearing aids provided no sound. Finally a team of doctors met with us. There was nothing else to try, except maybe a weird thing called a cochlear implant. One doctor said he could do the surgery, but did not talk about it in a positive manner. All we can remember is that he emphasized the dangers and the risks and said that Kyann might not benefit at all from a cochlear implant. It was a sort of doom's day environment in that room. I had hoped and prayed for a miracle. Instead I felt like all we had done was subject Kyann to four weeks of pain for nothing. We left feeling exhausted and worn down. Night after night we could not sleep, and I suffered from intense crying. Courtney was quiet and sad.

Yet we knew we had to continue to give 100% to Kyann. We kept putting books under her nose, acting out the stories in them. We used familiar books and were very animated in explaining the stories. Kyann amazed us. She kept talking to us, even though she couldn't hear herself. And being only 2 1/2, she had easily picked up lip-reading. Evidently, Kyann had been deaf for at least three months before we realized it. The neurologist explained that her hearing had probably been "turning down slowly day by day" until suddenly it was gone, making her very ill that June 6th day. We began pointing and using body language and facial expressions to communicate with her. Courtney and I couldn't believe that we'd misread all the obvious signs that Kyann had lost her hearing. Thinking back, for two or three months she had held our faces tightly and stared at our mouths. And I had dismissed it as affection.

We drove home to Ulysses, way out in Southwest Kansas, early in July, thrilled to be away from the hospital, yet wondering what to do next. We'd been home one day when Courtney called the Midwest Ear Institute in Kansas City, taking a lead from an audiologist at the hospital. We were invited immediately for a consultation to determine if Kyann was a candidate for a cochlear implant. Within 24 hours we were back on the road with a glimmer of hope in our bruised hearts. Again we were saddled with a long drive and only visual aids to entertain Kyann. She was given a bendable, funny-faced snake from her Aunt Leanna. That snake turned out to be a gem, playing peek-a-boo over the seats and "striking" its surprised victims, making Kyann roll with laughter.

I'll never forget our meeting that day with Dr. Charles Luetje. It was truly a wonder that we got to see him at all! He wasn't supposed to be available for the consultation, but we walked in and were told that he was "in"! He treated us with amazing love and concern and handled Kyann tenderly as though she were his! He viewed her CT scans while I held my breath. And then the words came, "Mom...your child will hear again. Kyann has just enough cochlea to hold the implant which will give her artificial hearing." Hot tears stung my eyes. It was hard to speak. He said Kyann's cochleas were underdeveloped, a common find in many deaf people, but that it didn't explain why her hearing failed. Then Dr. Luetje began to unfold for us the "best case scenario." He said that the perfect implant patient would be a 2 1/2 year old who had previously had normal hearing and who had learned full speech, as Kyann had! The child would be from a home where learning was emphasized and would have no other problems that would detract from the success of the implant. All of this was better than good news. Kyann was exactly 2 1/2 years old! It was as if he was describing her, our family, and our home! But when he said he could not fit her into his schedule for several months, we were worried. This was tough news, for in the month that had passed, Kyann's speech had deteriorated substantially. We couldn't understand her anymore. She was simply talking as fast as she was thinking, leaving a blur of sound that was meaningless to us. We explained this to Dr. Luetje, fearing Kyann would lose her ability to remember and regain normal speech. He listened intently and thoughtfully. It was evident he was bothered. Nonetheless, we were greatly uplifted by what he told us about the implants. All of the information we received was upbeat and promising. We were given videos, books and pamphlets, and were able to speak to a number of parents of children with implants.

We returned home, anxiously sharing the good news with everyone!

Then it happened! Midwest Ear Institute called when we'd only been home three days to say that Dr. Luetje wanted to implant Kyann in just one week! He couldn't bear to make Kyann wait, and had given up a non-surgery date to accommodate her!

On the morning of July 17, 1999, Courtney and Dr. Luetje lovingly carried Kyann into surgery. It was impossible to hold back the tears after they disappeared through the doors. We had signed all the forms, and were ready, but it was still very hard. The surgery took about two hours. Kyann's short blonde hair was shaved off behind her right ear to accommodate the surgery. The wait didn't seem all that bad. Our pastor made the long drive to be with us, and that helped a lot. When we were informed that Kyann was in recovery we rushed there to be with her and comfort her. She had a big bandage on her head, an IV in her arm, and was quickly hoisted into Courtney's lap where she bawled loudly while trying to paw at the big wrappings on her head. She was quickly calmed as a painkiller was added to her IV. Family and friends filled Kyann's hospital room in a show of support and love. Her recovery was remarkable! By early evening she rode the halls in her wheelchair, then progressed to walking. We gave her a present...a toy stroller. Midwest Ear Institute had given her a stuffed cougar, made available by the implant manufacturer. By late evening she was pushing her cougar up and down the halls, entertaining the other patients on her floor. Dr. Luetje visited Kyann the next morning and released her.

Within four hours we were on the road home, our little one sporting a swollen head, stitches and shaved-off hair. She managed beautifully. We were unbearably anxious to return to Kansas City in a month to have her device turned on. It was a big day for us when we returned to Midwest Ear Institute. Kyann had become accustomed to complete silence. The sudden noise was shocking to her, no doubt about that! It was a chore to keep her device on her. At first she kept yanking it off. But we knew she'd learn to love her "mousie" (our pet name for it) over time. And that is exactly what happened. The struggle with Kyann's acceptance lasted about a month. Suddenly one day she became very upset when we took her "mousie" off to change its battery. We knew then that she had arrived! Every day something wonderful happened. One day an airplane passed overhead. I have to admit that I didn't even notice it. But Kyann said, "I hear an airplane! Where is it?" One by one she noticed the sounds around her and she remembered them! The joy we felt and still feel is due to the fact that we do not take for granted the blessing of cochlear implants. How marvelous to be alive in this day and age, and to have a choice to help our child, instead of having to accept deafness!

Kyann began speech therapy a few weeks later, but her main success can be attributed to our reading marathons, and never-ending input and support from her family. Prior to her hearing loss, every day was full with learning experiences, reading and interacting, and since we were anxious to return to normal life, we resumed doing just that. She talks beautifully, listens intently, is happy and healthy, answers and talks on the telephone, and loves music. Her main limitations are not hearing well in a noisy environment and the inability to tell the direction of sound. Plus Kyann cannot use her CI when swimming or showering. The external components of a cochlear implant cannot be exposed to water. So we are very protective around water. When people stare at her "mousie" and ask, "What's that on her head?" we gladly explain. Kyann thinks nothing of it. She will start preschool in two weeks. We expect success for her. Kyann is worth the entire trauma that was experienced to get her to this point. It is our hope that other parents will not deny their children the benefit of sound. The earlier the better and the more books and teachable moments the better. And never mind the expense. It is a fact of life now, batteries, cords, programming appointments, traveling, and device insurance. We are spending a significant amount of money every year. Is it worth it? Is Kyann worth the expense? A great big audible "*yes*"!

Here we are 2 years later, reading up a storm. Kyann doesn't remember the frustration of the silence she once felt when she was frantically ordering me to "read the book"! We could not have chosen silence for Kyann. God did answer our prayers. Kyann knew exactly what she longed for during her months of silence. To her, sound is incredible! We don't take sound for granted, nor Kyann's implant. It is an awesome treasure! Our child is not deaf! She hears!

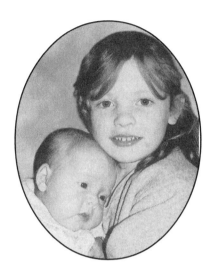

Amanda & Amelia's Journey..By Lisa Liebhart

Our daughter, Amanda, was diagnosed at nine months of age as having bilateral profound sensorineural hearing loss. We had noticed at around three to four months old she wasn't responding to things like her sister did at that age. I voiced my concerns to our family doctor and he did a few routine tests and referred us on. At nine months of age we received the diagnosis. For me, there were a lot of things running through my mind, mainly about how we were going to communicate and make sure she received the best education possible.

In our search for answers, I heard about the cochlear implant. My father had seen an article in a magazine and had cut it out and put it on his refrigerator and kept insisting that this was what Amanda needed. We started researching and got three different doctor's opinions, and she was a perfect candidate for the implant. At twenty-seven months old, Amanda was implanted. Six weeks later on May 14,1997, she received her external device and her initial stimulation. Just the look in her eyes gave us all the answers to all the questions we had racing through our minds as to whether we had done the right thing..

Now she is approaching her fourth year anniversary date and she is doing wonderfully. She is mainstreamed into a regular classroom and is not missing a thing. She is even on the honor roll. All of her teachers are just totally amazed with her and how the implant has worked. Most people don't have a clue she was born deaf. She has no problem communicating, not even with the other kids in her class.

We are now about to embark on another journey with the cochlear implant. Our four-month old, Amelia, was just diagnosed two weeks ago with the same type of hearing loss that her sister has. If all goes well, she will be getting the gift of sound for her first birthday, sometime around Christmas of this year. The news of her hearing loss was very disturbing, but this time we knew where the answers were. There is hope. That hope is the cochlear implant and seeing the success our older daughter has had and what it has done for so many people.

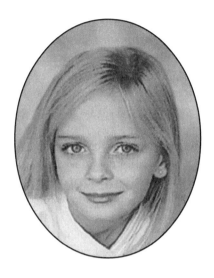

Ray of Light...By Beth Ray

April 1, 1998, began just like any other day. My husband had left for work, and I was busy getting my son Bo and my daughter Laura ready for school. I took a little extra time to fix Laura's hair just right and to pick out the perfect outfit because today was picture day. After spending the day with my youngest child, Lyndi, I picked Laura up from school. As soon as I saw her I knew something was wrong. She said she felt sick, and lay down in the seat. This was very unusual for Laura; she had never been sick a day in her life other than the sniffles. Laura stayed home from school the next day; she had started throwing up and running a fever. I was able to control the fever, but she continued to throw up and became very weak, so I took her to the emergency room. I totally expected to be told she had a stomach virus and to be sent right back home with a prescription that would make her all better. Little did I know this would be the beginning of the worst nightmare any parent could ever go through.

Laura was rushed by ambulance from our local hospital to the Medical Center in Columbus. They tested Laura's spinal fluid and told us she had contracted bacterial meningitis. Within minutes of arriving at the hospital she had slipped into a coma. We were then told that she probably would not make it through the night, and that we needed to prepare ourselves for the worst. During the night she developed a rash, and her urine output decreased. The doctors said that these were both signs that she was taking a turn for the worse. My husband and I prayed so hard. I remember sitting, staring at her, begging and crying "Please God, please don't take her from us. Please, God, just let her live." Our prayers were answered and she made it through the night. Laura stayed in a coma for several days, and then slowly began to wake up.

The doctors had warned us that there were several dangerous side effects of the high doses of antibiotics Laura was given to save her life, one being hearing loss. They also said that meningitis itself could cause hearing loss. At this point, we didn't care; as long as we still had Laura, we could handle any other obstacles thrown our way. To everyone's amazement, Laura had come through this with no signs of hearing loss. We were so blessed to be bringing our precious Laura back home. And just in time for Easter! We live in a small town where everyone, especially our local churches, had helped us make it through Laura's illness. She was on so many prayer lists and prayer chains; she pretty much had the whole community praying for her.

It felt so great to be back at home, back to our normal life. (Or so we thought.) Later that night Laura was coloring a picture when we began to notice she wasn't responding when we talked to her. My husband began to lean down closer and closer and louder and louder "Laura! Laura!" He then reached above him and set off the smoke alarm; she didn't move. I went all to pieces! How could this be happening now? Why, God, why?" After all of the begging and pleading with God to just let her live, and we could handle anything else, I was feeling very ashamed for feeling such anger and betrayal. It just seemed so cruel for this to happen so suddenly, and at this point when we thought our nightmare was over. Our precious Laura never got upset. She even consoled me, telling me "Everything will be all right".

When I was able to calm down, I realized we had already had one miracle (Laura surviving the meningitis). Maybe we could have one more. After all, it was the night before Easter! I figured the more people praying for Laura the better. We got busy and printed up flyers with Laura's picture that read, "We need an Easter Miracle. Please pray for Laura to hear again." And at 2:30 in the morning we were going to all our local churches, over 30, taping the flyers to the doors. That way on Easter Sunday, Laura would have thousands of people praying for her! On Easter morning, I awoke like a child on Christmas morning. I jumped up, so excited, ready to claim our miracle! I ran to Laura's room, knelt by her bed, and whispered "Laura, good morning, beautiful," then louder, "Laura, Laura, LAURA!! No response. They say God has his reasons for everything, but how do you explain that to a six-year-old? Especially when you don't understand yourself.

The next day we took Laura to Jamie Figueiredo-Howard, an audiologist in Columbus. She confirmed our biggest fear. It was profound loss, both ears, and it was permanent. She gave us phone numbers and names of several doctors in Georgia that did cochlear implant surgery. I started that day making calls, trying to learn all the information I could. I even ordered a video. After all, I had never even heard of cochlear implants. Meanwhile, I worked with her, using flashcards and we had a teacher and speech therapist coming to our home twice a week to try to maintain her speech. On May 5th, Dr. Wendall Todd performed Laura's surgery at Egelston Hospital in Atlanta. Although the thought of our child being put to sleep terrified us, there was never a question of whether to have the surgery or not. We knew we had to give her that chance. I, at my age, can't imagine being in total silence. I surely can't imagine being a six-year-old child and being in total silence.

Laura came through the surgery fine, and came home the next day. The next six weeks would seem like six months. Finally the day came, we were headed back to Egelston to meet with Jolie Fainberg, Laura's audiologist to "hook her up" with the outer device so she could hear again. We were so excited. I had the movie camera, I wanted to forever capture that look on her face when they turned it on. Our excitement soon faded as we watched Laura's face. It didn't light up, like we expected; instead it cringed. Laura wasn't hearing very well, and what she was hearing, she didn't like. Jolie was quick to remind us, like we had seen in that video; sometimes it takes weeks, even months, before you'll see optimal results. It was just so hard to be patient at this point.

With each day, I saw Laura's strength and determination grow. After a couple of weeks Laura was able to repeat words and sounds, then she began to answer questions and carry on conversations. After a couple of months it seemed as though Laura had her own hearing back. She could talk on the phone. She started the new school year in regular education classes. We finally had a sense of normalcy back in our lives.

Laura became close friends with a girl in the hearing/speech class who told Laura she had also had surgery for a cochlear implant. When we asked why she didn't wear her outer device we found out that her parents (like us) were also discouraged at first, and since the little girl didn't like the way it sounded, they just set it aside and never gave it time to work. To this day, that still breaks my heart. That little girl sits there in total silence and Laura's right next to her and can hear just fine. If they had only stuck with it a little longer and given her time to adjust to the different sounds.

Laura has continued to do well in school. She's a Junior Majorette with our High School Marching Band. She's won several beauty pageants, and even did some modeling. She even had the opportunity to meet Heather Whitestone, the first deaf Miss America. Laura loves to watch medical shows; she was so fascinated watching E.R. when their storyline had to do with cochlear implants. She said, "Mama, we need to go there. I can tell Dr. Benton that he needs to let Reese (his son) get an implant. When he see how well I can hear, he'll let Reese get the operation too!"

Laura has such a great attitude about her implant. She says, "Some people wake up and have to put glasses on; I have to put this on." She is very excited about the new smaller design that fits just on the head. We are really looking forward to that becoming available. The period of time that Laura had no hearing was so frustrating and heartbreaking. We thank God everyday that we have Laura and that she will not have to spend her life in silence, thanks to the technology provided by Advanced Bionics.

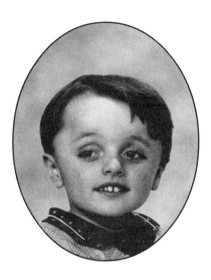

Ryan's Story...By Melanie O'Donahue

I was born January 4, 1997, at the Olathe Medical Center in Olathe, Kansas. Even though I was about a week and a half early, and my mom had to have a cesarean section, I was a healthy, happy baby! I was a much-anticipated child, so dozens of people came to visit me early in life and they brought me lots of presents. I know this because all of the toys still occupy my bedroom, often overflowing onto the floor!

At about six months of age, my mom and dad starting wondering why I wasn't sitting up yet. I had had lots of ear infections, so the doctor was pretty familiar with our family. It seems like we were at his office at least once a week, sometimes more. Because I was a first child to my parents, they were concerned about a lot of things, but the doctor told them not to worry, everything was just fine.

We continued to laugh and play. My mommy would read books to me and sing to me in the car. We went for walks and visited lots of friends and relatives - I was truly the apple of everyone's eye! By September, when I was nine months old, my mom and dad decided that I really wasn't doing everything that I should be - they loved me so much and thus began our "journey" that would encompass dozens of doctors, hospitals, tests, and finally a diagnosis. This was a very stressful time for everyone - me included. I didn't have any idea what was going on. My parents seemed very upset and my mommy cried a lot!

I was poked, prodded, stuck with needles. I had all kinds of tests with fancy names and lots of letters like: MPI, CAT and ABR. My parents missed a lot of work, and those friends who were so excited about me when I was first born, well, they kinda dropped off the face of the earth - funny how people can't handle it when someone else (like me) is in a crisis!

We went to lots of doctors. Most of them just shook their heads and sent me to another doctor, or wrote a prescription for another test. One doctor said I was retarded, another one said that I was "developmentally delayed." One even said that I would never be able to go to college. Boy, did my mom ever tell that guy off! Despite all of this turmoil, that lasted about nine long months, my parents never gave up on me. They knew that I was a smart kid and they knew that their love for me would get us through...

The final doctor that we went to, Dr. Gerald Tremblay, asked if we had had my hearing checked. I was very bright, he said (told you), and maybe I wasn't hearing. Now, why hadn't anyone thought of that before?

In July of 1998, eighteen months after I was born and one year after my parents had wondered, I had that ABR test, and the doctor's found out that I did indeed have a hearing problem. In fact, I was profoundly deaf.

My mother was devastated. My father was very sad. But, they never faltered. Teachers began coming to my house to help me learn. One even came and helped me learn to walk. Her name is Kristy, and we still see her and hug her whenever we can.

Another teacher, Jennifer, was teaching me sign language. It was a long process and very frustrating. I know my mom was sad. She wanted to talk to me, to sing to me, like before. She would tell these teachers these things. Her son had a voice, and she wanted to be able to hear it - she wanted to be able to tell me that she loves me (even though, I already knew that).

Jennifer told us about a new thing called a "cochlear implant." Had we heard of it? It was a pretty new thing, and she had a student in her classroom at school who had one. Maybe we could check into it. Kids who were deaf that had it could learn how to talk, and they could hear - wow, cool, huh? Of course, my mom got all excited!

So, that very day she got on the phone and made an appointment

116

with MEI (that's the Midwest Ear Institute) in Kansas City. We were told that we would have to meet all kinds of requirements in order to have the implant, and this would take some time.

My mom and dad filled out all kinds of papers. They had to promise that they would back me 100 percent in this endeavor because it would take lots of intense training in order for the implant to be effective. Whatever it takes, they said... (Good for Mom and Dad!)

The next step was to actually meet the doctor (oh no, not another one) and get his input. Do you know, he said that I was smart (told you) and a great candidate for the implant? Dr. Charles Luetje became a very important and impressive person in our lives. When my mommy asked him what the success rate of the implant was he said, "100 percent - guaranteed, he will talk." Well, you can imagine what she said - and they set-up the surgery.

On July 1, 1999, I had my implant operation at Trinity Lutheran Hospital, which was performed by Dr. Luetje. Did you know he called my parents every 30 minutes during the surgery to let them know how I was doing? I remember that my mommy cried when she left me with the doctor. Not to worry, he said, I'll take good care of your best friend.

I didn't care much for the hospital (remember, I had been to lots of them in my two and a half years of life). I had to wear this huge thing around my head, and I had no idea what was going on! My head hurt, and, well, those doctors just weren't my favorite people!

On August 2, 1999, we went to MEI to get 'turned-on.' I remember that there were lots of people there my grandparents, Kristy, another teacher, of course my parents, and the people at MEI. I just figured we were going to do another one of those silly tests where you have to look at the dancing bear or something.

They made everyone go into a little room where they could watch me on television. I was busy playing with these instruments and having fun with the audiologist named Jennifer. Barb (another audiologist) was also there, messing with some machine behind me. I didn't have a clue that I was hearing for the first time.

Then, my parents and everyone came into the room. All of a sudden my mommy leaned over and I heard her say something - for the very first time I heard my mommy's voice. I remember everyone was crying - me included. All I wanted was this strange thing off of my head! It wasn't very comfortable and it was kind of scary!

Well, let me tell you, my life changed right then and there! At first, I really didn't like my implant. I didn't want to wear it at all. But my parents weren't going to let me off that easy, and it soon became a part of my life and me.

I didn't realize that Barney not only danced, he also sang. Cars make sounds, and so does the rain! People say things, and they have feelings that they express with words. The world is a wonderful, noisy place!

I go to a school, the St. Joseph School for the Deaf, in Overland Park, Kansas. They teach me all kinds of things there. I can spell my name, I know all of my colors, numbers, and my friends' names. I know animal sounds, and I even count to ten.

It has not been quite two years since I had my implant, but it has made an incredible difference in my family's life. My mom doesn't have to follow me all over the place anymore, which was a real drag. Now, she can just call my name, and I can hear her and go find out what it is she wants. I can go across the street and play with my friend Jack by myself. I have gotten more independent because of my implant, because I can hear and understand what people are saying to me - to our family, this *is* a miracle!

My favorite thing about the implant is that everything makes sense to me now. Things used to just pass me by. I didn't know what things did, and didn't understand a lot of the world. Now, I can sing, I dance, and I am happy! I know that I have a long road ahead of me, but I love to learn, and I want to make my parents proud of me, so I work really hard in school, and take in as much as I can.

Sure, there are times when the implant is a real pain. In fact, being deaf is not too much fun. I can't wear my processor to the swimming pool, so, I can't play with the other kids there, and for some reason, that makes them mad. I can't wear my implant in the bathtub, that is hard because I like to sing to my toys or talk to my dad and ask him things. Some kids in the neighborhood don't ask me to play because it is hard for me to understand what they are saying sometimes, and they get really frustrated - imagine how I feel?

Also, some people have decided that because I have a disability, that they don't want to deal with me. That hurts. Maybe some day they will see that I am just the same as they are. I have hopes and dreams too. And with my cochlear implant, I have every opportunity to be whomever I want to be! Oh, and before I forget... I love hearing - especially my mommy telling me that she loves me soooooo much, and thanks to my implant, I can hear her tell me that and tell her I love her too, every single day!

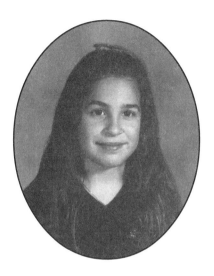

A Tool To Hear...By Patricia Pagano

At nine months our daughter, Stephanie, was starting to call me from her crib. She began to babble and would say "bye-bye" to me when I left her at daycare. At 10.5 months she had a high fever and ear infections that we had a hard time getting rid of. I knew something was wrong. We contacted the pediatrician who immediately referred us to an ENT. The ENT felt her lack of hearing was due to all of the fluid she had in her ears. After we finished the medication and went in for a recheck, the ENT felt we should give it more time. "After all, she doesn't look like a deaf person" was his statement. I knew then that I had to fight to have testing done. Our pediatrician sent us for an ABR at 18 months, which confirmed our suspicions. She had a severe to profound loss in both ears. We immediately fitted her for hearing aids and enrolled her at the local school for the deaf.

Our daughter rapidly began to learn signs, but was verbalizing less and less. I began to do research on hearing loss and available methods of communication. I read about Cued Speech in *Choices in Deafness* and asked everyone about it. The comments that were filtered back to me included, "It doesn't work, no one uses it, she will never fit in with her deaf peers." At that point I wanted her to fit into our family and use the same system of language that we were all using. The philosophy of

119

Cued Speech matched our needs. We felt our eyes twinkle again for the first time in almost a year.

Within a few months of using Cued Speech, Stephanie started to verbalize again. Her receptive language was increasing at a phenomenal rate. She understood that there were different brands of cereal and candy. She understood that people had first, middle, and last names. We could say virtually anything to her and she would comprehend it. Stephanie continued to grow in her receptive language, but her expressive language was not progressing. It was most likely exacerbated by the fact that she continued to lose hearing with each ear infection. She had an ear infection every two months even with multiple PTE tubes.

We attended the Helen Beebe Center and saw many children with her type of loss who were speaking due to the Auditory-Verbal therapy that they were receiving. We also saw several children who had received cochlear implants and were doing remarkably well. We knew then that if we wanted our daughter to speak, we needed to investigate the cochlear implant. At the time we were beginning to investigate the CI, most children were being implanted by two years old. At this point, her hearing was classified as a left corner audiogram starting at around 90-95dB and quickly dropping off between 250hz and 500hz.

The clinic where we chose to have her evaluated conducted extensive testing for about two days. Stephanie's testing showed that her receptive language (4.5) scores were much more advanced than her expressive (3.0). An excerpt from the initial speech and language testing shows how much impact Cued Speech had on Stephanie's early years. "Stephanie indicated age-level understanding of vocabulary and only slightly delayed comprehension of grammar and syntax. She was acutely tuned in to language and made language associations without prompting throughout the evaluation. Stephanie combined words in phrases and used articles, pronouns, simple verb and noun modifiers, negatives and the present and present progressives. Early concepts such as 'under, over, out, in, longest, and smallest' were understood." The amount of receptive language along with some of the key markers of the English language were key factors in helping the clinic decide whether she would be a candidate for the CI.

For her first year with the implant, we used Cued Speech all the time. Any sounds, words, concepts, everything was cued to her. At her six-month evaluation she was doing O.K. At her one-year evaluation, Stephanie's scores were amazing. She continues to make improvements.

Stephanie was mainstreamed in first grade at a parochial school. Her grades in first, second, and third grade average between a B and A. At the end of second grade, the Basic Reading Inventory, 6th edition (Jerry L. Johns) reading test, was performed on her and her comprehension level was a 4.5 grade level and her ability to decode was 7.1 grade level. She reads books voraciously. We take a weekly trip to the library and she reads about 10 third-to-fourth-grade level books per week. In school, she has a full-time translator, a teacher of the deaf, and an SLP as auxiliary services. She has learned some sign language from friends or providers. It is our intention to have her learn the system at a later age so that she can communicate with deaf peers. Stephanie is currently taking Tae Kwon Do classes where she must learn the names of her forms, kicks, and other exercises in Japanese. She must also be able to count, greet the instructors, and thank them in Japanese. She has also learned the names of the ballet steps in French, and the various steps used in tap and jazz. Stephanie has even learned a few words in Italian, as my family speaks it fluently. The cochlear implant is a tool that has helped Stephanie, and will continue to help her achieve many successes.

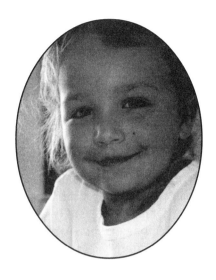

Nicole's Story...By Greg Hubert

When we confirmed our daughter Nicole's hearing loss at 15 months, my tears did not come from concern about her actual loss of the sense of hearing. Instead the tears came from the deepest depths of my heart, because this son of two deaf parents has seen firsthand the tremendous language, educational and societal disadvantages faced by the deaf. I could already envision the impact on Nicole's life and, beyond that, on her children. Since the probable cause of her hearing loss is genetic, I also deeply blamed myself for bringing this on my own child.

As the child of deaf parents, I learned very quickly about the cruelties that could be inflicted by hearing people on the deaf. It's quite an understatement to say what a powerful experience it is for a child to hear other adults saying such incredibly mean things about his own parents. Even more significant, I came to experience firsthand the dependency of my parents on their own hearing children. The oldest child quickly becomes the messenger and interpreter with the hearing world. As that child grows older and more educated, the role evolves into advisor and even decision-maker when the subject matter or language is too difficult for the parents to comprehend.

As we listened to the heart-wrenching details of Nicole's ABR results, my wife Shelley and I began a journey down a path that we were certain would be full of heartbreak and despair. The earmold impressions were taken immediately after the ABR, so we would be back in a week for Nicole to be fitted with her hearing aids. As we sat there in shock, we also scribbled down a list of names and phone numbers of resources that the doctor said we could contact for help. One of those names, Lynn Wood, a Certified Auditory-Verbal Therapist, would turn out to be the first of many and, at that time, unimaginable gifts.

Would it really be possible for Nicole to learn to listen using the amplification of powerful hearing aids? How could such an option be possible with a bilateral, severe sensorineural hearing loss? We only knew my mom and dad's world of speechreading and sign language, supplemented by our own improvised, family-only mode of communication. This family-only communication is best described as exaggerated pronunciations and mouthings and visual clues that evolved over time to make words more easily understood by both parents.

Nicole was so accepting of her hearing aids, almost as if she had some innate sense of their importance. It was only a few months later that our despair had turned to great hope as we celebrated Nicole's progress and we marveled at the many other children and families that really seemed to be living their lives in a hearing world. Everything we did with Nicole became an opportunity to bathe her in language. Shelley truly amazed me how she could always find the energy to read to Nicole before bedtime, even after a really brutal day at work.

Over the next year, this little physiologically deaf girl began to soar in the world of spoken language. She loved her newly developing language abilities. She loved to play with animal toys and make their sounds. Everyone in her life was so happy to work with her to encourage those skills to continue to grow. I sometimes wonder whether I would have developed such a close relationship with my daughter, if her hearing loss had not drawn me to her. Would I have taken her for granted?

Even Nicole's pre-school teachers were very actively involved in her language development. They each attended a therapy session so that they would become more knowledgeable in how to support her. They were not intimidated by her hearing aids and they learned how to put them on and take them off. They were happy to learn how to use the FM system to help her even more. We are so fortunate to have such a wonderful Montessori school and dedicated teachers supported by Shelley's employer Computer Associates International, Inc.

Since it was uncertain whether Nicole was able to hear the high frequencies "C's", "f" and "th," Lynn encouraged us to learn about cochlear implants. Lynn had seen such great results with implants and she knew that implant candidacy was changing to include cases such as Nicole's. But we knew "our" daughter would never have to rely on an implant! I can even remember times when the quiet anger raged inside me when Lynn would subtly mention another implant-related success in another family.

Some people call these things fate and many others see the work of a divine power in what happened next. Lynn held a parents' party on a Saturday night in April 1999, where Shelley and I had the opportunity to really talk in depth for the first time with another family about their implant experiences. They were one of the "pioneering" implant families in our area. Two days later, Nicole suffered the first of a series of sudden and unexplained hearing losses that threatened to take away everything she had worked so hard to achieve. A review of the CT scan confirmed enlarged vestibular aqueducts, and prognosis was a continued further loss of her residual hearing. Having been touched by the courage and success of another family, we were now emotionally prepared to make the decision on the implant quickly.

Grandma and Grandpa knew all the "horror" stories and were initially opposed to an implant. Grandpa never outwardly expressed much opposition, but Grandma was pretty vocal about her beliefs. Her opposition was surprising, given her oral education, compared to Grandpa's ASL education at a state school for the deaf. We were able to overcome some of their opposition by listening to their concerns and explaining the implant, using brochures and literature from the manufacturer. But I believe that what was most influential was their deep love for Nicole and the tremendous language progress that Nicole had made in the past year. They understood what would happen as Nicole continued to lose her remaining hearing.

July 29, 1999, began with a very early morning surgery at Carle Foundation Hospital in Champaign, Illinois. Activation day was August 25. All implant parents know how slow the days pass between surgery and initial activation, and they know about the fantasy that the day of activation will just magically switch your child back into a hearing world. For those who have lost hearing, the real terror comes over the next days and weeks as you wait for the proof that this implant and the brain are going to work together to provide some meaningful information. Until then, fear tugs and rips at your heart because it seems that your child's reaction is more like one of confusion. It's that wonderful plasticity of the young brain working to sort out the new signals that are coming from those auditory nerves. For us, the first real evidence came a week later at a friend's Labor Day party when we could tell by her responses that something was really starting to "register"

I am now so thankful everyday of my life for this incredible cochlear implant technology and for Lynn, who is also our biggest supporter, coach, and guidance counselor. (Sometimes Shelley does need to remind me not to forget, especially when Nicole is demonstrating that stubbornness and lack of patience which she also inherited from her parents.) There is no doubt in my mind that this implant gives Nicole a quality of sound that she never had before. Her language progress post-implant has been truly phenomenal!

Our physiologically deaf child is now able to live her life as a hearing child with a moderate hearing loss. She has the opportunity to be a part of this hearing world that surrounds her. She loves going to her preschool with hearing children. She can listen to her Disney videos and sing her songs. She can talk on the phone to relatives, and she will even be able to share in the experience of her younger brother's first words. Does any parent of a hearing child realize what a gift it is to be able to carry on a conversation with your child who is seated in the back seat of your car?

We have not been afraid to believe our daughter will soar as high as she wants. She will not have to trail her hearing peers, but she will instead have every opportunity to walk at their side and even lead if she wants. We have set goals and measured her progress in comparison to her hearing peers in every day life. One year post-implant, all of the language test scores placed Nicole equal to her hearing peers. Because of her spoken language progress, we have now begun to reintroduce some signs to her and she has shown some interest, especially when visiting Grandma and Grandpa. It's kind of ironic that we taught her some baby signs in her first year of life, before we learned of her hearing loss. We had suspended our use of sign when we first began " therapy," in order to ensure that we focused on her spoken language development.

Shortly after the birth of our second child, Grandma and Grandpa came to visit us for a couple of weeks to spend time with big sister Nicole and her younger brother Spencer. Within the past year, Nicole has finally come to understand that they cannot hear her spoken words. She has gotten a little better at looking directly at Grandma when she

126

talks. Grandpa can't understand her spoken words, but he and Nicole share an even more powerful language of love. They are so very proud of Nicole's accomplishments and they enjoy her speech even though they may not hear her. For the first time in my life, I heard Grandpa say that he wished that he could hear — because he wanted to hear the sound of his granddaughter's voice doing so much talking.

Due to early detection and intervention with today's technology, the opportunities for our physiologically deaf children are so tremendously different from those of just a few short years ago. Since our children are no longer functionally deaf, we must remain vigilant to ensure that they are educated in a manner that is consistent with their abilities. Since we have been so fortunate, we must also help to reach out to those parents who are today confirming their own child's hearing loss. The implant pioneers blazed a trail for us. Please help to make sure that today's parents are given the opportunity to see what is possible for their children. Let us all work together to share the miracle with those children who need it!

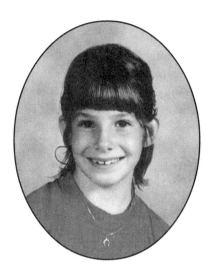

A Full Future With Sound...By Landa Colletta

"Sshhhh, I hear something?" (This is Monika's most famous phrase since acquiring her Nucleus 24 in 1999.) "What do you hear?" Monika's dad stopped what he was doing and actively listened. Dina, her older sister, and Viktor, her younger brother, held their breath, so they, too, could hear what it was. On this particular crisp winter day, there was no wind, no snow, and no sound in the bush.

Monika looked up in the sky, as did the rest of the family, but there was nothing there. As they looked around, their eyes finally rested on the only object making a commotion: the family dog. "Is that what you hear?" Riker's tongue was fully extended, and he was panting heavily. He had been running in the bush. She listened intently, smiled, and thought it was funny that panting 'made' a sound.

A few weeks later, another walk in the bush... This time it was quite windy. Again, her familiar phrase, "I hear something," and she looked everywhere to see where this new noise was coming from. The only sound's anywhere were from the tops of the trees, creaking and rubbing together from the strong winds .... Her eyes were like saucers as she watched the trees swaying back and forth, listening to them talk.

Another interesting sound discovery happened under our car. We were driving one day this past winter, and again her famous line " I hear something!" And, like clockwork, we stopped everything and listened intently to find the source of the sound she was hearing. "That noise, what's that? .... oh,, it's gone.....there it is again.....!" We looked at each other and started laughing. On the road there were slushy sections, dry sections, then more slushy sections .... she had always been able to feel the vibrations, but never knew there was a sound with it. These were only a few of the most memorable sounds she discovered within five months of her switch-on-date with her cochear implant. Needless to say we were impressed!

Okay, now let me tell you the rest of her story.

Monika was diagnosed at nine months with a severe bilateral sensorineural hearing loss. Why she is deaf will remain a mystery. Sound arrived for her on September 23, 1995, one week before her first birthday. She was at a moderate to severe level, when her hearing aids were switched on. In that week she started Auditory-Verbal therapy, and in those few days we knew we made the right decision. Airplane, boat, cowboy, bye-bye .... were words that came fast and easy for her.

In September 1996 she started junior kindergarden in a regular school setting, and loved every minute. She learned so much and was at par with her classmates. She had A-V therapy every week, and also had someone come to our home making sure things were on track.

By the middle of her senior kindergarden year, in 1998, things began to change for this five-year-old. At home we noticed her speech was changing, and she wasn't hearing the same. We started going three times a month to the audiologist. Each visit made it more clear that she was losing more hearing and it wasn't coming back. Her aids were at the maximum setting.

At dinner one evening, I noticed her starting to get teary eyed.... "What's the matter?" I asked. Everyone stopped talking. She looked at me and said "I can't hear what Dina's saying to Viktor." I held myself together and had Dina turn to her and explain what she had just said to her brother.

I had heard a lot of things about the cochlear implant, but had not researched it myself. By August of that year, her hearing loss was at profound levels, and still dropping. It was the audiologist who sat me down, looked straight at me, and said " We can't do anything more for her. She has a lot of potential, she is very bright, but this is as far as the hearing aids will go for her..... but.... I want you to look 'seriously' at a cochlear implant..... she could very well qualify for one."

My mom is a nurse practitioner, and I wanted as much 'true' information as I could get my hands on. I read periodicals, medical stories, talked to a few parents whose children had an implant, I even saw *60 Minutes* which featured an update of a cochlear implant recipient 10 years later. There was no negative, anywhere. So, in October, I called University Hospital in London, Ontario, and set up an appointment with their team of experts for December. I came in with a page of questions, and I was totally impressed with their knowledge, caring, and their positive attitude toward the device.

By mid January, 1999, things had gone from bad to worse. The audiologist found her left ear barely registered on the paper, and her right ear was below profound levels. Monika, as you could well imagine, was extremely frustrated, and kept asking us why her hearing aids 'weren't working'. She had picked up lipreading on her own and was doing a great job at it, because she fooled a lot of people into believing she could hear them!

I arrived home after this appointment, sat beside the fireplace and began tossing junk into it. I had become emotionally drained, and I knew we needed to make some tough decisions. I was about ready to toss the last envelope into the flames, when the corner of my eye grabbed the address of the hospital. Inside was a letter, which stated a time and date in February the hospital could see Monika for testing. I was ecstatic. I had no idea that they had put her on this 'list' for possible candidates.

The February test day came and went, and we would find out in April if she made the list. April came, and it was a very long month! Finally the call came with the news that Monika had made the list. There were so many emotions filling up at the same time, I'm sure Webster would have had trouble finding the words in his dictionary. To imagine, that this was something we would never had considered a year before ... and here it was in front of us.

Surgery was on June 21, 1999, and the implant of the Nucleus 24 was a total success. She was switched on in August, and life has been a roller coaster of knowledge for everyone in Monika's life to date.

She now hears between 20-25 decibels in both ears, and is in a regular school in third grade, with some assistance. This June will be her second-year aniversary, with her new hearing. Everything they said would happen has happened and she has excelled in it. She is an amazing little girl and has opened doors she has never been able to open before. She has the greatest attitude, she loves to hear, and is totally frustrated if something isn't working 'just so'.

She can distinguish between different bird sounds, or the frogs, or crickets. She can hear a dog barking in the distance, the refrigerator kick in and out, and she enjoys the sound of the flute and would like to learn, but she's learning on the recorder first (ouch). Most of all, she can play, fight, tease, and talk with the best of them.

I strongly believe in the advancement of technology, and because of this tool, many children and adults will have an awesome future! It has definitely made Monika, as well as thousands of other people, begin to have a full future with sound.

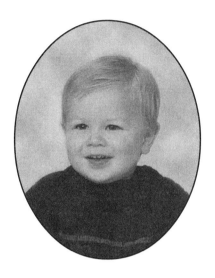

Nolan Listens, Hears, and Speaks…By Tim Green

Nolan Green was born almost five weeks premature. His birth was made somewhat difficult by his fairly large size, almost 8 lbs. for a twin! Due to his size, Nolan was allowed to stay in the room with Mom and Dad and did not have to be rushed to the nursery. Unfortunately, he had swallowed some fluid during the delivery and soon was under an oxygen hood in the nursery. He remained there for three days until they discovered a hole in his lung and he was transported to St. Francis Neonatal Unit in Peoria, Illinois.

During the next 10 days, Nolan's damaged lung was repaired; he was hooked up to a ventilator and required to take several medications. The doctors believe that it was during this time that the profound sensorineural hearing loss occurred. When Nolan left the hospital at 12 days old, his hearing was tested and we received a paper that said he had passed. It wasn't until approximately two weeks later that his mom received a call from a nurse at St. Francis, indicating that Nolan needed to return for a second hearing test because he had not passed the first time. Evidently a clerical error had been made on the first test, mistakenly indicating that Nolan had passed the test, when in fact he had failed. After frantic calls to the neonatologists and nurses, we were reassured that only about 1 in 1000 don't pass the hearing test the second time.

After we were given an explanation regarding how the testing works and what they should see for hearing responses, it became evident that he continued to fail the hearing test. He was then sent to see an audiologist who again provided another test. Again, Nolan failed, and he was then sent to an ENT specialist who referred him to the ECHO program at Carle Hospital in Urbana. Following additional testing of this now almost three-month-old infant, Nolan was fitted with bilateral hearing aids. He wore the hearing aids for five to six months, before the specialists conceded that the aids were not going to provide him with enough hearing for speech. At this point, it was determined that Nolan would be a good candidate for a cochlear implant. Following preparation for the surgery and life after the implant, Nolan finally received the implant on July 1, 1999. The actual microphone hookup four weeks later was an exciting moment for all of us. We have all been off and running ever since!

At first Nolan saw a speech therapist once a week in Urbana. This was eventually increased to twice a week with two different therapists. One of these therapy sessions occurs in Nolan's home. When Nolan was almost two, he started attending a preschool at the ECHO (Expanding Children's Hearing Opportunities) school once a week in addition to his therapy sessions. Nolan has continued with this program for over a year. Nolan will be three years old in August of 2001. On his 3rd birthday he will start school in the public school's early childhood education program. His vocabulary has increased by leaps and bounds over the past six months. Nolan can and will repeat anything that is said to him.

At his parent conference in December Nolan tested 10 months behind where he should be in terms of his speech and language. At a similar conference in April, he was reported as testing only eight months behind where he should be. Of course, like any two-year-old, he doesn't always perform on command, which is a source of frustration for his therapists and parents. But...it is amazing to hear him count to 10 as he walks up the stairs. Even though he may not need the extra food, it is wonderful for Nolan to say, "More fries, please." He knows and calls all of his siblings (five in all) by name. Wearing the "backpack" with the processor in it is the only way of life Nolan knows. As soon as he gets up in the morning, it is the first thing he wants on. He knows immediately when it come off, and replaces it instantly. When we go out in public, those who don't know Nolan, or children, of course, in-

134

quire about the device. However, it never seems to be done with malicious intent and in fact is perceived with awe once the explanation is provided.

We feel extremely fortunate that Nolan was born at a time when this device was gaining in popularity. Had this occurred a decade ago, Nolan would probably be using only sign language and would be preparing to go away from home to attend a school for the deaf. Our hopes from the beginning of this process have been that Nolan will be able to attend public school with his twin brother. Each day that hope becomes less of a dream and more of a reality. We hear our twin sons talking everyday. Nolan is just as verbal as his twin brother is. There appears to be very little difference in sound quality between the speech of the two boys.

Having a child with a disability like Nolan's has opened the hearts and minds of his entire family. Nolan's siblings are extremely tolerant of others with disabilities. Differences in others are no longer considered to make the individual "different" from us. As much as we hate to see what Nolan has gone through and will go through to varying degrees for the rest of his life, we are proud of the way it has helped our children grow as caring human beings.

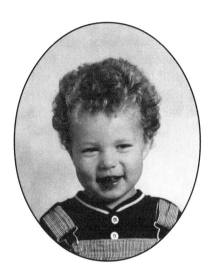

Ryan's Story…By Scott Weber

Ryan was born in August of 1997. Ten fingers and ten toes, thank goodness he is 100% healthy and normal, or so Julie and I thought. After one year I started to wonder when Ryan would say his first words. I asked a few people, and they didn't seem concerned, so I wasn't concerned. I was still wondering after a few more months, but I didn't want to be paranoid about this because he appeared to be a normal baby boy. In January of 1999 a concerned baby sitter said that she didn't think Ryan was hearing very well. My hidden suspicions proved to be correct.

My wife Julie had Ryan's hearing checked. This was a traumatic day for Julie because Ryan didn't respond to any sounds up to 100 decibels. At this point, I was not too concerned. I thought it was probably fluid in the ears so he would only need tubes to drain the fluid. The next day both of us took Ryan for further tests. The results were devastating. Ryan was profoundly deaf; basically he could not hear anything, we were told. My immediate response was, would hearing aids help? The answer was a pessimistic maybe. My wife started to cry. I tried to ask logical questions about what to do. First we had hearing aid molds made that day and we were given videotapes of success stories of deaf people. We left the hospital after about two hours with the worst news I had ever received in my entire life. Nobody had mentioned anything about a cochlear implant at this point.

That night we watched one of those videotapes of success stories. They were not very encouraging, to say the least. Our immediate thoughts were that our little boy was going to have a very tough life ahead dealing with society. We took the next steps to try and help our son. The hearing aids were fitted, therapy (sign and speech) was started, and our appointment for Children's Hospital and Dr. Wackym was made. The hearing aids and speech therapy were a disappointment. The sign language therapy was going pretty well. Our little boy could at least communicate with us, but what about the 99% of people who don't know sign language. How would he ever be able to communicate with them?

Children's Hospital confirmed the severity of deafness but, more importantly, Dr. Wackym was the only person in the medical profession who offered an optimistic outlook for Ryan with a cochlear implant. A couple of months went by and it was our opinion that hearing aids were of virtually no use. We scheduled surgery for a cochlear implant and we decided to use the latest Med-El implant. Dr. Wackym performed the operation in July of 1999 and the implant was activated one month later in August. Ryan was now 24 months old and had not uttered one word. Ryan's implant was adjusted about six times in August and September to get the right program for him. I remember wondering how well will (the implant) work? Will this be another disappointment like hearing aids? I hoped not, as this was the last thing the medical profession said they could do to help Ryan with his hearing.

Ryan has responded very well to his implant. He responded to sounds and his name in less than two months. He said his first word, "ball," in just over two months. Ryan's implant map was further fine-tuned and his response to sound and speech grew at an amazing rate. Our entire family was so happy to hear words like dad, mom, grandpa, and grandma. These were words that we very possibly could never have heard from our little boy. In February of 2000, only six months after activation of his implant, Ryan's speech and sound comprehension was only about six months behind that of an average hearing child. Speech therapist played an important part along with our efforts to achieve this.

Ryan is now just under four years old. He has had his cochlear implant for two years, and I can happily say that his latest evaluation puts his speech and sound comprehension as age-appropriate. It is so wonderful for us to hear Ryan using his ever-expanding vocabulary and to hear him using tonal variations correctly. I am still concerned about Ryan's perfection of his language skills, but not to the extent that I once was. Ryan talks and communicates with people every day and I believe that if a person didn't see his implant they would have no idea that he is deaf. This is a big relief for Julie and me compared to what we had faced a few years ago. Ryan seems to enjoy communicating verbally because he talks all the time. However, when Ryan's implant is off, he talks only about 25% as much as normal.

Julie and I would like to express our sincere thanks to Dr. Wackym, Med-El Corp., the speech therapists who work with Ryan, and the staff at Children's Hospital of Milwaukee.

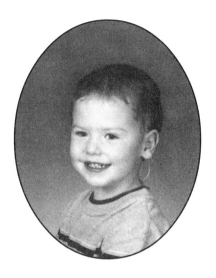

No Regrets...By John & Jamie Kelley

It seems like yesterday. December 24, 1998. Reluctantly, we had taken the last appointment available before the end of the year. We didn't really want to have our fears acknowledged on Christmas Eve, but here we were, sitting in a little room receiving the news. "The tests show that Ryan has a profound hearing loss. He is not hearing anything, and probably never has." Our hearts sank. I looked down at this precious little 2-½ month old, and just started crying. "I don't understand—he seems to hear me when I sing." I sat very still, almost numb, for the rest of the visit, not really hearing the options, the outlook, or the opportunities that lay ahead.

After the shock wore off, after the tears were shed, we finally started to look to the future. Four different times in the next two months, we saw TV shows featuring the cochlear implant. Shows that we normally don't watch would keep our eyes glued to the television. Friends would call and say, "Hey—there's a show on about this thing that might help Ryan." It was almost as if God was saying, "Here's an option to look into." We kept our new-found knowledge about this remarkable technology in the back of our minds and started to learn about how to raise a deaf child.

Ryan was our first-born child. He was a big 8-pound, 14-ounce baby

141

boy. All went fine in delivery. We checked out two days later, expecting no complications. Our hospital did not offer newborn hearing screening, and with no known hearing loss in the family, we felt no need to worry. About a month later, though, we began to wonder. Ryan was never startled when the dog barked; he never turned to our voices; he never woke at loud noises in the night. Fortunately, our pediatrician moved quickly and referred us to an audiologist when we voiced our concern. After the initial testing was complete, we wanted to know why this happened. A CT scan revealed Ryan had Enlarged Vestibular Aqueduct Syndrome. The damage had been done before birth, and it seemed to be "just something that happened." Looking into our history, we found a great-great-grandmother who had been deaf. But all who knew her were gone. Was she deaf from birth? Did she have an illness? No one knew. So, we trudged on, knowing that trying to figure out why this happened was not what we should be focusing on. One of the doctors we talked to told us that we, Ryan's parents, needed to decide whether we wanted to put Ryan into a hearing world or a non-hearing world. Without even discussing it, we knew that we wanted to put him in a hearing world if at all possible. We had to get Ryan on his way to hearing.

He was fitted with his first hearing aids on February 26, 1999. They looked so big on his little four-month-old ears. His response was not an earth-shattering one, so we really didn't know what all he was hearing. He wore them faithfully, but we knew he was not getting enough from them to hear all the speech sounds. We started looking into the implant.

We talked to lots of different people—some for the implant and some against it. We did quite a bit of research and finally decided to give Ryan the opportunity to hear. On December 23, 1999, almost a year to the day after learning about his hearing loss, Ryan was implanted with a Clarion cochlear implant. He was 14-½ months old. Holding his Pooh bear and sucking on his binky, he was given to me to hold after the surgery. My husband and I were wondering how we could've done this to our baby. He looked like a little war vet. I had to tell myself several times that we had just given Ryan so many opportunities in life by giving him the implant. We took him home that same day. He healed very quickly and enjoyed Christmas very much. People could not believe we would have him undergo surgery right before Christmas, but to us, it was the best Christmas present we could have given him.

A month later, on January 21, 2000, Ryan was "turned on" to sound!! It was an emotional day, but one of great joy. As his first map was made, we watched Ryan's expressions as he was trying to process the beeps he was hearing through his implant. He seemed to be in awe of the laptop computer that he was hooked up to. He knew it was doing some pretty neat things. The map was made, and the processor was finally turned on. Ryan looked around and smiled at us as we said his name. Tears filled our eyes in amazement. He began to turn to his name about two days after hook-up. This is unusual, I guess. I know the use of his hearing aids helped him develop this ability so quickly. He had been turning to his name with aids, too, but the implant sound was a different sound to get used to. Ryan began hearing Ellie, our dog. The first time she barked he nearly jumped out of his skin! Once he knew what this sound was he would sit and watch Ellie bark and laugh. They seemed to become much better friends after this exchange.

Ryan had begun speech therapy when he was eight months old. By the time he was implanted at 14 months, he was saying about 10 words. Almost all of these words were just representations of words ("ma" for more, "uh" for up). We continued the therapy and worked very hard at home after hook-up. He seemed to pick things up very quickly, and seemed very motivated to learn new words. "What's dat?," he would say as he pointed to everything in sight. He was very curious. From the very beginning of Ryan's experience with his implant, he has seemed to enjoy the sounds that he receives through it. The first thing he does when he gets up in the morning is walk to his battery charger and pick out a battery. Lately, he's been saying, "This one all right?" After nodding my head "yes," he gives it to me and patiently waits for me to get it in the processor and into a harness for him. Once it's on, it's on for the day. A very loud "UH-OH" is heard if the headpiece is brushed off his head by something. A look of wonderment is seen when the battery goes dead in the evening. "I need a new battery, Mom," is all he says as he marches to the battery charger.

One day in the summer of 2000, I remember sitting on our deck with Ryan. He was playing with a tractor, stopped suddenly, and said, "Fwee, fwee." I stopped to listen carefully and realized he was hearing a bird that was singing in the tree. This was a sound that so many of us, including myself, just block out. I said to him, "Do you hear the bird?" He said "Fwee, fwee" again. I started to cry. That was something that just a year-and-a-half before I just thought he would never hear.

I still get chills thinking about that day and what a miracle the implant really is. Many times a day Ryan looks at one of us and says, "Did you hear that?" His finger is almost always on his cheek when he says that. I'm sure that has evolved from all the conditioned response testing he's done in therapy! Many of the sounds he's hearing are things that we tend to tune out in our everyday lives: the furnace kicking on, a big truck going by our house, a train blowing its whistle in the distance. One day he even pointed out to us that he heard the "tick, tick, tick" of the clock on the wall. We were in a pretty small room with hardwood floors, so I'm sure the ticking was amplified compared to other rooms. But I was still amazed that a sound so small could have an impact on Ryan. We continue to do therapy and a weekly schooling at an oral school for the deaf. Ryan is doing extremely well. At the age of 26 months, he was testing at or above age level in all areas, including receptive and expressive language. He is a very normal thirty-month-old boy who loves to do the things that other kids love to do. He loves basketball, play-doh, the outdoors, and music. In fact, music plays a big part in his life. As much time as we spend on the road, music tapes have been a lifesaver. As he is beginning to sing, he is doing a great job stopping and starting at the right time. We are raising and lowering his pitch as the song demonstrates. I hope he continues this love of music.

The past year and a half has been full of victories for Ryan and our family. We have seen him go from being a fairly quiet child to a child who has so much to say and is so excited to say it. We feel very fortunate that the technology was available to us, and that we took full advantage of it.

A person once said to me, "You should let Ryan make the decision to get an implant or not to get one." As I look back on that bit of "advice" I feel that if we had done that, we would have missed out on these first three critical years of language development. I feel that we are giving him a choice. If he decides someday that he doesn't want to wear the implant, he can take it off. But as much sound and enjoyment from that sound as he gets out of his implant, I can't really see him ever wanting to be without it. It has certainly been a life-changing piece of technology that has benefited Ryan tremendously. This is one decision that I know we will never regret.

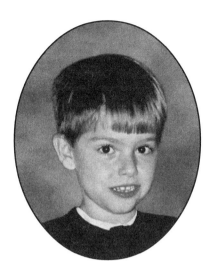

The Story of You…By Julie Bartel

Taylor's story begins on July 30, 1996. That is the day we held him in our arms for the first time. We, however, did not give him life. We were privileged to hold the baby boy we would be adopting only minutes after he was born. As we held him, we were almost speechless; we could only hold him and cry tears of joy. As we told him how very precious he was, we began to fall in love with him. He was our miracle, an answered prayer right in our arms.

We were told to return the next day and take him home with us. It all seemed so simple. But our well-laid plans were interrupted by an early morning phone call. We received word that in the night he had been transferred to the NICU unit at a local hospital. We arrived to find our little boy in the Neonatal Unit with an IV in the top of his head. We were told that some routine blood tests had come back abnormal; his white blood cell count was dangerously low and they were running more tests to determine the cause. They also began a test titled "TORCH", each letter of the word representing an infection that could be passed from mother to child.

After several things were ruled out and having Taylor examined by many doctors, we thought the problem would be corrected simply by a blood transfusion. But after the fifth day a nurse suddenly swept us into an isolation room. She said one of the tests had come back positive and we needed to be in isolation and wear gowns and gloves any time we entered his room.

We soon found out that Taylor had congenital cytomegalovirus, or CMV. (This represented the "C" in the TORCH study.) It is a virus that is only harmful to a baby if it is contracted in the womb. It is such a common virus that 95% of the population is CMV positive. It is very rare for a baby in the womb to contract it because usually by the time you are of childbearing age, you have already had it and have produced antibodies to it. But if it is contracted in the womb it attacks the nervous system.

Immediately we had questions; what would this mean for Taylor, is there a cure, will he live? These answers would not soon be answered. Because the virus attacks the nervous system, any damage that was done inside the womb was permanent and irreversible. Any further damage could happen as long as the virus was still in his system, and it was known to be progressive. Taylor would shed the virus in his urine and could do so for three to seven years.

Taylor was put on a strong medicine, which he received twice a day intravenously. "Gancyclovir" was known to stop the virus in some children. They didn't exactly know how it stopped it and so they were never sure which children it worked in and which children it did not work in until the child had grown through the developing years.

Taylor did receive a hearing test (ABR) before leaving the hospital. It was abnormal. While 50% of these tests can be abnormal at such an early age, the doctors felt, under these conditions, it was an accurate one.

We began our journey into deafness. Taylor had several doctor appointments his first year of life. A careful eye was kept on him so any deficiencies could be caught as soon as possible. But we still did not seek medical services for his ears until he was almost a year old. As we look back on it now, it probably took us that long to cope with the fact that our precious little boy whom we had waited so long for could be and probably would be deaf. We were not in denial, but test after test was inconsistent and so there was always that hope that it wouldn't be "bad." Finally, we knew that we needed to do something. Taylor was fitted for hearing aids and we also began sign language classes. We loved him so very much and wanted to be able to communicate with him no matter what. We do believe that his hearing loss was progressive. When he received his hearing aids, he did seem to respond sometimes and it seemed his audiograms were a little bit better. After a year or so with the hearing aids, his audiologist suggested we go to an adult hearing aid because they would be a bit stronger.

During this time, we adapted at home. To get his attention, we would stomp on the floor or flash the lights on and off. We were learning sign and, of course, concentrated on the words we needed most: drink, more, mommy, daddy, go, sit, walk, etc. Taylor was very visual and caught many concepts by watching us. He explored many things through sign, and we found him to be very mechanical minded. He was always a happy child, but as he grew, we saw that other kids would try to play with him by talking. When Taylor didn't respond they gave up. He began playing alone more and more. We had started reading books about deafness and the options opened to deaf people. We had heard about the cochlear implant, but we were relieved we would never have to "make that decision for our child." Our child wasn't a candidate for it. Many people had said it was very risky, no guarantees it worked, and lots of training afterwards. No doctors had ever mentioned it to us, so surely it wouldn't be for us.

As he continued to grow and his hearing seemed to dwindle away to nothing, we thought about his future. Here was a deaf child in a hearing family. No one in either of our families was deaf; we didn't know anyone who was deaf. What would his future hold? How happy would he be? How *safe* would he be? How would relationships outside our home be if he couldn't communicate with other people and most could not communicate with him? It was at this time the audiologist mentioned that Taylor could be a candidate for the cochlear implant.

We were scared! Thinking about putting this small child through a surgery like that frightened us. We tried not to think about it. We needed to research the implant and what it meant for our family. Later we met other families with hearing-impaired children, as well as talked with several professionals through therapies, sign language classes, and early-intervention resources. I began asking everyone what his or her opinion of the implant was. I took both positive and negative responses. We received only one or two negative responses, so I continued our research. I was given the names of families whom I could call and speak to about their own experience with the implant. I eagerly called these families to see what they could tell us. All of these families had children with severe hearing loss and hearing parents and/or siblings.

We knew there was controversy among many groups of people concerning the implant. Without exception, each family told us the benefits of the implant far outweighed any controversy they had encountered.

After hearing their stories, we thought again about our family situation and decided to go ahead with the cochlear implant. We came to the conclusion that we really had nothing to lose. If we had the implant and Taylor lost total hearing in one ear, there was so little there anyway, what would it hurt? We had been under the opinion that we would wait until Taylor was old enough to make the decision for himself. We learned that to be most effective, it needed to be done at an early age. The decision could still be his when he was older, but we would rather him say to us, "I choose not to use it," than "Here was this opportunity, now lost, why didn't you give it to me?"

We were very happy with our decision. We chose what was best for *our* family and we were following through with it. We had done our research and we would begin proceedings to make the implant possible. Taylor was implanted in December of 1999. Were we scared? Yes. Any surgery was risky, but we knew that he was in good hands. We had prayed about, and for, this decision, and knew God would be with Taylor. We were also confident that he was with a very competent doctor. We were unsure, however, on how to prepare Taylor for the surgery. How do you explain to a deaf three-year-old what is about to happen to him? We took a stuffed dog with him into the hospital, and the staff was very helpful. They did everything first to the dog to show Taylor what they needed to do with him. When we saw Taylor in recovery, they had even put the same bandage on the dog's ear that Taylor had. Even though the surgery was long, it was probably harder on us than it was on Taylor. He was in some pain for a few hours, but by the next morning he was simply on Tylenol. The following day, he didn't even require that. His ear healed quickly and he was very curious about the stitches. He would put his hand up to the scar several times, and you could see his little mind trying to figure out what was going on. Now we anxiously awaited the day it would be turned on so we could see if the implant was successful.

January 10, 2000, is a day we will never forget. Just as memorable as the day he was born, this was the day that Taylor's hearing came to life. There weren't any big accomplishments that day; Taylor didn't begin speaking in sentences or singing songs. The simple flutter of his eyelashes when sound was introduced was all the audiologist needed to know that he was getting stimulation from the cochlear implant. A new phase in his already full little life would begin. Over the next few months

148

as his implant power was increased and programmed, we saw many things. In fact, we have labeled that year as the one we witnessed miracles almost daily. This child who we once could stand behind and yell his name at the top of our lungs without any recognition was experiencing sounds for the first time. He still communicated to us in sign, but he was telling us he heard the birds, he heard cars driving by, he heard a train whistle. Soon he recognized his name. I would often call him several times a day just to see him turn to me. When he would look, I would sign to him "I love you" back without looking up so his play would not be interrupted. He had caught on to my little game. Taylor went from not hearing us at all, to now responding to our call from his room upstairs…and we were *downstairs.* He no longer had to be in a world by himself!

Today, after a year and a half, Taylor is detecting speech at 15dB. He didn't hear speech before, and only heard the low frequencies at 85+ dB. The once faint sound of a jet engine was now loud enough for him to turn the implant off because it was too loud. He hears the phone and can recognize who is talking on the other end. He hears the meow of our cats, often teasing them to get them to meow more. He hears us *say* "I love you" and returns it by *saying* "uh ooh." He tries to mimic our words and wants to know the words for everything. A whole new world has opened up for him. Has our journey been easy? No, pain and tears have accompanied it. Has it been fun? Not always, but everyone must make the choice to deal with the things that God allows in their life or wallow in pity. One thing is for certain, we wouldn't trade this journey with anyone, for the joy we receive from this little boy experiencing everything new for the first time will never be matched by anything. He has shown us to appreciate every little thing, nothing is taken for granted. Our lives are not limited by disability; we have been given the ability to experience it more fully and appreciate it every step of the way!

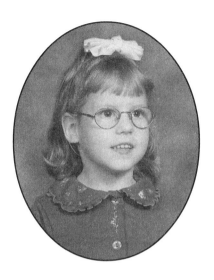

Kathryn's Story...By Pam Pulse

"Your daughter has a severe hearing impairment. Step into the next room and we will pour molds for hearing aids." WHAT? I felt hot, like I was going to pass out. This was my 12-month-old baby she was talking about! OK, so she had barely responded as we sat in the sound-proof booth, listening to progressively louder tones. We had been suspicious of hearing loss since she had been about six months old. My husband wondered, "Could she have a hearing loss, she's so loud?" My response had been, "I'm loud" (no denial there, huh?) After all, Kathryn made "baby sounds" all along. The speech language pathologist had meant no harm as she delivered the news. What had become "routine" for her, was the blow of a lifetime for us.

An ABR one week later confirmed the fact that our daughter did have moderate to severe loss in the right ear, severe to profound loss in the left. By the age of 13 months she had her first pair of hearing aids. We also met with a genetic counselor because we were interested in having more children. There is no history of deafness in either of our families. As part of the quest to determine if she had a "syndrome" which may include other impairments, Kathryn had a number of tests. An EKG was "questionable" so she saw a pediatric cardiologist who ordered an echocardiogram. She had a head CT scan and lab work. A gastroenterologist had confirmed a diagnosis of GE reflux as a baby but she seemed to outgrow that by about 12 months (just in time for our new challenge, hearing impairment!). APT/OT evaluation showed some gross motor delay and sensory integration problems (we later learned this is common with hearing impaired kids). When Kathryn was 14 months old, we noticed her eyes didn't always seem focused; the possibility she was having seizures led us to a neurologist and an EEG. We later learned what we thought were seizures, was farsightedness, corrected with glasses. I became very familiar with the wonderful staff at Children's Mercy Hospital in Kansas City, Missouri. Although she was only 15 months old and just starting to walk, it seemed that every cell of her body had been evaluated!

Once we knew she was essentially "only" hearing impaired, I submersed myself in learning communication options. We were given a list of programs by the hospital. Our First Steps case manager expanded on those options. First Steps is a statewide program that provides support, education, and funding for services for children up to age three who are at risk for developmental delay. I read everything I could get my hands on, and talked to many people, both professionals and other parents of hearing-impaired children. What I learned is that:

a) The more people you talk to, the great variety of opinions you receive.
b) What "works" for one family does not necessarily "work" for another.
c) People are passionate about their opinion of oral vs. signing.

We decided, if possible, we wanted Kathryn to learn spoken language, and we felt that she would have greater opportunities in a mainstream environment if her primary mode of communication were speech. We chose an Auditory-Verbal program and at 15 months Kathryn started speech therapy two times per week for one hour through St. Joseph Institute for the Deaf. Her progress was slow, but her AV therapist taught us a lot and she was very optimistic. We also enrolled in the (free) John Tracy Clinic correspondence course, which was wonderful. In December of 1998 when Kathryn was 2-½ we noticed that her speech seemed to be at a plateau. We also had a "feeling" that her hearing had deteriorated. In January of 1999 we saw Dr. Charles Luetje, an otologist known for his work with children and cochlear implants. He recommended a cochlear implant for Kathryn because, as he explained, although she had made progress, he felt her speech should have been much better than it was. We were referred to Midwest Ear Institute in Kansas City, MO. Their audiogram confirmed our suspicions – Kathryn's hearing loss was profound bilaterally. This time, instead of shock or denial, I had a sense of relief, and hope that she would be a candidate for an implant.

My husband did not initially share my enthusiasm. Although he knew her hearing had deteriorated, it took a few weeks for the idea of invasive surgery on his daughter's head to sink in. From the day her hearing impairment had been diagnosed, we have dealt with our situation together, as partners. However, we have rarely dealt with issues pertaining to Kathryn's disability on the same time line emotionally. I was the one who took Kathryn to her appointments, made the contacts, etc., and he learned and read everything "second-hand" (OK, one of us needs to work in the family!).

The process of "qualifying" for the implant took about six weeks. On April 15, 1999, Kathryn was implanted with a Clarion-S series cochlear implant. It would change her life (ours too!). Although she did have some temporary post-surgical labrynthitis (rare), her incision healed beautifully (I'm a nurse, -it was a beautiful incision!).

That summer we visited the John Tracy Clinic (JTC) in Los Angeles, CA. They have a free preschool program and a simultaneous program for parents. I cannot say enough about the staff and facilities at JTC. I can say that the 3 weeks at JTC was the most empowering experience of my life.

In the fall of 1999 when Kathryn was three, she attended St. Joseph's Institute for the Deaf in Overland Park, KS, in their full-time oral preschool program. She adjusted slowly but did make progress and we felt very supported. By then, her gross motor delay was resolved, but she had been identified as having significant oral motor "challenges" (poor breath control, poor lip strength and tongue mobility). In the summer of 2000 she completed a five-week session at Central Institute for the Deaf (CID) in St. Louis, MO. That oral program seemed to "fit" her needs to a great extent. Kathryn started school as a full-time residential student at CID in the fall. She currently lives in a dorm during the week and comes home every weekend. Although emotionally it is a daily challenge for us to deal with, Kathryn has adjusted well, is happy, and is making tremendous progress. She will continue to attend CID until she can be fully mainstreamed. For us, the cochlear implant has been a blessing. Kathryn is learning new sounds and language daily.

Her zest for life is contagious to those who come in contact with her.

I will never say that I am grateful for my daughter's deafness. However, I will be eternally grateful for the support my husband and I have received from our family, friends, and church. If it takes "a village" to raise a child, then it takes "a very special village" to raise a child with a disability.

Advice to parents of hearing-impaired children:

1. Give yourself permission to grieve and to "re-grieve." Yes, it is very sad. No, it is not your fault.
2. Become knowledgeable. Know your options.
3. Join professional organizations. AVI, CIAI, JTC and especially AG Bell Association for deaf and hard of hearing.
4. The House Ear Institute and Advanced Bionics have great newsletters.
5. Be flexible (in our family, we call it the "F-word"). Be willing to give up a little control (this was particularly hard for me).
6. Network – no one knows what you are thinking or feeling except other parents in similar situations. You are not alone.
7. Trust your instincts. If you don't understand, ask questions. If it doesn't "feel" right, it's not. No one will ever know more or care more about your child than you.
8. Be organized. Keep copies of all medical and speech records.
9. Know this: Having a child with a hearing loss will change your life. It will not ruin your life.

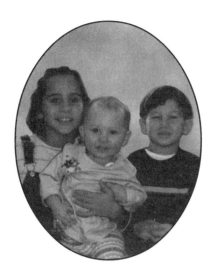

Triple Crown...By Andi Hill

In late summer of 1994, my husband Steve and I learned that our precious daughter Jessica had a congenital severe sensorineural hearing loss. Hearing loss is characterized by categories, not percentages, and a severe hearing loss meant that without hearing aids Jessica heard no speech and only very loud environmental noises (like a chainsaw or a jet engine at close range). Sensorineural hearing loss meant that the origin of Jessica's hearing loss was the inner ear (specifically the cochlea), and hence not surgically correctable. Like 94% of parents who learn that their child has a significant hearing loss, neither Steve nor I had known anyone with a hearing loss like Jessica's. Our hearts ached with fear and disappointment, for all that we had dreamed of for our daughter and our family seemed at great risk. The tears that fell from both of our eyes that morning in August in the audiologist's office arose out of feelings too deep and distressing for words. As I held my bubbly nine-month-old, I had a thousand questions - like, *what* do all those numbers on the audiogram mean?' 'Can a child with a hearing loss like this ever hear speech?' 'How can we learn sign and simultaneously teach it to her?' 'Are there any other options for her to use to communicate?' 'Will she be able to attend regular schools?' 'What about our church and our faith ... how will she ever come to understand it?' I can remember distinctly the depth of pain I felt realizing that Jessica had never heard me say her name, much less 'I love you' or 'You are beautiful'. In spite of five months of suspicion and raising my concerns to anyone who would listen, I was still completely unprepared and over-whelmed by the realities that were hitting me as the audiologist delivered the news. Jessica was deaf. I had never known anyone with a hearing loss like this. My only awareness of deafness was my love for the play *The Miracle Worker*, that I had seen performed at Helen Keller's birthplace several times. Tears, disbelief, doubt, and confusion were a very regular part of our lives at that time. We grieved her loss and ours. My faith was deeply shaken, and yet in the final analysis, my faith was all I had. It wasn't until we began to educate ourselves that we began to heal, slowly and painstakingly, step by step. We began to look into programs that could help Jessica, and made several calls as suggested by our audiologist. We were surprised and disappointed by the difficulties we experienced with the agency in our state that was designated to help children with hearing impairment, and found that our experience with the system that was supposed to help us through this process to be another source of stress, frustration, and additional grief. So, we chose to go this route with Jessica alone, and made choices that went against the opinions of the 'experts' with whom we had mostly been in contact.

Jessica began wearing hearing aids at the age of 10 months and si-multaneously began Auditory-Verbal therapy. After much research on the many opinions and options for educating a child with a hearing im-pairment and meeting with other families, we decided that the most appropriate choice for Jessica was to teach her to use her residual amplified hearing (through hearing aids) to listen and speak. I immersed myself in reading, attending therapy (we found a local therapist who was familiar with the AV method), and learning how to work with Jes-sica at home to promote natural language development. We worked with her at home, and our therapist worked with Jessica weekly in therapy. Jessica's initial progress in therapy was slow. By the age of 18 months her progress was not commensurate with her intelligence and other factors; moreover, it became obvious that we would not meet the goals we had set without additional intervention. At that time Jes-sica was attending therapy twice each week and receiving lots of lan-guage stimulation at home, but her progress was laborious.

In October 1995, Steve, Jessica, and I attended a one-week program at the Helen Beebe Speech and Hearing Center in Pennsylvania. The program is designed to accommodate one family per week, with an extensive, busy schedule of intensive therapy sessions, hearing and language evaluations, and parent education. Our trip to the Beebe Center was a turning point in our understanding of hearing loss and Auditory Verbal therapy. It was there that we came to understand that any choice relating to how we communicate is a lifestyle choice. Auditory Verbal Therapy was more than a method ... it was a lifestyle. It was at the Beebe Center that we learned for certain what we had suspected but had been unable to successfully diagnose with the audiologists in Alabama: Jessica had a profound hearing loss. This explained part of the building frustrations we had all experienced with therapy, and the slow progress we were making. Jessica's hearing loss was profound, and not severe. This 15-20 dB difference in her diagnosis made all the difference in her aided hearing, and she had been significantly under-aided for over a year. Again I grieved another loss, and, at the same time, experienced intense anger for not trusting my own intuition. For some time, I had suspected that Jessica's loss was greater than the original diagnosis and follow-up testing had shown. This experience of misdiagnosis and under-amplification demonstrated to me the essentiality of having a pediatric audiologist ... one who loves, is patient with, and has experience testing *children*. Jessica was immediately fitted with the most powerful hearing aids available and with a personal FM system. Jessica made steady progress in her power hearing aids, but time became our enemy. Her language skills were significantly delayed. As her frustration level (and ours) continued to increase, Steve and I, fueled by the urging of our therapist, decided that it was time to consider a cochlear implant. The power aids gave Jessica a lot of decibels, but my guess is that in amplifying sound adequately, the power aids caused too much distortion. Even with the most powerful hearing aids, Jessica did not have access to sound in all of the speech frequencies. The cochlear implant appeared to be our last hope for Jessica to hear, speak, and have the opportunities we had always hoped for, dreamed of, and expected for her. For the severely to profoundly hearing impaired, the technology is a phenomenal option.

We chose to interview cochlear implant teams in Atlanta, GA and in Birmingham, AL. Regardless of the CI center we chose, this was to be a decision that would involve extensive travel and commitment, as the closer of those two centers was a 200-mile round trip. Although still in the process of making our final decisions about the cochlear implant, we decided on our trip home from Birmingham that should we choose for Jessica to receive an implant, we would choose Birmingham. We were very impressed with Dr. Audie Woolley, the cochlear implant surgeon, and with Nancy Gregg, MS, CCC-SLP, Cert AVT, the cochlear implant program director, and felt so assured and encouraged by all of our meetings with them. Dr. Woolley had received his medical training at Washington University in St. Louis, MO, which is partnered with Central Institute for the Deaf and St. Joseph's Institute for the Deaf, both of which are internationally renowned oral schools. The experience, expertise, and expectations for children with hearing impairment that we found at the Birmingham program exceeded what we had hoped to find. We were also very impressed with the post-implant audiological care and Auditory Verbal Therapy program available under one roof through Children's HEAR Center. After interviewing both teams, extensively researching cochlear implants, attending the AG Bell International Biennial Convention's cochlear implant symposium in Salt Lake City, Utah, talking with parents of young children with cochlear implants and with one adult who herself had received an implant, and observing numerous cochlear implant kids, Steve and I decided that the cochlear implant would give Jessica the best opportunity to reach her potential and to be able to someday open the doors of opportunity for herself.

For such a miraculous technology, the cochlear implant has generated a significant amount of controversy. As part of our cochlear implant candidacy process, our center required that each implant family read the position papers of several leading organizations that serve the needs of people who are deaf and hard of hearing. In reading through those papers, we were surprised that what we viewed as a technological tool was to many a threat. We also found that some of the claims in those position statements to be erroneous based on what we had seen with our own eyes. For us, the controversy over the cochlear implant technology was no different from the controversy we faced in choosing an oral method of communication for our daughter versus a manual method. In the end, we are the parents, and we have every right and responsibility to make decisions for our family and for our daughter's future that reflect our goals, values, and beliefs. After all, these decisions impact our family and our lifestyle more than any professional or theorist, for we are the daily practitioners, and on our backs and by our hands come success. In addition to an article by Dr. Thomas Balkany, I was reassured of my thoughts on this subject of controversy by the words of another parent, David W. Hewlings, in his article for a Helen

Beebe Speech & Hearing Center newsletter:

Not surprisingly, such an abundance of solutions generate a fair amount of disagreement among proponents and practitioners, and new parents of deaf children get swept up in the 'controversy'. But we're willing to try anything that might allow our children to bridge the communication gap and function independently out there in the big world. That is, after all, our job. So while we're grateful for the number of options, we've come to believe that controversy exists only in the minds of the practitioners and in the media, and that it does not exist for us. You can't wage war when only one side fights. From this parent's point of view, the attacks coming from the Deaf militia require no response. The real story is, and always has been, that parents have not just the right, but the duty to choose the manner in which their children will be educated. And that choice must be made with the individual child's abilities and interests in mind. There is no controversy in this house. There is only love, resolve, and incredible faith and trust in our children's abilities.'

After numerous trips from Madison (outside of Huntsville, AL) to Birmingham during the summer of 1996 for audiological, medical, and speech-language evaluations, Jessica's surgery was approved and set for August 29, 1996. Jessica was the first child at Children's HEAR Center with a severe-profound hearing loss and who was audiologically a 'silver" hearing aid user to receive a cochlear implant. Jessica's surgery was 'textbook'. Three weeks later we celebrated Jessica's 2nd 'hearing birthday', which came on September 19, 1996. As the cochlear implant team worked with Jessica to program the cochlear implant, Steve and I were on pins and needles, excitedly and nervously awaiting the end of the initial stimulation, when Jessica would hear for the first time. As the 'mapping' (the term used for the individual programming of the CI) of Jessica's implant was completed, and she heard for the first time, Jessica cried. So did I. So did Steve. Her crying response to the CI signal was normal, and not unlike an infant who cries in response to unfamiliar sounds; after all, she *was* a newborn with respect to hearing! Our tears fell out of a profound thankfulness and joy. We held and comforted Jessica as she gradually grew accustomed to the sounds she heard. We were assured that Jessica's responses to the implant were very positive: she had instantly connected the sounds of the implant with the sounds she had heard in hearing aids. We went back the next day for a second check of the cochlear implant 'map' and then to the Birmingham Zoo to celebrate. We were beginning yet another journey, this time with the cochlear implant. To us, the cochlear implant is only a tool, not a miracle cure, and appropriate therapy strategies that complement the auditory potential of the CI must be undertaken to insure successful use. We knew this, and were ready to get to work. The miracle comes with time and hard work, and we desired more than anything else to have a miracle unfold for Jessica.

Prior to the cochlear implant, at age 2-1/2, Jessica understood about 20 words and could say five. In just one year of cochlear implant use, Jessica's vocabulary went from under 20 to about 500 words, and she was speaking in two-word sentences. By the end of the second year of implant use, that number had doubled, and so had the length of her sentences. By the end of the third year of implant use, we could not keep track of Jessica's vocabulary, as it exceeded 1500 words. Those three years were filled with challenging, intense, and frequent application of the Auditory-Verbal method. For every one session with our Certified AVT, we did three sessions at home. Jessica also attended weekly articulation therapy with a speech language pathologist from our local public schools and did school preparation work with a teacher of the hearing impaired. We changed our lifestyle, adapting the AV philosophy vigorously, and using everyday language situations deliberately to benefit our daughter's speech and communication development. We had hoped that the implant would give Jessica better auditory access to speech than she had received in hearing aids, and our hopes had been more than realized. We have been amazed by all that Jessica hears with the CI: the phone ringing and oven timers buzzing, birds singing, rustling leaves, the wind blowing through the trees, the soft wind chimes that hang on our deck, a whisper, a soft rattle, and so many more fantastic noises that most of us sadly take for granted. One of the more interesting things Jessica liked to listen to with her CI in the early days following her initial stimulation were the bubbles in her coke!

The miracles of the CI technology continue today. Jessica is now in a private elementary school where she is the only child with a hearing loss. She participates fully in the regular curriculum without academic support. Jessica reads above grade level and is on the All 'A' Honor Roll. She is artistic, outgoing, sensitive, generous, caring and athletic. Jessica has participated in ballet, gymnastics, art lessons, soccer, and church activities. She has sung in two musical performances at her school, as part of a group ... something that in my wildest imagination I would never have thought she would have had the opportunity to do, even with a cochlear implant. Jessica's success has come through her determination and positive attitude, through the use of a technological tool, the cochlear implant, and from a commitment to her needs on our part and on the part of all those professionals who have guided, directed, assisted, and encouraged us in our journey.

But our story does not end with the miraculous experience of Jessica's cochlear implant. Between Jessica's cochlear implant surgery and her initial stimulation, I learned I was pregnant. Given my complicated history of trying to conceive the first time, this news came as a shock to Steve and I both. Throughout the pregnancy we wondered if our son would be able to hear or if we would face this journey a second time. Fortunately, I was so busy with weekly trips to Birmingham for Auditory-Verbal Therapy and with implementing and emulating our AV lessons at home that I had little time or energy to dwell on 'what if?'. Jared Christopher was born in May 1997, and the day after his birth, through newborn hearing screening, we learned that he also had a hearing loss. Vivid in my mind is the image of our hospital room after our audiologist left. Steve and I cried and prayed together, asking God to preserve our joy and to give us strength. This time my grief was not selfish and focused on what I had lost. The grief I experienced after learning of Jared's hearing loss was for Jared and for all the additional challenges he would face for a lifetime. My grief was still real. It was still deep. It still cut like a knife through the heart of a mother in anguish for her son. But I had hope. I knew what to do, and knew that God would somehow provide a way for me to do this again. We already had a dedicated team of professionals that we trusted and loved. We took Jared to Birmingham one week later to see our pediatric audiology team, and his hearing loss was confirmed as severe/profound. Even before he received his hearing aids I would sing and talk directly into his ear in hopes that he would hear at least some sort of auditory information. Jared began wearing hearing aids at five weeks of age, and I began to stimulate his listening skills immediately. He wore his hearing aids all waking hours from the onset of hearing aid use; still, his benefit was marginal. Given the level of Jared's hearing loss and our parallel experience with the growing miracles of Jessica's cochlear implant, we knew what we wanted for Jared ... a cochlear implant.

Shortly after Jared's birth, the FDA lowered the minimum age for cochlear implantation to 18 months. Still, 18 months seemed like an eternity for our precious son to have to wait to hear. Had it been possible, I would have had Jared receive a cochlear implant at 5 weeks of age instead of hearing aids. Our surgeon was willing to do Jared's cochlear implant at 12-15 months of age, pending insurance approval, and we were thrilled that our agonizing waiting could end 6 months earlier than originally expected. Our joyful hope was quickly extinguished. Our insurance company denied Jared's cochlear implant three times, each time claiming that to implant at under 18 months of age made the procedure experimental. We wrote letters, emailed, and made phone calls. We appealed, appealed, and appealed again. Our cochlear implant team did likewise. I sought the advice and counsel of other parents who had successfully procured insurance approval for their children's cochlear implants outside of FDA protocols. I talked to insurance reimbursement specialists at three different CI manufacturers. It was so disappointing, frustrating, and downright maddening to know that there was something that could help Jared, and that in all likelihood would help prevent some of the language delays that Jessica was enduring and yet to be denied access to it. I recall telling someone that to make Jared wait until 18 months of age to receive a CI was like telling a family whose child had moderate loss that "Your child has a hearing loss that makes it difficult for him to hear speech, and will cause a delay in his language. You can put hearing aids on him after waiting the prescribed 18 months. Ludicrous!! The only remaining recourse for us was to pursue formal legal proceedings. Given the length of time that a legal process would take and Jared's age (now 15 months), with our CI team, we decided the best way to circumvent the insurance company's denials was to set Jared's surgery for one week following his 18-month 'birthday'. We went ahead with the surgery, and our insurance company did cover it. In early December 1998, Jared became our state's youngest cochlear implant recipient. Our dream for Jared to hear with a cochlear implant became a reality shortly after Christmas 1998, when he heard for the first time. What a Christmas gift that was!

Jared's cochlear implant has been a remarkable success. Once again, that success has come through a determined commitment to provide for Jared's needs by utilizing a method that complements the technological potential of the CI. We made a 200-mile round trip weekly for Auditory Verbal Therapy with two small children for four years. We have diligently applied what we have learned in AVT and followed through at home with our 'lessons'. We have been to 30 different lectures and conferences on the subject of AVR and hearing impair-

162

ment. This journey has required extensive commitment and teamwork from Steve and me both, as well as help from family and friends. Jared recently turned four, and his vocabulary is so extensive that it cannot be counted. He speaks routinely in 6-10 word sentences that are mostly grammatically correct. I continue to be amazed by his progress, at the speed with which he acquires new and complex language forms, and the degree of retention he has for vocabulary. I have been granted the joy of the 'cute little things that children say' in this journey with Jared; something I felt deafness stole from Jessica and me. How incredible it is to be witness to everyday miracles, and to be keenly aware of it!

Jared had his cochlear implant a little over a year, and Jessica three years when I was again taken by surprise and learned I was expecting a third baby. My plate was full and I had all I could handle meeting the AV therapy, hearing loss, and other CI-related demands of two children. The thought of having another child, with the possibility of hearing loss a third time, was more than I could bear to consider. Fear and anxiety raged within me. Unlike my pregnancy with Jared, 'what if?' plagued me. How could we possibly manage three children? How would we cope if this little one was also hearing impaired? Surely this baby would hear! During my pregnancy, we were continuing weekly trips to Birmingham, so I was still in close contact with our CI center. I talked with our CI surgeon, who was reassuring. Even though we knew that the type of hearing loss we carried was recessive and that each child had a 25% possibility of having a hearing loss, the actual *probability* of Steve and I giving birth to a third child with a hearing loss was 1.56% (we later learned the actual etiology of our children's hearing losses to be associated with Connexin 26). I clung to the hope that our baby girl would hear, unwilling to truly internalize the possibility of deafness a third time...after all, she had a remarkable chance of being born with "typical" hearing.

Julianne Grace arrived in September 2000. The joy I felt as my beautiful baby girl lay on my chest, our eyes locked, erased the fears and anxieties that had plagued me the preceding months. I knew in that moment that the love I felt for this baby girl would in time transcend the outcome of her hearing tests. Our audiologist came the next day to perform the newborn hearing screenings. Like her older siblings, Julianne had a severe to profound hearing loss. I wish I could say that I was accepting of the realities before me from the moment I knew of Julianne's hearing loss. I was devastated. I was overwhelmed. I was ransacked with grief. I was filled with selfish self-pity. And yet I knew that love has the power to heal, to restore hope, and to transcend. I knew that it was only through a dependence on God that we would be able to have the strength, hope, help, and support we would need to practically meet the challenges of three children with profound hearing loss. God had again taken me to the end of my rope so that my need for His providence and grace would be my only hope. My locked eyes with my beautiful, blessed, baby girl and my faith would go a long, long way in seeing me through a very difficult year.

Before Julianne was born, I had talked with our surgeon about whether or not he would consider doing a cochlear implant on a baby less than 12 months of age (which was the latest FDA age protocol). Perhaps something deep inside, my maternal intuition, was still trying to prepare me for what I would face, even though I had attempted to shove the 'what ifs?' from my mind and deny the possibility of deafness for a third time. I had told our surgeon about a baby I had read about in North Carolina who had received a cochlear implant at seven months of age. Dr. Woolley assured me that if this little one had a hearing loss also, that he would indeed consider very early implantation. I remember emailing him not long after Julianne's birth, with a one-liner.. "Can I hold you to your word?" He emailed me back with an encouraging and uplifting message saying yes, he and the CI team would begin the evaluation process when Julianne was three months old. In my heart I knew that all the testing would be completed easily and that Julianne would be an excellent CI candidate. But the almighty insurance company loomed in the future, and that hurdle was one I feared.

We completed the testing and evaluation process for Julianne's cochlear implant in early April 2001, when Julianne was six months old. Our audiologist and surgeon both wrote letters to the insurance company detailing Julianne's need for a CI, and disclosing their awareness that she did not meet all the current FDA protocols. They clearly outlined the FDA's provisions for the application of clinical judgment on behalf of the implant team. We wrote a persuasive letter, pleading with the insurance company to allow Julianne to hear and citing our previous experience with our other children's cochlear implants. My husband enlisted the help of the insurance service representative who sold the policy to Steve's company, and she helped to push internally for the approval of Julianne's surgery. Our insurance company had 30 days to review Julianne's case, and I thought that if we heard anything by mid-May, we would be fortunate. One week after our submission to the insurance company, Steve called me and said, 'Are you ready to do

Julianne's surgery?' The approval had come in an unprecedented seven days. I cried in relief, thankfulness, and amazement at God at work in the midst of our trials.

On May 31, 2001, Julianne became one of the nation's youngest cochlear implant recipients. She was eight months old at the time of her surgery, and 8-1/2 months at the time of her initial stimulation. It was the first day of summer, and we were beginning our third cochlear implant journey. I could not contain my emotions as Julianne heard for the first time. I told her that I loved her. That she did not understand those words mattered little to me, for I knew that in time she would. Tears of joy turned quickly to sobs of thankfulness, relief, and closure. I am amazed, thrilled, and thankful at what Julianne is already doing with her cochlear implant. At this writing, she has had the CI for three months. Julianne hears everything, just as her siblings do. It is fun to see her wide-eyed and listening to the sound of something as soft and benign as a ceiling fan. To encourage her development, we are pointing out environmental sounds and doing lots of language stimulation. We have begun work with a Certified AVT with Julianne as well. She is baby-babbling constantly, and already has three true words: "da da" for Daddy, "adutff " for duck, and "ba ba" for bye bye. This will be an interesting journey again, unique in all facets, unique just as each child is a unique and marvelous creation of an incredible and loving God.

It took me a while to realize that our little family is riding a wave of change in the potential of children born with profound hearing loss. For quite some time, I was easily frustrated and annoyed by the number of supposed 'professional experts' who were unfamiliar with the term "cochlear implant" and who hadn't a clue as to what the 'speech banana' was. As I began to realize that the reason for this apparent ignorance was due to the fact that the cochlear implant REALLY was new technology, and that its potential was only beginning to be realized, that I was able to enjoy the task of educating those I came across about cochlear implants. I suppose this reality should have been evident to me, as each of our children was a 'first' of some sort: Jessica was the first child with a severe-profound hearing loss to be implanted by our center. Jared was the youngest CI recipient in our state at the time of his implantation. Julianne was the youngest CI recipient in our state, and one of the youngest in the nation at the time of her implantation. Each child broke a barrier of some sort and, for at least some period of time, was a first or only within a domain. By the hand of God, may they continue to break down barriers, and may the barriers of cochlear implant controversy within the deaf community eventually fall. Children born with hearing loss in this millennium have untold opportunities ... remarkable opportunities ... real opportunities.

My path to emotional and spiritual acceptance of the physical and pragmatic realities of coping with our challenges have stretched me beyond the borders of all I hoped, feared, imagined, or expected for myself and for my life. The day-to-day challenges of raising three children with cochlear implants in the Auditory Verbal philosophy is often overwhelming and exhausting. Many days I feel inadequate, as if my very best is never enough. And yet, each day I just get up and try again. Ultimately, any sacrifice I make pales in comparison to the additional challenges my children will endure for a lifetime. Facing hearing loss in each of my children has been an exercise in faith and trust. It has required me to refocus my time, energy, and commitments. It has required me to look deep inside myself and to come face to face with the realities of my own deafness, that being a deafness to the voice of my Lord that guides, lovingly directs, sustains, and cares for my deepest needs. I am indeed thrice blessed, and at the end of this race I hope to bear a triple crown.

Stories by Teenagers and Twenty-Somethings

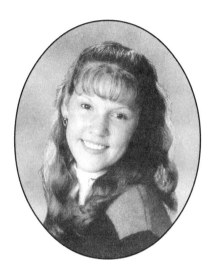

I'm Loving Life...By Rachel Ruhl

Last night, I *heard* my boyfriend tell me how glad he was to have met me ... I *heard* my brother and sister arguing in the next room about what television show to watch ... I *heard* our puppy barking in the backyard. Nine years ago, I made a decision to have a cochlear implant and it was the best decision of my life!

I can remember wanting to be a part of the hearing world and dreaming of obtaining certain goals in my life. I wanted to graduate from my home school rather than the high school 20 miles away where I was a member of the deaf class. I wanted to get a good job at our community hospital and help people feel better. I wanted to meet and fall in love with a great guy - a hearing guy.

Along with the love and support of my family, I believe I've accomplished these goals, and more, due to my decision to have a cochlear implant. I also believe that, because of the cochlear implant, I can make a difference in other people's lives as well.

I work in the health information resources (medical records) department at a small rural community hospital. Last week, a deaf patient came to the emergency department, alone and scared. She used sign language but no one understood what she was trying to say. The doctor contacted the medical social services department requesting an interpreter STAT.* The social worker asked me if I would try to talk with the patient. (She had taken an overdose and time was crucial.) I spent the next two hours in the emergency room interpreting for her. She would sign to me and I would verbally tell the doctor and nurses what she had said. I would then, in turn, sign to her the messages from them.

When I left work that day, I felt exceptionally good. I had been told that I was a valuable member of the healthcare team and had performed a special service to someone in need. I love my life and my cochlear implant!

* STAT means immediately in medical terms

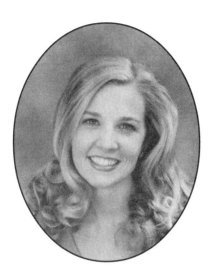

The Wonder of Sound...By Allison Wilson

After just four months of an exhilarating adventure with a Med-El cochlear implant, I wake up each morning, praising God for a new day full of sounds and excitement. I can now hear birds chirping as I walk outside, bacon sizzling on the stove, and coke fizzing in my glass as I pour a drink to take onto the patio. I sit and listen to the birds and crickets chirping, the dogs barking throughout the neighborhood, and the rustling of the leaves. Each time I take a sip from my glass, I hear ice clinking, and I am reminded of what a wonderful blessing it is to hear with a cochlear implant. Even though I have not been able to understand words on the telephone, I am thrilled that I can hear the phone ringing and the beeping of the keys when I dial a number. The microwave's beeping captures my attention while I prepare breakfast. As my mother cuts a hard loaf of bread, I am shocked that I can hear the knife sawing into the bread. I chuckle as I hear the squeaking cabinet door and make a mental note to remind my father to fix it, along with the fan in my bedroom that squeaks. As I dress, I hear the clock ticking in the bathroom, and water running in the sink reminds me of how much *I thought* I could hear with hearing aids. This is all so much more. There is so much more depth to my life. I turn on the computer and hear the modem dialing up, and then the wonderful words of "You've got mail" that I have grown to love, and the keyboard clicking away as my fingers dance rapidly. I listen to the *Sound of Music* CD as I type, and suddenly catch myself singing "Do-Re-Mi" along with Maria! I am startled by the sounds I hear from another room, and I yell to my mother, "Be quiet putting up the dishes!" and she laughs excitedly and makes even more noise. As we drive to church, I hear the seatbelts clicking into place and the blinker repeating its unique sound over and over. In church I am often distracted by people coughing or sneezing. The music is indescribable. The violins, the drums, guitars, and piano all sound so strange, yet so good. I can distinguish my father's deep voice from my mother's gentle voice, and I am learning to understand their words without lip-reading. Each time I understand a word or sentence without reading their lips, we all shout for joy. When we arrive home, I hear raindrops rhythmically tapping on leaves hanging over the door. As I listen to the comforting sound of rain, it seems as if each raindrop represents a single blessing in my life. There are far too many to count. Even as a 23-year-old and a graduate from Baylor University with a degree in Journalism, words fail me when I attempt to capture the beauty of learning to hear.

When I was two years old, I had spinal meningitis, and it rendered me profoundly deaf, as well as extremely weak. When it got to a point where death could be possible, the doctors told my parents that the following three days would be crucial. Yet, miraculously I lived, only to lose my hearing. My hearing loss was not a progressive one; I lost it overnight. Despite my hearing loss in the 100-120 decibel range, I began to lip-read without instruction, out of necessity, and my speech began to change. The doctors believed I would have ataxia (problems with balance), and I had surgery on one knee that developed septic arthritis. There was a question of whether that knee would continue to grow. (I am now 5'11"!) After a few years of speech therapy, I was mainstreamed in kindergarten, where I learned to read by lip-reading my teacher as she taught me during naptime. I took in speech therapy until I was in junior high school, and communicated solely by reading lips. I wore hearing aids in both ears until I received the cochlear implant, which brought my hearing up to 70 decibels.

My family and I prayed persistently for God to heal my ears, and we still continue to pray for a day when I will not even need a cochlear implant. There were many nights that I fell asleep believing that I would wake up and be able to hear. I have a great faith that God, in His great power, can perform awesome miracles. I struggled with whether to have the cochlear implant and allow God to use doctors to "heal" me or to continue to pray for healing. I decided to do both. After spending almost a year researching cochlear implants and praying for healing, I made the decision to have the surgery. Even though that decision was made, I still faced a series of hard decisions: Which brand of implant should I choose, and which ear should I have implanted? I did further research into the three companies and chose Med-El. Secondly, I decided to have my "good ear" implanted, meaning that I would implant the ear that had the least amount of damage from meningitis. The night before the surgery was highly emotional—filled with great excitement and expectation, a fear of the unknown and many questions. I had a hard time "giving up" my hearing aids and the way I had been hearing for 20 years. The way I had been hearing with my hearing aids was so unique to me, and I wanted to somehow savor it because it played such a role in fashioning me into the person that I am. I wanted to somehow capture the way I was hearing, but it was not possible.

On March 19, 2001, Dr. Peter Roland performed the surgery at Southwestern Medical Center in Dallas, Texas. The surgery was a great success. It lasted two hours, and I went home within a few hours afterwards. I also had a post-op appointment the next morning. The nurses sent me home with a bandage on my head, and I was told I could wash my hair that day. I was also worried about losing a lot of hair when the area was prepped for surgery, but I was happy to see that only a tiny amount was gone. Because my doctor used glue to seal the incision, I did not have to return until "hook-up" day, when the implant would be fitted and turned on for the first time.

After four weeks of silence and healing, I was anxious for April 12 to come. We traveled three hours from my hometown in Shreveport, Louisiana to Dallas, Texas, where Pam Kruger, my audiologist, fitted and mapped (programmed) the new device. She hooked the external portion of the implant into a machine that programmed the implant. The device produced a series of tones, and she asked me to tell her when I heard a sound, but it was difficult to recognize a sound because it was such a different way of hearing than I was accustomed to hearing with my hearing aids. It was more of a feeling or vibration in my head, but I learned to listen for those "feelings" and my first map/strategy was created! When she turned it on, I was surprised at how poorly voices sounded compared to the way I remembered with my hearing aids. Even though the hearing aids were a far cry from reality, it was all I had known. Everyone's voices were muffled, flat, and faraway. I cried in the office because it was so different than I had expected. When my family went around and told me they loved me, and I listened to their voices, it sounded incredibly beautiful despite the strangeness of the actual sounds I was hearing. I had heard stories of horrible hook-up days and stories of rapid progress, so I tried to prepare for whatever I might face. Yet, nothing could have prepared me for the days that followed. Just hours later, I began to truly love it! I was hearing thousands of sounds, but had no idea what I was hearing! I remember opening an accessory kit that was sealed with Velcro as we drove away from the hospital and the sound of the Velcro was so incredibly loud to me! Many sounds were out of proportion at first. Loud sounds such as the car motor were faint and muffled. Tiny, high-pitched sounds were very loud and distinct. For example, I could hear in another room, yet I couldn't hear the TV. It was just a matter of hours and days before my brain began to accurately interpret what I was hearing.

I do get frustrated with others who think the implant is an overnight process and believe that I can hear perfectly. It takes time and patience. It is frustrating and challenging, but it comes naturally and beautifully. I never could comprehend that learning to hear was a process until I walked through the mall and heard music playing on the intercoms that I never once heard in the four summers that I worked at the Gap. The first time that I heard words without lip-reading, I was sitting on my floor wrapping a present for my mother for Mother's Day. She knocked on my door and asked me a question ... and I replied! I did not realize that I had answered her without reading her lips at first. Moments of joy such as these give me such great hope and excitement for the days to come.

At this point, I am hearing in the 25-40 decibel range with a cochlear implant. It is amazing that my hearing has gone from approximately 100 decibels to 30 decibels! Just four months into this adventure, I look back and marvel at this great miracle. Voices are now clear and sharp, and I am learning to understand what others are saying without lip-reading. I listen to audio books and write down the words I can hear, and the list grows longer and longer each time. I can easily tap my foot to the beat of music, and was thrilled that I could recognize what particular instrument was playing as I watched *Phantom of the Opera*. I am looking forward to what will come in the next year as I continue to learn to hear with a cochlear implant. What a wonder, what a joy this journey has been, and putting this into words does not compare to capturing how my heart truly feels. Words fail me.

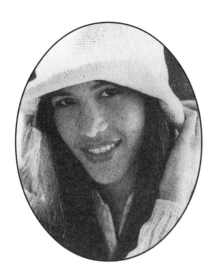

The Gift That Keeps On Giving…By Elisa Roberts

In the last few months of my pregnancy, as I sat in the rocking chair in which I would soon coddle my newborn son, I finally decided that a Nucleus cochlear implant would be right for me. I thought about the gurgles and coos my baby would make for me, even direct at me, and I couldn't imagine not being able to hear and answer him back with soft encouraging motherly murmurs of my own. I knew my son would be special. I was determined to hear him. My son was almost two months old the day I went in to be 'hooked-up' and receive my first Nucleus mappings. As soon as I was "turned on" I looked over at my baby nestled sweetly in my husband's arms as he cooed and chirped in soft little breaths. The sound of him gently stimulated my new hearing and my heart melted with love and remembrance. Is there anything sweeter than the sounds an innocent new child makes? That night, I heard and understood the gentle tunes of my son's s baby mobile hung over his crib.

My son is now a balking and screeching toddler. He is learning to speak and sign. I am learning to hear and listen too. Together we play piano and sing to the songs on his favorite shows and videos. My son knows that Mama cannot hear without her Nucleus processor. I bought him a Cochlear Corp. koala bear with a toy Nucleus processor. He knows his koala needs his processor on to hear, too, and that we don't chew on Mama's or bear's processor.

Since I've had my implant my speech has become so much more clear and confident. I've always had a dream of being an actress but feared my deafness might hold me back. Amy Ecklund, a Nucleus recipient, who played Abigail Bauer on *Guiding Light*, is a huge inspiration to me. A month ago, I auditioned for a role in a local independent film. I am proud as ever to say that I got a callback.

I'd like to thank everyone at Cochlear Corp., as well as my implant team for giving me the chance to hear again. To be able to hear my son's first words and to listen to all the sounds in the world is such a golden opportunity. My cochlear implant is truly a gift that keeps on giving.

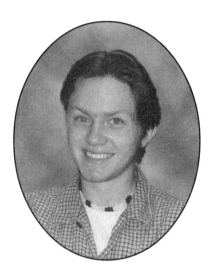

Here's the Scoop...By Jonathan Gutierrez

My name is Jonathan. I was born hearing, and could hear normally for about 18 years. Just after I had graduated from high school, I suffered a traumatic head injury, which left me profoundly deaf. I was completely deaf for almost a year and was told by the audiologists I saw that I'd be deaf for the rest of my life. They had said that the regular kind of hearing aids simply amplify sound, but that wouldn't work for me, as I couldn't hear even the most amplified sounds. They also said that the tests showed that the nerve damage in my brain was so extensive that they would not be able to hook up a cochlear implant.

A year after the awful accident I had, my family and I went back to the House Ear Institute to have more tests done to see if perhaps my brain had healed enough for them to give me a cochlear implant. Indeed, as it turned out, our prayers were answered, and the test results were positive! Soon we had scheduled an appointment for cochlear implant surgery, and I was told that shortly after that, I would hear again.

In August of 1997, after the surgery had been successful, the day finally came when they would turn on the device which would allow me to hear again. At first, I heard my mother laugh, then cry tears of joy, and I myself couldn't believe it! Remember, I was told I'd NEVER hear again, so this all came to me as a "dream-come-true." Immedi-

177

ately after the sound came on, I knew that hearing would be different. As I wrote earlier, I could hear for 18 years; what I was hearing with this new device was not exactly like it was before.

Over the next year, as I continued to adjust to this new kind of hearing, I definitely enjoyed it very much. Music was a great thing to be able to hear again, and I could still sing along to my favorite songs I knew from when I could hear normally. Learning new songs could be hard, especially if the music was noisy, but with a lyric sheet, I could sing right along.

As I became familiar with hearing different sounds, voices, words and phrases, hearing got easier. Today, nearly four years after I received my implant I am doing very well. Whenever I see people I haven't seen in a while, they often exclaim, "You're doing much better with your hearing!" When I'm in an environment that is not too noisy, hearing is a real joy for me, though lots of background noise can make hearing difficult. Sometimes I have to ask people to repeat certain words or phrases, and though some people tend to be impatient with me, most respond kindly and try to help me understand what they are saying.

Now that I can hear again, I have a much wider range of employment opportunities, and right now I am planning to become a youth-pastor. All in all, my life is MUCH BETTER having a cochlear implant! I am so thankful that, though my hearing is not perfect, I can hear very well, and I am very happy with what I have. I could not imagine living the rest of my life and not being able to hear my loved ones say "I love you," or hear laughter, my favorite song, the waves crashing on the beach, and all of the other beautiful sounds I love to hear. And, if there is ever a sound I do not want or like to hear, like heavy-metal music, I can always turn my cochlear implant off, and then I'm as deaf as ever! Being able to turn it off at night, also, allows me to get a good night's sleep (I use a vibrating alarm clock to wake up in the morning).

So many of us take for granted some things in life, like our natural senses. Only when we lose them do we realize how very precious they are to us. For those who were born deaf, I understand that hearing may seem like a great challenge, but I can assure you, it is worth it!

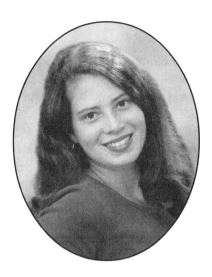

Sound at the End of the Tunnel...By Tatum Wilson

Twenty-three years ago a plump little baby girl was born in Lawrence, Kansas. The doctor said she was healthy, her parents thought she was beautiful, and her brother and sister wondered if that red and wrinkled baby would ever be "cute." However, within a few months it was determined that this baby was different. She had no hearing in one ear and a severe to profound loss in the other ear. Countless visits to otologists, neurologists, and audiologists provided no answers as to why this baby was deaf.

My name is Tatum Wilson and I was that baby who could not hear. When I was 18 months old, my parents were advised that I would probably never be able to speak, but they made the decision to vigorously pursue oral communication in spite of my limited hearing. I attended public schools, with minimal assistance from the speech therapists and lots of extra work at home. I was co-valedictorim of my class, on the pom-pom squad, and was an officer on the student council. My hearing aid and lip-reading skills worked well for me.

During my freshman year in college, I developed Meniere's disease and lost all of the limited hearing I had. My whole world changed. I still had the ability and desire to be an "A" student, but I could no longer be a full participant in the learning process because I was deprived of so much information and interactive communication. I could not talk on

179

the phone, and I was afraid to go out because I could not hear what everyone was talking about. I became dependent on others to 'hear' for me.

When Dr. Luetje, my otologist, suggested a cochlear implant, I was skeptical. Could it work, or would it just make me more different? I received the implant and on the day before Christmas in 1997 a miracle occurred. When the implant was 'turned on', "I COULD HEAR," even better than I had ever heard before!! It was truly a miracle!

I graduated from college Summa Cum Laude and even won the Outstanding Public Speaking Award. I will have a master's degree in physical therapy this May. My cochlear implant has given me a huge part of my life back and has made it possible for me to enter a profession where I can help others as so many have helped me. How fortunate I am to live in a time where technology and the medical profession have combined their talents and skills to make a difference for those of us who cannot hear.

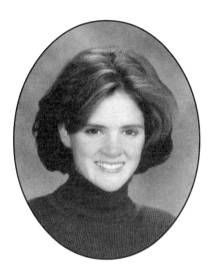

My Cochlear Implant, Success at Its Best...By Jacklyn Light

One of my favorite ways to unwind is to put in my favorite CD, such as Billy Joel or Shania, crank up the volume and sing along! One might be surprised to know that I am deaf; but with the help of the cochlear implant, you would never know! The implant is a miraculous device that has brought sound back into my life after losing my hearing to meningitis at age six. Now, 15 years after receiving my cochlear implant, I can honestly tell you that if it weren't for the implant, I wouldn't be where I am today. After successfully completing four years of college, I landed a full-time job in a corporate fitness center. I actually teach all of the aerobics classes!

Without my cochlear implant, I would not be able to hear the beat of the music or hear myself shout at my participants to "Get moving!" I wouldn't be able to hear their groans of enthusiasm as they are pushed to their limits. Another part of my job that I enjoy so much is presenting educational workshops. I love getting up in front of a group — teaching them something, and being able to easily communicate with them. The cochlear implant enables me to carry on a successful professional and social lifestyle. The fact that my job was located in New Jersey - away from my home in upstate New York - was another challenge. However, my cochlear implant allows me to stay in touch with my family and friends by allowing me to talk on the telephone. This is another challenge I have overcome with the help of my implant. One would assume that my deafness would prevent me from talking on the telephone, but with my CI, I actually have to work to keep myself from running up a big phone bill! Also, in New Jersey, I have my own apartment. My cochlear implant allows me to live independently and feel safer. I can hear the doorbell, the smoke alarm, the oven buzzer, you name it and I'll hear it! My implant has helped me to become the successful, independent, and confident person I am today.

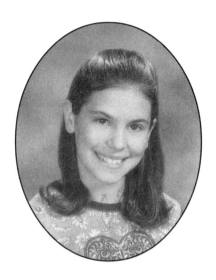

Remy's Story...By Remy Glock

My name is Remy Glock and I am 13 years old. I received a cochlear implant when I was 10 years old. I've had hearing aids most of my life, since 10 months of age. I am deaf because I was born with profound sensorineural hearing loss. I don't know what it's like to have normal hearing, but I can tell you about some of the differences between hearing through hearing aids and hearing with a cochlear implant.

It's hard for me to remember what it was like with hearing aids because I've adapted to my cochlear implant so well. I didn't hear many sounds with my hearing aids. I heard loud environmental sounds like airplanes and loud lawn mowers. I couldn't really hear nature sounds like birds, crickets, waterfalls, dogs barking in the distance, and emergency sirens. Speech sounds were a problem for me too. I couldn't hear s, sh, st, and generally the mid-high frequency sounds. I would not be able to hear someone calling my name in the distance or the school bell. In softball my teammates would yell my name, but I couldn't hear them. That was one of the major problems. If a ball came towards me from out of nowhere, then I might have been hurt. Most of my friends were irritated that I couldn't hear as much as they could. I'd end up asking too many questions about what was going on. They didn't make fun of me or tease me. They were just tired of my questions.

With my cochlear implant, I have made many more friends, because I can follow along much better with sounds and hear my name. When I first got the cochlear implant, I thought it was a mistake because not everything was familiar. The sounds would be loud or scary. Most of the environmental sounds hurt my ears, like the airplanes, trains, and birds chirping. When my headpiece falls off, I put it right back on, then these sudden sounds shocked me because it was so loud! I started to realize several months later that the sounds and voices I was hearing were much clearer because my brain gradually learned what type of sounds they were. I heard like 60% more than with my hearing aids. The cochlear implant helps my speech become more understandable and I can realize what mistakes I'm saying in a conversation.

With hearing aids almost everyone had to get my attention but not anymore. The cochlear implant has made me become a better athletic. I hear more calls and follow the coach's instructions and plays better. In a basketball court, it is very noisy with all the fans cheering and players yelling for plays, the ball bouncing on the court floor and the buzzer. I can still hear the official's whistle to stop a play or when there's a foul. I can hear some things on the telephone. I have to concentrate for the key words. If the person changes the subject or if the question is too long, I get confused. But it just takes practice. I believe my telephone use will improve in two-three years from now.

If you are profoundly deaf, I recommend that you get a cochlear implant because your life can be safer and more enjoyable. There are lots of sounds in the world and I appreciate what I can hear with my implant.

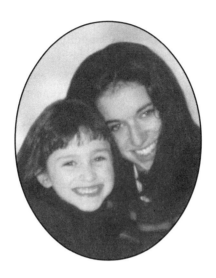

Rachel & Jessica's Story... By Melissa Chaikof

When our older daughter, Rachel, was born in May 1987, little did my husband and I know what challenges the future held for us. When Rachel was all of a week old, I had already begun to suspect that she couldn't hear. Our apartment was very small, and we kept her infant seat on our dining room table right near the front door. When this heavy door would slam, she wouldn't startle. I voiced my concern to our pediatrician at our first office visit when Rachel was not even three weeks old, but he dismissed my fears, telling me that I was "an overly anxious new mother who didn't understand how newborns react to sound." By Rachel's next visit at age two months, I insisted she be tested. While my husband and I had tried to mentally prepare ourselves for bad news, nothing could have prepared us for the agonizing two-and-a-half hour wait while the audiologist performed an auditory brainstem response (ABR) hearing test. At the end of the test, she confirmed our fears, telling us that Rachel had a bilateral severe-to-profound hearing loss. The next two-and-a-half years had us on an emotional roller coaster as we tried to find the best approach to teach Rachel spoken language. We were living in Boston at the time, which was a bastion of Deaf culture. Thus, oral programs were not plentiful, but we very much wanted Rachel to be able to take advantage of all the opportunities the hearing world had to offer. At the age of three months, Rachel received her first set of hearing aids, body-worn aids, which consisted of two boxes with wires running up to button-like earplugs. Because the microphones were on the boxes, Rachel had to wear the boxes on the outside of her clothing. To see one's baby outfitted like this was very difficult, but we wanted her to hear.

When Rachel was 10 months old, she cooperated for the first time for a hearing test and proved to have more hearing than we had initially thought. At the same time, she began to show definite responses to sound and received her first set of ear-level hearing aids. We thought things were looking up. However, we began to see Rachel's response to sound diminish shortly after that hearing test. Thinking we needed a better program, we traveled to the Helen Beebe Speech and Hearing Center in Pennsylvania to spend a week there learning about the Auditory-Verbal approach. We left so impressed by the children we saw there that we returned home with renewed enthusiasm and motivation and transferred to Jim and Lea Watson's Auditory-Verbal Communication Center in Gloucester, Massachusetts. Unfortunately, Rachel's diminishing responses to sound were a result of her diminishing hearing and not a result of her program. By the age of 18 months she was totally deaf.

We were faced with a difficult decision at that point. We could attempt to keep Rachel oral, using visual and vibrotactile cues, or turn to sign. We chose the former, reasoning that we still had time to turn to sign if it didn't work. Fortunately, while an oral, vibrotactile approach was a new challenge for Lea Watson, she agreed to keep working with Rachel.

When Rachel was two, Lea was speaking to Judy Simser, an AVI board member and Auditory-Verbal therapist in Ottawa, and learned of the cochlear implant. (AVI is Auditory-Verbal International. It is the association of Auditory-Verbal professionals, parents, and others who follow the Auditory-Verbal Approach to teaching language to hearing impaired children.)

While we knew of the implant's existence, the professionals we had encountered up to that point had told us that it was something to keep our eyes on for the future, but that most users heard only static at that point. However, Judy Simser told Lea of the remarkable progress she was seeing with one of her students who had received an implant. With her referral to the cochlear implant team at New York University (NYU) Medical Center, we made the trip in October 1989. They quickly identified Rachel as a candidate, introduced us to other children whose performance bowled us over, and scheduled Rachel for surgery eight weeks later. While the cochlear implant was not yet FDA approved for children but was in clinical trials, we decided to make the leap to facilitate Rachel's development of spoken language. We also reasoned that, even if she only heard environmental sounds, it would be more than she currently had.

On December 21, 1989, Rachel became one of the first 200 children in the country to receive the Nucleus 22, the first multichannel cochlear implant available in the U.S. We were guinea pigs at the time, as no one yet knew what to expect from these children. Since then, though, we have never looked back. Whereas prior to her implant Rachel had only mouthed words, within two months post-implant, she found her voice. Soon, she began to demonstrate beginning language. With her newfound hearing, we could also return wholeheartedly to the Auditory-Verbal approach.

In June 1991, when we moved to Atlanta for my husband's new job, we transferred to the the the Auditory-Verbal Center of Atlanta (AVCA). Rachel was four years old but still had the language of a two-year-old. What followed were six more years of hard work for us and for Rachel, trying to close the gap between her chronological age and her language age. Because she had had no auditory exposure to spoken language until almost the age of three, closing that gap was going to be difficult and would take a long time. When Rachel finally graduated from AVCA at the age of 10, she had caught up in all areas except vocabulary and auditory memory.

When Rachel was almost four, her little brother, Adam, was born. We held our breaths as, at all of five days old, the same audiologist who tested Rachel's hearing tested his. This time, though, the outcome was very different. In all of two minutes, she pronounced his hearing normal in both ears. Previously the "experts" had all told us that Rachel's deafness was most likely the result of a virus I had had when I was five months pregnant. Thus, we took Adam's normal hearing as further proof of this theory.

When Rachel was almost eight years old, her little sister, Jessica, was born. She was not yet 24 hours old when her hearing was tested. Despite repeated attempts, the audiologist could get no response to sound in either ear. Rachel's "viral" hearing loss had turned out to be genetic. Not only that, this time it was worse as Jessica never had any residual hearing. Although she was fitted with hearing aids at age three weeks, she never demonstrated any response to sound until receiving her cochlear implant.

Of one thing we were certain with Jessica, we didn't want to wait two years to get her hearing and start feeding in language. Despite the reward of watching Rachel's language develop, we knew the hard work it entailed and the difficulties she still encountered because of her language delay. Thus, we trekked back up to NYU, this time all the way from Atlanta, when Jessica was 14 months old, as they had already implanted a 20 month old. While FDA guidelines for implantation specified age two and up, because the device was now FDA approved, surgeons could use their own discretion to implant at younger ages. I will always remember sitting with Jessica in the surgeon's examining room. He asked me, "So, when do you want to do this?" I answered whenever he was willing, hoping he'd say age eighteen months. I almost fell off the chair when he replied, "How about next month?" I remember beaming and telling him he had a patient! Whatever it took, we were back to commuting to New York for a few months to get Jessica hearing as early as possible.

Jessica's surgery was in May 1996, when she was 15 months old. At the time, she was either the youngest congenitally deaf child or second youngest (by a week) in the country to receive a cochlear implant, depending upon whose statistic we believed. Jessica received her implant when she was sixteen months younger than Rachel was when she received hers.

We jumped right in with Auditory-Verbal therapy at AVCA with Mary Ann Costin, who had also been Rachel's therapist, as soon as Jessica received her speech processor. The speed of her progress soon amazed everyone. Within two months, she was already demonstrating a clear understanding of language. Her receptive language continued to progress at such a rapid rate that, just past her third birthday, it was already age appropriate.

The one remaining concern we had with Jessica was her expressive language, which lagged severely behind her receptive language. While Rachel's receptive language always exceeded her expressive early on, the disparity had never been as great as Jessica's. Being proactive parents, we couldn't simply sit and wait for the expressive language to come. Having lived through this once before and having now seen so many other implant children at AVCA, we knew that something was not right. Consequently, we visited a pediatric neurologist, who diagnosed Jessica with oral motor apraxia, which she explained to us is a scrambling of the signal from the brain to the mouth. She assured us that, with oral motor therapy, Jessica would be fine.

Mary Ann referred us to Sharon Wexler, an oral motor therapist, and we started oral motor therapy in April 1998. Within just four months, the difference in Jessica's speech and expressive language was tremendous. Where before she might utter one highly unintelligible word, she began to speak in two to three word phrases with continually increasing intelligibility.

Rachel is now in the seventh grade in our public middle school. She is almost fully mainstreamed, receiving resource help only for language arts. She spent two years working intensively with her resource teacher to increase her vocabulary and close the remaining language gap. She has made honor roll every semester in middle school as a straight "A" student. In addition, she has run for and won one elected office at school and is currently running for another. Who would ever have thought that my totally deaf daughter would have the self-confidence, clear speech, and social ease to stand up in front of a large group of people and make a speech?

Jessica's annual language evaluation at age 5.9 in November 2000 showed that her language scores, including her expressive language, are between ages 6.0 to age 7.9. Her voice quality is totally natural and she enjoys singing. She has been and will continue to be fully mainstreamed in school.

While lobbying for additional state funding for the Auditory-Verbal Center of Atlanta recently, Jessica didn't hesitate to speak to the state senators and representatives, walking up to each one who came to meet us, holding out her hand and saying, "It's nice to meet you." For the legislators, hearing was believing.

We are thrilled with and proud of both of our girls progress. However, we have seen the difference in ease of learning language that Jessica's early implant has made for her. The early implant, in combination with Auditory-Verbal therapy, are a perfect match. Since Jessica's surgery, surgeons have implanted children at younger and younger ages, including a six-month-old in Europe. In addition, the FDA has lowered their guidelines to age 12 months for one brand of implant. Because of Jessica's progress, we have become vocal proponents of early implantation, so much so, in fact, that, when speaking to the cochlear implant audiologist at NYU the other day, he teasingly said to me, "If it were up to you, we'd do them in utero! " The sooner the better!" It's never too early to give a child hearing.

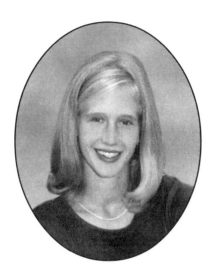

A New Path…By Sarah Jones

Shortly after I turned 18 years old, I began a new path in my life. For the first time ever, I was starting out on a new path of hearing sounds that I could not hear before. I now can hear almost anything, from a refrigerator humming to the clock ticking, from people calling out my name to people whispering to me, from dogs barking to birds chirping. Even today, I am still learning new sounds and it has been a wonderful and fun experience for me.

I was born on January 13 of 1982 on a snowy day in Washington D.C. Despite the fact that I was born on 1/13 at 1:13 PM in room 113, everything went well and my parents named their baby girl Sarah Ann. However, my first two years were spent going from doctor to doctor. My parents had noticed that I was not responding to noises, such as the door slamming, people clapping or people talking. After many tests, doctors would continuously tell my parents different excuses each time. A few doctors would just tell my parents that everything was fine and that nothing was wrong with me. One doctor even told my parents I had a brain tumor. As I was approaching two years of age, my parents began teaching me sign language as a way to communicate with me. One day, not long after that, while I was in speech school, an audiologist pointed me out and said, "That child is deaf." From that point on, I began my foray into the hearing world.

After the audiologist pointed me out, my parents took me in for hearing tests. The hearing tests showed that I had a severe-profound hearing loss. As I was given hearing aids, my parents decided that they wanted me to be able to speak. Except for those few slip-ups, all three of us had to drop sign language completely so I could learn to talk. When my family moved to Connecticut, I was placed in a deaf pre-school with other hard of hearing students. Through the many grueling and long hours of speech lessons, I eventually began to learn how to speak.

When I was seven years old, my family moved again to Marietta, Georgia. After a long debate with the pre-school I attended in Connecticut, I was mainstreamed and attended a public elementary school. After been told that I wasn't going to make it past the third grade in a public school, my family and I were just more determined to prove them wrong. For 11 years following my move to Marietta, I continued using my hearing aids and living a life that most other hearing people live. I played softball, ran crosscountry and track, rowed on the crew team, took piano lessons, and participated in Girl Scouts. I went through elementary, middle, and high school with a hearing impaired teacher to help me when I needed it. In high school, my friends often took notes for me to help me out in class. My teachers were aware of my hearing impairment and often helped out when they could. My life was complete at this point and I did not feel left out because I was hard of hearing.

When I was 17 years old, one of my best friends sisters was implanted with a cochlear implant. I was often amazed with her progress and so I began to research about cochlear implants and learn about what they can do for a deaf person. At this time, I began losing some more of my hearing and was advised by my audiologist to get an implant while I still had some hearing left. My only concern was when would I have the time to go through with this? I was starting my senior year of high school and applying to different colleges. My parents and I began researching into the different devices available and talking to Dr. Wendall Todd and audiologist Jolie Fainburg, we decided to go with it and have the operation over my Christmas break. After many endless hours of research we decided to go with Med-El. We were satisfied with their battery life, the BTE and the size of it, the different programs they offer and, most of all, we were impressed with their customer service. We received insurance approval only three days before my surgery.

I will never forget the day I was hooked up to my implant. The days following that, I remember being so tired and worn out from just wearing my implant. At the end of the day, when I would take out my implant, it was a huge relief that it brought me to tears. For the first year I wore my hearing aid in my other ear to help me when recognize the sounds that I could not recognize with my implant. For the first few months all the new sounds going through my head were more a sense of feeling than hearing. As the months went by, I began to slowly 'hear' the sounds instead of feeling them. One day, about six months after my surgery, I was in Florida visiting my grandparents. As my grandmother and I were standing outside, I heard a very quiet noise. When I asked my grandmother what that noise was, she got tears in her eyes and replied "a bird." It was then that I began to realize what a difference my implant is starting to make in my life. A year after my surgery, I was a freshman at the University of Tennessee, Knoxville. I was still wearing my hearing aid but in the dorm rooms I would try to leave my hearing aid out and practice with my implant. As I was waiting for the elevator to go to class, I heard a noise and reached up to fix my hearing aid so I could try to tell what that noise was. I realized that I had forgotten to put in my hearing aid and since then, I have not worn it. A short time after that incident, I lost my implant at a crew race and I had to wear my hearing aids for a few days. I was completely lost without my implant and could not hear anything. I often wonder how I could hear before my surgery.

Today, I continue to fascinate others and myself with my implant. Even after a year and half after my surgery, I am still hearing new sounds. My friends and family often laugh when I ask them what a sound is, because I think it opens their eyes to sounds they often take for granted. Only two years before my surgery, I was content with my life and satisfied with what I had. Now I wonder how I ever lived with just hearing aids and I am truly content with my implant.

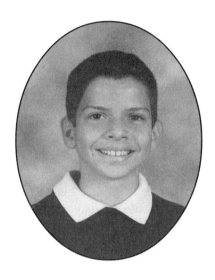

Danny's Story...By Ana & Danny Morales

Favorite hobby:	Listening to music
Favorite sport:	Roller Hockey
Favorite Subject at school:	Science and History
Likes to do:	Kickin' Back
Likes to eat:	Pizza and Japanese food

How I feel about cochlear implants vs. hearing aids? The CI's advantages are that: it helps me to understand people very well, to engage in conversation without interrupting, to pay more attention to what people are saying, and a long list of helpful advantages of the CI. HA's advantages are that I can locate where the sounds are coming from and I like music better using both, the CI and HA. Bolesta inspires me to listen better, more attentively, and helps my pronunciation to improve better than everybody expected. I see myself as a person who strives to listen, and talk better. I'm also a sensitive person who cares for people around me. I am very family-oriented and I love to play sports. I push myself to have a good life and to be a better person. What worries me today: shootings that are taking place in high schools and I hope it doesn't happen anymore. What I want to be: As a profession, an Architect, but what I really want to be is a person who's having a successful life, happy and away from trouble. (This section was written by Danny.)

Danny Morales was discovered to be profoundly hearing impaired at the age of seven months. At age one he was properly fitted with a pair of powerful hearing aids. Since we as a family are Spanish speaking, we decided to start his therapies in Spanish. Living in Miami, that was not hard. He always liked to wear his aids. At that time, our big family, the professionals, and a great circle of friends helped his progress.

We had to make a choice of selecting the approach and language, as he was ready to go to school. We decided to stick to the oral approach and started the verbotonal program, which was given to him in English. We weren't 100% sure about it, but we followed our instincts. He knew the difference in both languages already; he grew up to be bilingual. Danny had therapy almost every day. He started to go to a pre-school in the mornings, while mom went back to work. He liked to play and made friends everywhere he went. We were part of a group of families with deaf kids. We had so much fun together.

Danny was almost four years old when we had to move to Venezuela (where we are from) and he had a brother on his way. He adapted very well to the new school and made a lot of friends. He was mainstreamed 100% and had help in the afternoons with therapy and tutorial sessions. He enjoyed playing with friends and cousins a lot. Our family is very large, and he had plenty of opportunities to talk and practice his listening and lip-reading skills. After six years, it was time to get back to the States. As usual, Danny adapted very well to the changes. The English language was a challenge to him and still is. He loves to read and has a vast vocabulary. In my search for a good therapy, I found out about Bolesta. I met with Ellen Rhoades and all my thoughts about the cochlear implant changed. Up till then, I had been opposed to implantation for Danny; maybe I was misinformed. Danny was 10 years old now and was receiving therapy from Tina. He was mainstreamed again, adapted very well, and finished his elementary education in a public school. He was very afraid of needles and doctors in general without any reason. He refused to have the implant done and didn't want to even hear about it. It took him two years to make the decision on his own and undergo the surgery. Danny was implanted by Dr. Loren Bartels in St. Petersburg, Florida. He has the Platinum series by Advanced Bionics. Now he is using the body speech processor, but he is waiting anxiously to wear the BTE.

His unaided hearing is 95dB, his hearing with hearing aids is 55dB, and his hearing with the CI is 30dB. His old audiograms looked more like a straight inclined line with less hearing level in the high frequencies. The new audiograms with the CI looks more like a boomerang shape with a better gain overall. I am pretty sure these results will keep changing for the better with Danny's hard work.

At the age of 13, Danny received his CI and is very happy with it. It is however, taking longer than I thought it would take. With Danny being primarily Spanish speaking, the progress made in Spanish is faster than in English. He is still adapting to it in class, but he feels more confident now among his friends. He goes to therapy weekly and continues to improve his listening skills. Now, we know we made the right decision for him to be oral.

There are a lot of people that worry that the deaf community eventually will disappear. I think that if there is anything that science can give you to improve anyone's adaptation to society, why not benefit from it? Danny will always be a deaf person. God decided that for him and his role in this world is to teach whoever is around him what a deaf person is, and what a deaf person can be.

I think that Danny's personality had made my job much easier. He is a very sweet and a very caring person. He is very family oriented, has high self-esteem and is very responsible. He likes to do things right and tries hard to obtain his goals. He does not mind asking 100 times to repeat things in order for him to be 100% sure. He knows that it is okay to ask for help. He loves sports; he would play them all if he could. He likes to be well educated, so he reads a lot. He loves to travel. Well, Danny can also be very stubborn. He can bother his brother for hours. He turns his processor off when he doesn't want to hear you, etc, etc.

Well, I can write pages and pages about Danny. We are very proud of him. We know he tries very hard and we will always be there for him. We give thanks to God to have chosen us as his family. From my point of view, the finished product of any child, handicapped or not, is attributed to a group of multiple factors, but the most important one's are family and love.

(This section written by Ana)

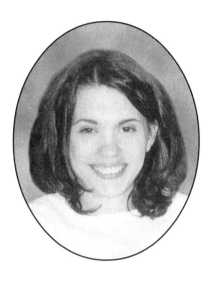

No Longer a Deaf Girl...By Crystal Lanclos

At the young age of four, I was diagnosed with a brain tumor. We weren't sure whether it was benign or cancerous, so quite naturally we were scared. When the doctors ran another CT Scan the tumor had disappeared; however so had most of my hearing. When you can't hear, it is a very scary feeling, I should know, I've lived most of my life either hearing impaired or deaf. I went through 18 years of wearing hearing aids.

My senior year in high school I woke up one morning for school and I could not hear anything, not even my own voice. It was one week before graduation and I was terrified. All of my life had been one obstacle after another. I dealt with teasing, embarrassment, among other things for being hearing impaired, now I would have to face being deaf. It was always a challenge for me to keep up with the other students, but I was determined I would make it. Well, my determination paid off and I graduated in the top 10 percent of my class and went on to college. My deafness didn't hold me back.

Soon after high school I learned about the cochlear implant surgery, but I was very afraid to go through with it. So I kept putting it off; I just kept doing the best I could with what I had. I couldn't get a decent job because everyone wanted someone who could answer the phone. I always worked hard at whatever I did, because to me I was more than just a "deaf girl." My parents kept pushing me to go through with the surgery and finally I gave in. I was implanted with the Nucleus Esprit in October of 2000. Little did I know what was in store for me.

In December of 2000 I went through the hook-up process. Feelings of nervousness overwhelmed me as I waited to be "turned on." Finally, everything was connected and I was sent on my way. As I walked out of the doctor's office I decided to give it a try, so I went into the ladies room and flushed the toilet. Can you believe, I HEARD IT! It was so exciting for me; in my 22 years on this earth I had never heard the toilet flush. After four months now I am hearing more than I ever dreamed possible. I hear birds and music, but most of all I can hear my family and friends tell me how much I mean to them.

If I could give one gift to a hearing impaired or deaf individual it would definitely be the cochlear implant. It has had such a wonderful impact on my life. Now I'm no longer viewed as a "deaf girl." I now have a wonderful job working for the Sheriff's Office and guess what? I ANSWER THE PHONE! It is such an amazing discovery that the medical profession has discovered; they will now be able to prevent babies from growing up without being able to hear. I want to thank the medical profession for the gift of sound as well as a new beginning in my life.

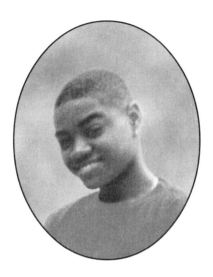

My Life is Different Now!..By Lavell Jones III

My name is Lavell Jones III and I attend T.F. South High School in Lansing, Illinois. I wear a Nucleus 24 cochlear implant. I lost my hearing in February of 2000, and had my implant operation in April of 2000. My external device that enables me to hear sound was activated shortly thereafter in May of 2000.

My family and I went to see my audiologist, April Hahn of the University of Illinois at Chicago Eye and Ear Infirmary. She programmed my speech processor two weeks after my surgery. After the programming was over she turned a switch and then asked me if I could hear what she was saying. Then she asked my parents to say something, and I heard my father's voice. At that time it sounded a little mechanical and somewhat robotic. About a week later I started to understand voices better. I also heard sounds like the doorbell, telephone ringing, people talking, car horns, fire trucks, police sirens, and other sounds around me. One day I heard the phone ring and I answered it, it was my dad calling and I heard him talking to me. He was so happy that I could hear him on the phone. I didn't have a phone adapter at that time. Now I can understand voices with greater clarity.

The implant has made a tremendous difference in my life. I can do more things now than when I wasn't hearing for those four long months.

I can become a veterinarian, I can play basketball for my high school and perhaps for the NBA someday. I can hear my dog bark, hear my mom and dad when they call me as well as hold a conversation with them, I can also talk and argue with my little sister. I can now attend the movies with my friends and hear what is being said, I can also go to parties and listen to my favorite CD's. They are not as clear, but I can hear the beat and some of the lyrics as opposed to hearing nothing at all. I have to adjust to talking in a crowded room or in a noisy area. I can adjust my implant to filter out background noise but I still can't catch everything that is being said. Sometimes I ask my friends or the person that I'm talking with to speak a little slower and look at me when they are talking to me. I am learning to lipread to enhance my ability to communicate. Hearing what people are saying without seeing their faces is becoming easier every day.

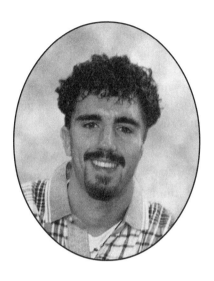

All Things Are Possible With My Implant...By Joseph Gill

Special Talents:

My ability to use sign language and understand it has helped me tremendously throughout my life. I learned it when I became profoundly deaf at age five. There have been instances where I see people trying to communicate with deaf people and I have stepped in to interpret because I also speak clearly. This has given me such insight with regard to other handicaps. I usually throw myself into situations to help people because I know how I have felt all these years of being handicapped.

Leadership:

Since becoming deaf I have always strived to do better. I made a promise to our school's Director of Curriculum that if he allowed me to transfer back to the school in our town, I would prove to him that I could make the honor roll. That was five years ago, and I have remained on the honor roll since. I never liked the label put on me at the other school I went to. It has been quite a challenge at times but I would not change things at all. People look at what I have accomplished and respect me for that. I also worked toward my 2nd degree brown belt in karate and became an inspiration to many.

When I was five I went into respiratory failure twice and had a herniated brain stem and also was in a coma for five days. They didn't know if or when I would be able to come out of it, or if I would ever be able to walk again or breathe without support. Up to this day, I walk and breathe normally. I've also joined our cross country and track team when the doctors permitted me to. My mother was so pleased when I made it across the finish line; I guess in her eyes I am a winner after all I have been through.

Obstacles Overcome:

As I said in the previous statements about my deafness and coma, there are many other things that happened. I have spent the last 15 years of my life in and out of hospitals. I have suffered eight bouts of spinal meningitis, five bouts of pneumonia, 20 operations, many of them minor craniotomies. I also lost my external ear during one operation. I also have had a cataract and had a lens implant. Despite all of this, I remain very optimistic in my abilities to live a normal life. I attend Westminster College, which is near us. I am mainstreamed with an interpreter. I feel that I can be a good role model because I have overcome many obstacles, including receiving my Eagle Scout recognition at age 15. I have also received the Silver Bronze recognition since then. When I wanted to join Scouts, the leader was afraid that he would have to adapt things for me to be able to receive this honor, but to his surprise he never had to do that. I did everything without special accommodations, even the mile swim. For my award project I installed permanent markers on the track field to mark the finish and starts for each track event. We marked them all off, did a diagram of the field, and proceeded to dig each one out and pour concrete into each hole. When that was done we painted each one, there were a total of 78 holes to mark the events.

Unique Endeavors:

This may not be what you consider a unique endeavor, but from a deaf person's standpoint it is. From the time I was little I always wanted to sing. But when I became deaf that was the last thing I ever expected I would do. I am now able to talk to my mom on my cell phone and understand some of what she says. To get to the point, none of this would even be possible without my cochlear implant, which has had a profound, positive effect on my life.

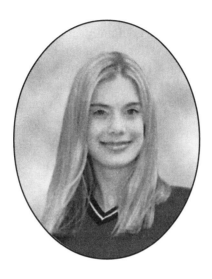

Determined to Hear With a Voice to Tell…By Lauren Day

My name is Lauren Day and I'm a 14-year-old Nucleus 22 co-chlear implant recipient. I was born with a profound hearing loss that was detected when I was three months old. I tried hearing aids, but they didn't help at all. My parents looked for other options to help me hear. They chose to send me to DePaul Institute, an oral school for the hearing impaired. There I met Pam Dickinson, the audiologist for the school. She told us about the cochlear implant and helped us throughout the treatment process.

Being 'hooked up' was the most exciting day for me as it was the first day I heard sound. The implant has changed my life so much; before I was implanted I would wistfully wish I could hear like my cousins. I didn't want to be different. Well, with the implant I don't have to feel different, I can finally fit in, and communicate with them. I feel so free with this device. It has not only allowed me to hear, but it has also opened a new world of communicating for me, such as talking on the telephone. I have wonderful friends who accept me for who I am; they have allowed me to gain self-confidence and they make me feel so loved. I have also been involved in many activities and clubs since being implanted. I have been mainstreamed since the age of 11 and have made the honor roll every report card period. The implant has made me realize that I am special and God gave me a very special gift when he gave me the implant. Not only has this device been a miracle for me, it has also benefited my family and our daily interactions. My cousin Natalie has decided to pursue a career in audiology because of her involvement with me. The cochlear implant was the best thing that has ever happened to me; my life would not be the same without it. If asked would I do it over again, my response would be "Absolutely!"

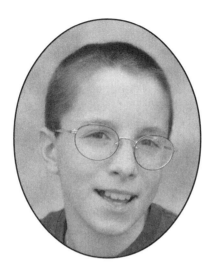

My Story…By Jacob Landis

When I was two years old my mom thought that I was slow in my speech development. Because of this, I had my first hearing test. It was determined that I had a hearing loss in only my extremely high frequencies. My parents were told that "it was no big deal" because my problem would not interfere with my speech development. But my parents continued to monitor my hearing.

My hearing loss continued for the next three years and I got my first pair of regular hearing aids when I was in kindergarten. I remember that my teacher warned my classmates that if sand got in my hearing aids they would break, so my hearing aids protected me from those "sand-throwing bullies." Back then my classmates didn't really understand that I had a hearing problem. They thought my hearing aids made me hear long distance. I thought my hearing aids were cool, because my classmates called them *"Power Ranger"* ears!

In the middle of 1ˢᵗ grade my teacher and I had to use an FM system. By then most of the kids knew I had a hearing loss. Suddenly, my hearing loss wasn't cool. My hearing was slipping away, and it became harder and harder to do the things in the 2ⁿᵈ and 3ʳᵈ grades. I could not hear the whistle to come in from recess, and I would have a hard time understanding the movies that I watched. I could not understand my baseball and soccer coaches, the most frustrating thing was that I could not understand my teachers. During 4th grade my teacher would sometimes have me sit in the corner of the room and read all day because I could not understand what she was saying. During this period I became angry and frustrated. I didn't want to go to school. I begged my mom to "home school" me so I could be at home away from those things that made me mad and sad. It was easier to be at home where my family understood my problem.

My hearing took a big drop in 3rd and 4th grades. Even though my second set of hearing aids were programmable, I was told that they wouldn't help me much longer. About this time my dad told me that I was being considered for a cochlear implant. I thought that a cochlear implant was an artificial ear that would sit on the side of my head and that if I got one I would be immediately be able to hear normally again. While my hearing aids didn't do much good I still hadn't qualified for the cochlear implant. At this point I became really angry and depressed. Mom and Dad had me go to a psychologist during the fall and winter of my 4th grade school year. Finally, the programmable hearing aids could no longer be adjusted to benefit me. In addition to being mad, I often felt scared too. I was afraid to go to sleep at night because I knew I could no longer hear the smoke detector in my room. I remember one night at dinner I looked up and saw Noah and Sarah running toward the telephone. I cried because I realized that I could no longer hear the phone ring. Its ring was in a frequency that was then out of my hearing range. It wasn't fair! I took out a lot of my frustration on my best friend and brother Noah. There were times at school that I would just turn off the hearing aids since they did not help much. I just didn't want to hear anything. I think a part of the problem was that the neighborhood public school that I went to had never had a hard of hearing student before.

While I was very angry that hearing aids wouldn't help anymore I was also angry that I couldn't really do the things that I used to enjoy. I dropped out of soccer and baseball. I usually just wanted to be alone or at home with my family. I spent a lot of time reading. Sometimes I would read three books in a day. I remember that fall I decided that I just didn't want to live anymore. Life was not fair. Life was not as fun as it used to be. Life was just full of frustrations.

For eight years I had gone to ENT doctors, hospitals, audiologists, dentists, orthodontists, and psychologists more than 600 times. I had received more than 60 audiological exams, with each one showing that I was hearing less and less. Although I had all these tests, the doctors never found the reason that I lost my hearing. My hearing aids were not helping me, and now I found out that I had to go through even more tests just to see if I could have one of those implants.

During September 1998, I started taking the tests at Johns Hopkins to determine whether or not the cochlear implant would help. I liked going there because I got out of school and my dad always bought me treats on the way to and from the hospital. Also, on most of the days that Dad and I went to Baltimore, my brother Noah had to do my share of the paper route. Finally, sometime in March 1999, the doctors, various testing people, my parents and I agreed that the cochlear implant would help.

On June 2nd, 1999 the operation was performed. That evening was pretty rough. The next morning my parents had a meeting at the school and I felt well enough to go to the school with them. I got to go and see my class. I wanted to show off the scar to the boys and gross out the girls. Within a few days I was climbing trees, playing basketball at Sean's and even swimming at the pool. Dad was always telling me to take it easy and constantly saying "safety first."

On July 6, 1999 the audiologist at Johns Hopkins turned on the implant and programmed the Clarion S Series processor. I had been told that some implant users said that everything sounded like *Mickey Mouse.* The first words I heard with the implant were "Jake, what does it sound like?" from my dad. Dad's voice sounded the way that I remembered it. The amazing thing is that I could hear it!

The next few weeks were both fun and hard. I had fun figuring out what all the sounds were. I could hear the highest note on the piano again. I could hear the birds chirping. But it was hard to understand everything that was going on. When I was with a lot of people and they were all talking, it was hard to figure out who was saying what. I remember when I was three years old I would always hear the microwave go "beep beep." For several years, I thought it was broken. When I first heard the microwave after the implant was activated, I asked my mom, "Who fixed the microwave?" I remember that she looked at me with a confused look, but then she realized that now I was hearing things that for many years I could not hear. My dad tells me that when the implant was activated he felt like he got his boy back. He says that he could see the "sparkle" back in my eyes. I remember one day I heard the phone ring and I answered it. It was my dad. We hadn't talked on the phone for two or three years. He later told me that as we talked he was sitting in his office at the bank with tears running down his face. A few years earlier I cried because I couldn't hear the phone ring. Now my dad was crying because I COULD hear it ring!

For the next year I went to rehab every week. I liked rehab because I got a break from school and got to have lunch at Johns Hopkins and get a treat for the ride home each time. Also, Noah still had to do my part of the paper route. I liked the rehab sessions because they were fun. Sometimes the sessions could be hard and frustrating, but overall they were fun. During the past two years I have made friends with several other kids who are deciding whether or not they should get an implant. They always ask me if the surgery hurts.

On August 28, 2001 I will begin 7th grade. I have had my implant for a little over two years. In our county there are over 75,000 students enrolled in the public school system. One hundred two (102) of them are deaf and hard of hearing. Of the 102 HOH kids, only ten of us are classified as being deaf. The other deaf students have either cued speech transliterators or sign language interpreters. I think I am the only one who doesn't have an adult following me around all day. I am fully mainstreamed and the only time I get special attention is when the speech therapist works with me twice a week. When I went deaf, the clarity of my speech deteriorated. I sort of like school but I don't like homework. Most classes are pretty easy. Last year I made the Honor Roll in all four marking periods. At school I have to work with my teachers. I have to make sure that they understand that I still need some help in getting all of their information. For the most part the help I need is pretty simple. I need to sit in the front of the class and ask the teacher to face me when they are speaking so I can see his/her lips (when I went deaf I learned to lipread). I carry a portable FM sound field from class to class, at the beginning of every class I have a brief moment with each teacher when I give them the microphone. I think this also reminds them every day that I still am hard of hearing. Another thing that I do is meet with all of my teachers before school starts. Mom and Dad cater a lunch and we have a brief meeting where I get to speak to all of my teachers at once. I tell them how I need their help and they can ask me questions.

I still don't like going to the movie theaters though. None of the theaters in our town have captioning. Plus, many of the movies are so loud and there are bad echoes. I just wait for the movies to be released on videos because then the movies usually have the closed captioning feature. I still don't really like to talk on the telephone. My parents say that I have to practice. Most of my friends live nearby, so if I need to talk to them I just walk over to their houses. Dad says that when I get a girlfriend I will wish that I had practiced a lot more than I have been. Last week, our family went to the beach. Mom forgot to pack my battery charger and rechargeable batteries for my processor. Well, that made me think. The hearing loss is my problem and I guess that I need to be responsible for those things now. Basically, my life is pretty normal. I know that I will probably always have to work at listening. I know that I have to be my own advocate to be sure I get the information. I will still need to ask some people to repeat themselves. I think that my best benefit is that I know that I can make it in the hearing world.

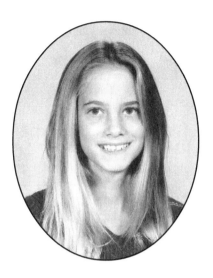

What Difference Does It Make?...By Kristin Pierce

Hey, I hear music playing! What beautiful songs I can hear! Without my cochlear implant I wouldn't be able to hear music, laughter, conversation, and everything else. I think my life would have been so much different. I'm here to tell you that hearing is a wonderful part of my life!

When I got my cochlear implant, I was only five years old. The first time I put it on, it sounded weird. At first I didn't like it at all because it was a totally different world. Soon after that I started to recognize sounds. I was so amazed that I could hear things and loved to make new discoveries!

The biggest difference my cochlear implant has made in my life is that I can talk and listen to my family and friends. I always share lots with my friends- jokes, secrets, conversations, and stories. I never feel left out. At home, I talk with my family all the time. I like talking to my grandparents and other relatives and friends on the phone. I understand what they are saying and it helps us keep in touch. I also enjoy playing the piano. I have studied piano for three years. Being able to hear has given me the gift of music. I dream of becoming a singer some day. I would love to sing to crowds! I've also thought about being a model or actress too. I was featured in a video about cochlear implants when I was seven years old. I believe that I can be anything I want to be. I have the determination and faith that I can do it! How different my life would be if I could not hear...

Adults' Stories

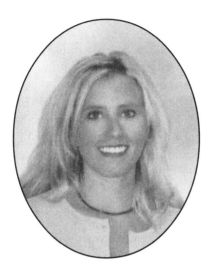

Full Circle...By Angela Wieker

It's amazing how things in life come full circle; things that were the most devastating and terrifying to us turn out to be blessings. That's how I feel about life since the implant; not that I feel that having a hearing loss is a blessing in any way, but maybe it has been, maybe the heartache that accompanies it has built my character into something it would not have been otherwise.

When I was in 1st grade, I went along with the rest of my classmates to have an annual hearing exam by the school audiologist. My parents received a phone call from her telling them that it looked like I might have a very mild loss in both ears; she recommended that they take me to a professional. The doctor confirmed their fear that I did indeed have a mild loss, but assured them that it would not progress. Following his recommendation, I was seen annually to monitor any changes. At each of those visits the disappointing news was given to my parents that my loss continued to progress. I feel very fortunate to have been mainstreamed throughout all my schooling. I was never fitted with hearing aids, although it wasn't from lack of trying. Every summer my parents forced me to try 2 or 3 types; which I got for a few weeks each. Each time, even though I didn't want them, I had high expectations of them improving my hearing. Each time I was greatly disappointed. My type of loss was the culprit; it was mild to moderate

217

sloping to severe. All the hearing aids would do was amplify what I already heard so that I was blasted with those sounds, while giving me no benefit where I needed it.

Even though I was mainstreamed, that didn't mean that the loss didn't impact me. I would have done anything to prevent people from finding out about the loss. As a child, the last thing you want is to be viewed as different, especially when you're living in a town in South Dakota with a population of 1500! I didn't know anyone who had a hearing loss let alone who was deaf, I was shy by nature and having this loss certainly didn't help my self-confidence. If we were reading aloud in class, I would count ahead to know exactly what part I would be reading; I learned to anticipate what people might ask in conversation. I thought that I had the solution to answering all questions with "yes" or "no" answers regardless of what the question was. What I didn't realize until I got a puzzled look to "What grade are you in?" can't be answered with a yes or no! It's easy to see how people with hearing loss are so quickly associated with low intelligence. Because of my young age, a hearing loss would be the last thing people would have thought was the reason why I didn't answer questions correctly!

Throughout those years I certainly thought about what I would do if the loss continued to progress. I think it's possible to be in denial and acceptance at the same time. I would think about it often, with my biggest fear being that I would wake up one morning and be deaf. That usually weighed on my mind the heaviest around the time of my annual hearing exam. I would have much anxiety over it during that time, and then think that somehow, even though evidence clearly pointed out that this loss wasn't going to stop, I believed that I would never experience life as a deaf person.

One thing that this loss has taught me about myself is that when told that I "can't" do something because of it, I can be certain that the person will eat those words. I can vividly remember in 5th grade the son of one of the elementary school teachers telling me that my parents told my teacher that the doctor said I would never graduate from high school due to the progression of the loss. To this day, I can remember exactly where I was standing on the playground when he delivered this shocking news. He may as well have punched me in the stomach, which would have hurt much less. I never mentioned it to my parents, and they certainly never mentioned it to me. I was very fortunate in many ways to have such wonderful parents. They never tried to stop me from participating in anything or made me feel like I couldn't do something; they treated me like a normal child in that regard, just always saying that I couldn't quit something once I started it. I was always active in sports, band, choir, and other activities.

It was during high school that I first became aware of cochlear implants. As much of the country, I was introduced to implants through the showing on a "*60 Minutes*" segment. My parents seemed optimistic that maybe this would be something that could help me in the future. I vowed then and there that I would NEVER get a cochlear implant! Despite the doctor's prediction being in the back of my mind all those years, I did graduate from high school, with 3.5 GPA, no less.

I did go on to college and, despite the urging of my parents and professionals, chose not to inform my professors of my loss. I admit that I struggled more and more with each passing year. That didn't stop me from maintaining my usual active life. I was a cheerleader for Men's Basketball and Football for three of my four years of college. I was able to perform dances in the middle of the basketball court in front of 40,000 fans without even hearing the music at times! On graduation day, that prediction from the doctor so many years prior still stuck in my mind as I graduated with a 3.75 GPA!

I had known for years that I wanted to relocate from South Dakota. So following graduation, I packed up and made the move to Colorado. I experienced a significant decrease in my hearing a few months after the move. I think it is still an arguable point, but some professionals feel that the change in elevation could have been the cause. Whatever the reason, I was suddenly cut off from all my friends and family because using the phone was just too frustrating. I could hear voices, but could not decipher what they were saying, so I just gave it up completely. I was difficult for my family as well. I can remember several times my mom telling me just to talk when she called so that she could hear my voice; I could always make out her crying on the other end. I could slowly feel myself slipping away from my once active personal life. I didn't want to go anywhere or do anything that involved interaction with people. If I saw people that I knew at a store, I would literally hide in the aisle to avoid having to endure the stress of a conversation. My independence was going along with it, always having to rely on others to make simple phone calls for me.

Throughout this very frustrating period, my family kept mentioning cochlear implants. I was very stubborn and stood my ground. I had no interest in thinking, hearing or speaking about implants. I was 22 years old; I certainly didn't want to walk around with wires sticking out all over, looking like a robot! The loss continued to progress and I know my co-workers were becoming more and more frustrated, as was I. At this point I was still in denial, still believed that someone was going to wave a magic wand and make this whole thing disappear. I had horrific visions of losing my hearing totally, moving back to South Dakota, and living as a recluse in my parents' basement. As ridiculous as that sounds, I truly believed that was my only option. I had never learned sign language and didn't know anyone who used it anyway, so that didn't seem like an answer for me.

I had lived my entire life in the normal hearing world and wanted to continue that. My mom took it upon herself to contact an implant center in Denver to get information. Theresa McGinn-Brunelli, an audiologist there, was very enthusiastic about my candidacy for an implant, and her excitement spread to my family. My parents came to Colorado for a visit, so, to pacify them, I agreed to go the center to hear about the process. I probably didn't hear most of what was said that day because my mind was already made up, the thought of the surgery alone stopped me from considering it. I had been disappointed so many times with hearing aids that I thought this would be just another disappointment. One day at work I was venting to a co-worker about feeling pressure from my family in regards to getting the implant. That wise person turned the tables on me and agreed that the decision was mine, but also challenged me if I didn't get the implant what would I do? Did I really have any other options? Just having it pushed back to me really made me stop and think. At the same time, Theresa had arranged for me to meet a lady, Diana Fuller, who had an implant. I can remember my friend talking to her on the phone. My friend gave her my address and phone number and didn't repeat it. When she got off the phone I questioned my friend as to who was taking down the information on the other end. My friend informed me that Diana was. That was the first glimmer of sunlight that I received about implants. I didn't want to get my hopes up as I had so many other times with hearing aids, so I totally downplayed the fact that this woman who is supposedly deaf just took down a series of numbers over the phone and didn't ask to have them repeated. I am so grateful for that meeting; Diana and her husband gave me so much information and recognized the fears that I had. I left the meeting finally allowing myself to believe a tiny bit that this device might actually help me.

Of course I still had many fears about the surgery and doubts about the implant, but, regardless, I went through with it on May 19, 1997. Dr.

Robert Feehs implanted me with a Nucleus 24 device, The surgery went fine; I was released the next morning. I'll never forget how awful I felt those first two days following the surgery. Fortunately the recovery period was quick and I was back to work full time within one week of the surgery. Now the waiting began! I was hooked up one month later and began the long journey of testing. I felt fortunate as to the timing of my surgery because I was able to be involved in Cochlear's clinical trial for their two new coding strategies, as well as their new BTE.

My progress was slower than I anticipated; I was extremely disappointed at the way things were going. I really hadn't shown much improvement at all. I still had about 40% hearing prior to the implant; I was told that people who had hearing prior to the implant seem to perform better than those who have never heard. I was getting frustrated with my lack of progress. By January I was so disappointed and frustrated that I stopped wearing the implant. Fortunately, my parents came out for another visit and dragged me back to the center saying that I didn't go through all of this to have the processor sit on my dresser. I felt that I had hit rock bottom, my last hope was not materializing and I had given up completely. I felt it was only a matter of time before I made the move to my parents basement. Luckily Dr. Feehs happened to be in the office that day and came in to talk to us. I was crying and upset because I thought something had gone wrong. He assured me that from a surgical standpoint everything had gone well. He recommended to the audiologist that they give me an entirely new processor and headset to see if that made a difference. I returned to the center two weeks later and scored over 85% on sentence and word recognition. I was elated! I knew that I had improved, but wouldn't have guessed it to be that much. We figured out that I had a bad microphone the entire previous nine months, which was why I wasn't improving.

It has been nothing short of a miracle since that day. I am truly in awe of this amazing device. Each day at work gives me a gift of hearing something I hadn't previously heard: the printer beeping when it is out of paper, people talking behind me, people talking from across the room and me understanding. I was very slow to try the phone. I guess that it had stressed me out so much in the end before the implant that I was scared to try it again. I will never forget the shocked look on my grandma's face when I was in South Dakota visiting and I took a phone call. I knew exactly what she was thinking. "How in the world is that possible?" I enjoy every day of the process. After 23 years of losing more and more hearing each year it was truly a miracle to have that situation reversed and hear more and more things each week.

I can't adequately express on paper how much this device has impacted my life. I simply couldn't live without it. Gone are the days of hiding the implant and the hearing loss! I want everyone to know about this amazing technology. What is unique about it is that I never take it for granted. Each day the realization that I am now a deaf person, because the loss has continued to progress since the implant, is very real. Each morning before I put it on and each evening when I take it off, or when then battery needs to be changed, there is a startling silence and I can't wait to turn the device back on. That silence is a very real part of each day and I thank God everyday for giving me my life back. Since the implant I have resumed my social life and do not stress about being in noisy situations when having a conversation. It's amazing how much stress and anxiety I put myself through over the years and how free I feel now that I don't have it anymore; I certainly didn't realize the degree of it at the time. My independence returned along with my hearing. I live an active life and still have yet to deny myself doing something because of the loss. I don't even think of myself as a deaf person because of what this implant has given me.

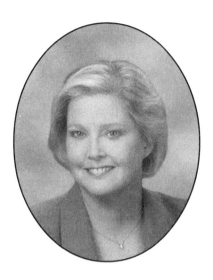

The Power of Words…By Nanci Linke-Ellis

The power of words. They can move, inspire, enlighten, and enhance our lives. This is something we are taught from the very first day of school. I'm not going to tell you how I went deaf. It's not important. It has never been what defined me. Nor am I'm going to tell you about how or why I hear again. What I am going to try to do is demonstrate the power of testimony. My words and those of others who have been similarly blessed with a modern medical miracle known as a cochlear implant. (I prefer "Bionic Ear.")

In late summer 1994, 34 years after being diagnosed with a bilateral nerve loss and fitted for hearing aids, one year after going completely deaf, and two months after being "turned on" to sound, my husband and I took a power walk on Montana Avenue in Santa Monica, headed towards Ocean Avenue and the beach.

My husband Steve is a something of a jock and he kept goading me into going faster, increasing the pace. There were two men strolling just ahead of us. Steve, naturally, wanted to go around them and I, of course, slowed down. Suddenly, I heard two words: "Advanced Bionics."

Startled, we both turned to each other and said, "Did he say Advanced Bionics?" We both slowed to match the rhythm of the men who walked ahead deep in discussion. I heard a smattering of words. "Clarion," "cochlear implant," "incredible technology," and the like. Eavesdropping is "unheard" for deaf people. (Now there is a pun I couldn't resist.) Fascinated, I leaned closer to the two, narrowing the space between us.

Finally, I couldn't stand it any longer and literally jumped in front of them. "Excuse me," I interrupted. "Did I happen to overhear you two talking about Advanced Bionics?"

Taken aback, they shook their heads and said "Yes." I apologized for interrupting, but I explained that I thought I overheard them mention the Clarion implant. "Yes," they said a touch surprised. Cochlear Implants and Clarion were hardly household words even in the deaf and hard of hearing community in 1994, much less on Montana Avenue, a tony food and restaurant district in LA's fashionable Westside. "Well, I overheard you discussing it" I declared. Unimpressed, they nodded their heads. "And the reason I overheard you is because…." I continued, whipping back my hair to reveal the newly implanted, partially fuzzy patch behind my right ear. "My God!" they said. Neither one had actually met anyone with an implant, much less seen the new Advanced Bionics technology up close. "How do you like it?" they asked.

I explained that my whole world had just taken a 360-degree turn. For the first time in my adult life, I had used the telephone. I could now do anything I wanted. I could work at any job that I wished to do. This wonderful device had, in one fell swoop, given me independence, privacy, confidence, and a newfound sheer joy of life. The window of opportunity had just flown w-i-d-e open for 42-year-old Nanci Linke-Ellis. What else was there to say?

Well, there was one aspect of this life-altering device that I had to share with them: that being, despite my own obvious exuberance, the cochlear implant was yet to be accepted in the deaf and hard of hearing world.

"It is actually quite controversial," I explained. "And for many in the deaf community very threatening." Within the deaf culture, people who use American Sign Language as their primary means of communication were up in arms about implants. They believed it to be a form of cultural genocide that struck at the very heart of their community. They were particularly concerned that providing children with implants would ultimately destroy deaf culture, as it now exists.

It was a brief encounter, a two-minute conversation. We shook hands, wished each other well and proceeded on our separate ways. This was the first time anyone had asked me to describe what it meant to be able to hear in a new, immensely superior way. To share these feelings with total strangers was a bizarre moment, to say the least.

Fast forward to 2001. Thousands of people received implants and some of the fear and suspicions have subsided. I was sitting in an auditorium up at Universal City Cinemas waiting to see the much-heralded "*Sound and Fury*" documentary. Nominated for an Oscar in the Best Full Length Documentary category, its director and writer Josh Aronson was there to make brief remarks on the making of his film.

The film tells the story of two brothers who deliberate as to whether or not to implant their respective deaf children. The resulting decisions permanently fractured the families, who no longer speak. One of them eventually moved out of state.

Excellent in its execution, the documentary itself left me slightly irritated. As the executive director of TRIPOD Captioned Films, I had tried to book the film into my existing circuit of theatres, but the distributor of the film blew me off. I had also made attempts to attend screenings, but, for some reason or another, I always managed to miss them. I had arranged for this evening's screening at the behest of Advanced Bionics as part of their hosted evening at a Cochlear Implant Conference held annually for hearing professionals, medics and manufacturers. Come hell or high water, I was going to see this film.

After Josh discussed the incredible drama that had unfolded before the eye of his camera, he mentioned that he was always asked, "Where did you come up with the idea to do this? How did it come about?" And then he told the story of meeting a woman in a brief encounter seven years before. It suddenly dawned on me – I think he's talking about me! I whispered in a nudge to my good friend Mary Ann. My husband, who, sitting in a different part of the auditorium (we never arrive at the same time for the same event – more to do with his being male than my being deaf!), had the same reaction. As Josh continued with his story (most of the recollection was surprisingly accurate for a two-minute encounter so long ago!) It was I!

I had invited parents of deaf and hard of hearing children, and other friends intrigued with the idea that a truly modern medical miracle was causing such a stir. To say the film is powerful is an understatement. Yet it's not just a story about to implant or not to implant; it's about families, who create belief systems that sometimes go head to head under the same roof. A modern day Cain and Abel parable with a King

Solomon technology twist to it. Moving and unforgettable, two families tragically unravel in a struggle to do the right thing and make their own disparate choices. So aptly named, it is about Sound and Fury.

Afterwards, there was a reception at the House of Blues. Josh (the director) recognized me the instant I arrived. He and his wife mentioned that they often wondered about what had happened to me, if I knew about the film, etc. My sense of awe had not waned in seven years. We exchanged business cards after I told him that without my Clarion implant, TRIPOD Captioned Films would never have existed. My reasons for relating this story is not to engage in any Hollywood name-dropping purpose. Just to demonstrate the amazing power of words; of their testimony and ability to change or affect the lives of others.

That's why this book was written. Not to persuade legions of deaf and hard of hearing people to run and get an implant. This is not a medical panacea. It is not for everyone; not everyone achieves my incredible level of functionality. At that time, I was the ultimate CI success story. Yet it had nothing to do with me. Rather it had more to do with what others envisioned for people like me. The best news of all is that, from this point on, I have been reduced to merely being just one of them.

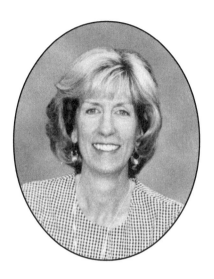

Journey Back To Hearing...By Linda Funesti-Benton

Imagine being 20 years old and being told you have a permanent hearing loss, that it will most likely continue to worsen over the years, and how much and to what degree is uncertain. I am sitting in the office of an ear, nose and throat specialist in a town in New Jersey where I was attending college in 1970. I made the appointment because I had been having recurrent strep infections that were not clearing up. Coincidentally, I'd been noticing that I had difficulty using the telephone lately with my right ear and wasn't hearing my apartment roommates when they spoke to me from another room. I asked the doctor if it was related to the strep infections. When his audiology testing uncovered a moderate sensorineural loss in my right ear and a mild one in my left ear, I was surprised and confused. How did this happen, what caused it, will it stabilize, what can be done about it? I had a lot of questions, and unfortunately the doctor had too few answers. His recommendation was to try a hearing aid. No one else in my family had ever had a hearing loss. Even my elderly grandparents on both sides of my family still heard relatively well for their age.So began a long, and oftentimes depressing, gradual decent into deafness over the next 15 years. The analogy of water torture comes to mind

227

about these years. With each passing year, my ability to hear, together with my self-esteem and independence, were being worn away little by little, drip by drip. I found the process of constantly adjusting to my changing hearing loss and adjusting to the "new me" difficult. Added to that was the fear of the unknown. Will I go completely deaf? If so, when? How will I manage? No doctor seemed about to give me a prognosis except to say that sometimes the loss stabilizes at some point. Well, mine finally did stabilize – at rock bottom. By the time I was 35, I was profoundly deaf in both ears. Realizing I was finally "deaf" was a curiously liberating experience. I was no longer in between being hard-of-hearing and being deaf. The fear and anxiety had abated. I had reached the bottom (literally) of the audiogram chart – but, hey, I was still here, alive and even kicking. During this 15-year journey through hearing loss, I had traveled around the world for two years, married, had two children, and picked up my teaching career again. Was it easy? Not by a long shot. But I don't consider it a negative experience either. Losing my hearing but continuing to live, work, and socialize in a hearing world taught me much about myself. It also taught me a lot about other people. Most difficult life experiences are like long, dark tunnels. Either you emerge into the light or at the other end a stronger and more aware person – or you don't emerge at all. I remember reading once that when it comes to having a disability you have two choices. Either you dominate the disability, or it dominates you. I chose to live as gracefully and fully as possible with my profound and irrevocable hearing loss.

I used a hearing aid, which gave me some help in the lower frequencies, and I was blessed with an innate ability to speechread well. Did I use sign language? We tried. My husband, and I and our two young children took a beginning sign language course. But, by that time the three of them were too adept at knowing how to get my attention and communicate with me. Our lives were very busy with two careers and two young children, and sign language just didn't work for us. All my friends, family, and co-workers were hearing. Who would sign for me?

I had captioned TV, captioned videos became the norm, and finally the voice-carry-over relay system was available for phone calls after five long years of not being able to make phone calls. I continued to be fairly adept at "faking it" in social situations. Friends, family and co-workers understood and sometimes made extraordinary efforts on my behalf. However, opportunities for career advancement and professional growth began to require more and more use of oral interpreters, which was extremely fatiguing. As my children began approaching the teenage years, and I myself entered the mid-life years, I began to feel more stress, more fatigue, and less enjoyment in every area of my life. But it was the social isolation I found most painful. When it became difficult to enjoy even old friends across a dining room table, I realized how much my quality of life had deteriorated. Others may not have realized how hard I was working to hear them, but I always came away from social situations drained and exhausted.

I actually found out about cochlear implants while living in Australia in 1978 – during the early research and development phases. For me, it was never a question of "if" I would have an implant, but rather "when." Through those years, I followed the development of implants and instinctively knew that the longer I could hold out, the better the technology would get, and the better the results I would experience with an implant. Still, I did not make the decision to get an implant quickly. Even after determining that the results with patients with similar degrees and type of hearing loss as myself were increasingly better, I still spent the better part of a year researching this. I called major medical centers around the country with implant programs and directly spoke with many leading audiologists about both of the implants then available in the United States in 1995. I read as much as I could find, including the National Institutes of Health Consensus statement on implants. I also met other implanted adults with both implants, and asked them a lot of questions. I knew that implant patients invariably heard environmental noises. In a local article I read at that time, the patient waxed euphoric over being able to hear the bacon sizzling. Frankly, I wasn't interested in hearing bacon – I wanted to hear, and understand, people.

At that time – and still presently – doctors and audiologists are not able to predict exactly how much and how well a potential implant candidate will hear in different situations. Research is still ongoing to determine how different personality factors, processing skills, and mental abilities might account for differences in performance post-implant of persons with similar hearing loss histories and etiologies. In addition, research is also ongoing to determine what electrode designs and what processing strategies offer the most promise for increased performance of implant patients. The pace of change in implant technology in the five years since I was implanted has been astounding. So, too, many patients' results have improved, and the time frames to reach that improvement have shortened. But during the late fall of 1995, I had determined that for me, given the quality of life as I defined it, and given the fact that no hearing aid was going to be of any benefit to me, it was time to "go for it." Dr. Patricia Chute of Manhattan Eye Ear and Throat Hospital in New York City told me that, although she couldn't tell me exactly how well I would hear with an implant, that it would definitely be better than the way I was currently hearing. I had nothing to lose, and potentially a lot to gain. I was then comfortable making the leap.

Interesting enough, when I discussed the operation with my two children, then aged 10 and 13, they didn't think I should have it. They thought I was fine as I was. Part of their feelings stemmed, I'm sure, from the fact that I would be undergoing surgery with an uncertain result. But basically they had only known me as a "deaf" mother. I found it reinforcing that for them, being deaf was merely an inconvenience for us all, not a defining feature of me as a mother or a person.

So, what was it like that day in February 1996 when I was finally fitted with the processor and "turned on"? I think I was more anxious that day than the day of the operation one month before. For me this was D-day. Did I make the right decision? Would it work? I deliberately went into this with low expectations. I did not expect to be able to use a telephone or understand speech without speechreading. I just hoped that speechreading would be easier and less strenuous. Above all, I wanted my children to be able to communicate with me more easily. I didn't want to add more stress to the parent-child relationship during their teenage years. Audiologists had forewarned me in the past that learning to hear again with an implant would be a long, arduous process of retraining the brain to interpret these new sounds. But for me, from the beginning, I could hear AND understand more than I could with a hearing aid. In addition, the quality of the sound was much more pleasing and less distorted. Yes, it was a gradual process and I hear today much better than I did during those first few months after activation. But instead of describing it as an arduous process, it was more like regaining paradise, little by little, one lovely step at a time.

I remember being so overwhelmed by the new sounds I was hearing that I just couldn't return to work after the initial two-day activation and programming in New York City. I felt I had landed on an alien planet. I discovered that microwaves beeped (!), my feet made noise on the carpets as I walked, and the doors in our house squeaked (a lot). It was as if layers and layers of gauze were being peeled away and the world suddenly became a much richer tapestry now that I could hear so many of the sounds that had eluded me for so long. To my surprise, I could actually distinguish voices on the car radio those first weeks. I held off trying the telephone till almost four weeks post hookup. For people who have gradually lost their ability to use a phone, the process is usually a struggle and fraught with anxiety. I had no desire to relive that struggle. But my husband convinced me to try a prearranged call at home, with him calling me from his office at a particular time. I gingerly picked up the phone, expecting to hear only a blur of sound. Remember, with a hearing aid, I couldn't even tell if there was a dial tone, let alone a voice at the other end. To my utter amazement, I could understand him. Not only that, but his voice sounded to me exactly as I remember hearing it on a telephone some 13 years before. It was quite an emotional moment. The next experiment was with my children, whose voices I had never heard on a phone. That worked, too!

Looking back over these five years, it seems like another life when I could not hear, when life itself sometimes seemed so stressful and so devoid of the important human connections most people take for granted. I now use a telephone for all my calls anywhere. Being able to page my roaming 17-year-old son not so long ago, and being able to receive his call back to me regardless of where he was, was a big anxiety reliever. I enjoy being more involved at my children's high school functions, serving on committees with other parents and teachers. It has made me feel much more a part of my children's everyday lives. It also has enabled me to be a role model for them about the importance of volunteerism and involvement in school and community issues. Carrying on "no eye contact" conversations with my teenagers while driving them endlessly from place to place has made a positive difference in our relationship – for them and for me. My husband and I now socialize much more with others – going out to dinner, plays, concerts, and movies. Professionally, I no longer use oral interpreters at all – even at conferences and large group meetings. My current job is a management job that requires a lot of phone contact and personal interaction – one that I doubt I would have applied for prior to my implant.

Do I hear everything all the time? Of course not – but neither do hearing persons. On occasion I need to ask persons to repeat on the phone or in noisy environments. Am I still deaf? Definitely. I get a not-so-subtle reminder of that each day when my battery in my implant suddenly dies. It's very quiet. But recently, a colleague who is an interpreter told me that a local interpreter group was putting together a panel of successful professional deaf adults and wanted me to be on the panel. For a minute, I almost asked why they wanted me. Then, I remembered…of course, I still am deaf. But obviously, with the implant, I rarely think of myself as such anymore.

Having a cochlear implant these past five years has changed my life – and my family's life – in so many ways. A year after my implant, my then 11-year-old daughter was asked in her language arts class to make a list of the 10 most important things in her life. She wrote: "The most important day in my life was when my mom had her hearing operation." Having an implant is a very personal and individual decision. It is a decision that should be made with the best and most accurate available information and by taking into consideration all the factors that are involved. It is not a decision that should be made lightly. But for me, unquestionably, it was the right decision at the right time. If I could sum up my personal feelings about having an implant in one sentence, it would be a paraphrase from Martin Luther King – "Free at last, thank God I'm free at last."

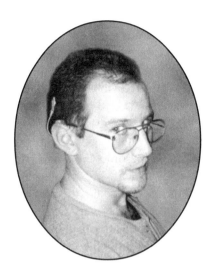

Analyze This…By William Southworth

I've tried to analyze this from many different perspectives in a logical manner. I've reached a conclusion: There is no logic to it. Accidents happen to good people for no apparent reason. There's no fighting it, no plea-bargaining. It suddenly happens and you have to pick up the pieces. I've never been so morose as to ask "Why me?" I was doing something that I've done hundreds of times before. Perhaps I became accustomed to it, overconfident and careless. Maybe my number was just up. Whatever the circumstance, the result was the same. A three-story fall off a roof to the pavement below. When asked what happened I tell people, "I lost an argument with gravity."

Fresh out of a coma, I had no recollection of recent events. At first I thought everyone was playing some kind of joke on me. I just couldn't get rid of the massive ringing in my head. Later I found out the ringing is called tinnitus. My ears didn't work. My vision was all screwed up. I was surrounded by strangers. I had trouble thinking and remembering events from one moment to the next. I was poked, prodded, and injected. I reached what I thought fit the description of what I was going through. I was being kidnapped! I fought back as best I could. When I did see a familiar face, their lips moved but no sound emerged. This added to my confusion. Eventually, they explained that I was in a hospital and to please stop hitting the nurses. What I wouldn't have given just for someone to hold up a sign for me saying "You are in a hospital." It would have made everything easier. I had a test later that week. How was I going to make up my work and finish my college classes? Anxiety over missing my classes merged into the rest of my life. Could I still do my job? Did I still have a job to go back to? How is my family surviving without my income? Will I ever be the same person I was? The realization of my predicament went far beyond what I've ever experienced. What about my marriage? 'For better or worse' took on a whole new meaning. At the time I was half paralyzed with a traumatic head injury as well as deaf. It was unclear as to what I would recover and what I wouldn't. The doctors thought that I might be a vegetable. For someone who was very active before, unable to do basic things by myself (like eating) seemed like a fate worse than death. Having someone feed, clean, and wipe me was something I wouldn't wish on my worst enemy. Being physically fit enabled me to survive.

When my wife came and visited I had a big speech prepared. I told her that I could see how this was a big change in our relationship. Vocal communication was an important part of how we dealt with one another. My heart would be broken, but I'd understand if she wanted to get out of our marriage. Her response was immediate: *"Don't think you're getting out of this that easily."*

Any feelings of being sorry for myself disappeared after that. I have been told that any injury like mine puts a strain on a marriage, but in our case it strengthened ours. My family couldn't have been more supportive. Both my wife and mother started to learn ASL. They arranged for me to meet with a speech specialist so that I could learn to read lips more effectively. It touched my heart to feel the love and support from them. My friends' reaction was a slightly different story. Some felt uncomfortable around me, others helped me to embrace what life had dealt. Those friends who rose to the challenge to communicate with me I am forever grateful to. Those who didn't went their own ways. One friend described it as he was sitting across from me at dinner one time. *"It's as if you suddenly spoke a different language."* He admitted that it was different, even difficult to talk to me. However, he was willing to overcome this obstacle. It spoke great things about his character and why I am proud to count him as a friend. On the other hand, others felt uncomfortable talking to me on the phone. They didn't have the patience to accept me with a disability.

Some weeks after my initial injury, when I became, as I call it, cognizant, it sank in that my hearing wasn't coming back in any shape or form. I would never hear my baby cry. I would forget what my wife sounded like. I wouldn't experience things like music or car alarms. Depressing thoughts that hit you when you lie awake just before dawn. I asked my cousin what was the big deal with Ricky Martin. He explained that I wasn't missing much. One of my favorite bands released an album shortly after I got out of the hospital. That tugged at my heart in more ways than one. I longed to hear music. *"But you can read the lyrics"* someone said. They were trying to cheer me up, but it's hard to explain the longing to hear a guitar or keyboard.

I wanted nothing more than to crawl under a rock. It was difficult to imagine going through life without experiencing sound in some form. No more movies or drive-thru fast food. All the daily things that were a part of my routine were changed. In ways that I took hearing for granted and used it in daily life. A big part of restructuring my life was a friend who reached out to me. He and I had always shared a love of computers. I hadn't spoken to him in many years, but he flew down to see me in the hospital. Eventually he offered me a job fixing computers when I got out. In part, this was to give me a bolster of self-confidence, and make me feel like I could still contribute to society. I realized on another level that I wanted to prove to everyone that my mind still functioned just as well as before the accident.

I call that stage of my life reclaiming my humanity. I was very grateful for what I had heard and seen in my life so far. The rustle of thousands of bats flying out of a cave, a wolf cry in the wilderness. My baby crying in the middle of the night because her diaper needed changing. I focused on being thankful for what I had heard before the accident. Then I took a fateful trip to the ear specialist.

"You would be a good candidate," I read from my audiologist's lips. She went on to tell me about the implant and what it did. Once it was done, it couldn't be undone. I felt any chance to hear my family, in some form, was better than not at all. I told her to go ahead and arrange the surgery.

At first, it was similar to getting a workout, learning to hear again. There were days when I was relieved to turn the implant off; 'blessed silence' I referred to it once. In many ways it was like learning another language. Everything sounded different. That wasn't a glass breaking, it was a toilet flushing. It became easier as time went on. I scared my mother one day and answered the phone. She honestly never thought she would speak to me in that form again! I continued to push the envelope. I truly appreciate having the implant. It allows me to communicate with people quicker and on many levels. There are many precise concepts when you are dealing with computers. I am glad I can hear exactly what I need to hear with little margin for error.

Seven weeks after I got my implant turned on, I surprised the audiologist by telling her how I had been using the phone. My relationship with the world had improved exponentially. Months later I stopped by the audiologist's office to pick up some battery replacements that I had ordered. A woman stopped me in the office. *"My doctor recommended that I get an implant, can you tell me about it?"* The quiver in her voice was clear even to me. I went on to tell her it has made all the difference. Some people don't notice that I have it. People that I have 'incidental' contact with: the bag boy at the grocery store, or the girl selling cookies door-to-door. Let's face it, we communicate with one another pretty rapidly. That is, a lot of information gets passed onto one another in a very few words. The implant picks up that for me so I can communicate with the world. My father pointed out that I'm not really deaf now that I have the implant. I shook my finger at him. When the battery runs out, when I take a shower, or sleep, I'm still deaf! During the waking hours, I shift gears. Yes, I'm deaf. But now with my implant I can hear.

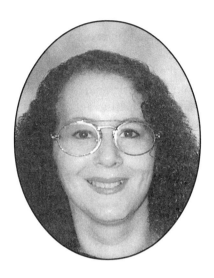

Hearing is Better…By Gwen Cooper M.D.

I think my earliest memory of hearing is outside the hearing aid store in 1961 with my brand-new hearing aids. How loud the trucks lumbering down the street were! I was scared and overwhelmed. We really don't know how I lost my hearing, maybe medications? My parents realized something wasn't right when I was four or five years old. I managed to evade discovery probably due to excellent lipreading skills.

I am now 44 years old, and I have had a cochlear implant for two years. How did this happen? One day I realized that I could not hear out of my right ear; first we changed the batteries, the hearing aid, and then went to the ENT. I am a busy solo obstetrician-gynecologist and this was a major problem because I felt I could not function as maximally as possible. First we tried steroids, then antibiotics, and finally the conclusion was irrevocable hearing loss from an already dismal 70 dB to worse. Well, that was terrible because, although I am an avid lipreader, hearing is important to my function in the practice, both the office and the operating room.

So that's when I started exploring the option of a cochlear implant. At first I was not thrilled with the idea of having my head shaved, an incision in my head, possible facial nerve damage, loss of all residual hearing in that ear, and possibly failure of the whole process. It became

237

apparent that I did not have anything to lose and a lot to gain from the procedure over the next several months. The physician and staff that I consulted were very supportive and helpful in providing me with information and options.

So, we did it, and the recovery was somewhat uncomfortable because I had to sleep on the "wrong side" until the incision healed. Of course I was told that when the implant is first hooked up, that it can sound "Mickey Mousey," but I thought that would not happen to me, and I would "hear" right away! Being the perfectionist and overachiever I was WRONG!

They hooked me up and it was awful. I recognized nothing. It was like a bad record, horrible. I thought I had really messed up now. Fortunately, thank God, after weeks and months of practice and encouragement, sounds finally made sense. I can truly say at this time that this was one of my better decisions! I love the implant, and I do wear the implant and the hearing aid together for bilateral sound, but I have walked out of the house and forgotten the hearing aid! I hear better with the implant than I do with the hearing aid, and it has preserved my perception that I function better professionally and personally with the enhanced hearing the implant provides particularly, in situations in which lipreading is impossible. I can hear people talk to me from behind me and know what they said. I am not as "deaf" in a dark room, like movies, bars, and parties, including darker restaurants. The only inconvenience is the bulk of the apparatus; however, as I write, the behind-the-ear version is being tested and used.

As a parting thought, if you don't hear, you don't know what you are missing – I didn't. No one is supposed to be blind, deaf, crippled, or mentally handicapped. Things happen to people, and I feel that for the gift of life a person should do everything they can to maximize the opportunities for a happy, fulfilling life for themselves and their children. I have two children, and that is my job – to turn them into independent happy, fulfilling adults, to function at the best they can be with whatever assistive aids they need.

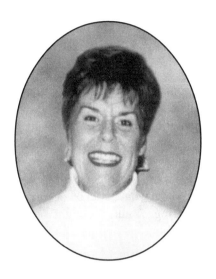

Best of Both Worlds...By Joyce Adams

Have you ever *thoughtfully* listened to the sounds around you? Ever become aware of the amount of sound, albeit noise, that bombards and inundates your senses daily? If you were hearing impaired or deaf and been blessed with technology that "fixed" the problem, you certainly have given this conjecture a lot of consideration. But the rest of the world probably never gives it a second thought.

As a hearing person, I was absorbed in society's new phenomenon, noise pollution. Noise is unwanted sound; the word is derived from the Latin "nausea," meaning seasickness, and noise is among the most pervasive pollutants today. Noise from road traffic, jet planes, jet skis, garbage trucks, lawn mowers, leaf blowers, blow dryers, and boom boxes, to name a few, is so constant and pervasive, we hardly recognize the elevating level of noise until it is gone. From the perspective of the hearing individual, it is one thing to be the perpetrator of the noise, but when the noise comes without our consent, it is definitely irritating and stressful. Even at night when most people are asleep, the loudly snoring person contributes to the cacophony of sound that is in the air. Spending time at the ocean or forest or places away from the city and hubbub of daily life allows us to experience the lack of noise with which we live and revel in the peace that results. My awareness of the increasing levels of noise sharpened along with the realization of its effect on each individual's health and well-being. I contemplated how we as a society could work to decrease noise and increase tranquility in order to eliminate at least one cause of society's burgeoning stress.

Then came the silence. A brutal headache, some aspirins, and a decision to stay home from work were the beginning events that would change my life forever. On October 6, 1997, I was hospitalized, in a coma, and diagnosed with meningitis. Three days later I awoke in the ICU of Memorial Hospital. I awoke on Wednesday and all seemed to be well so I was transferred to a room of my own. As the hours passed I noticed that I asked people to repeat things and this seemed to be escalating. No one told me what could be occurring. By Friday of that week, I had lost all hearing. A nurse brought me the Physician's Reference Guide and I read about meningitis. As I read about the disease, I realized that I could have died. So, I was happy to be alive with everything else intact! The article stated that the adults in the study lost their hearing, which is a side effect of meningitis, but that in most cases the hearing of the group studied returned. The doctors also felt that my hearing would return and I believed them. At the time, the condition of silence was perplexing, but the inconvenience of not being able to hear had not yet penetrated my psyche and my reality. While in the hospital, the staff and I communicated by me trying to read lips or by writing on a small board that the staff located. I was released from the hospital after two weeks but could not return to work. I took a six-week leave of absence hoping that at the end of six weeks all would be back to normal. As weeks turned into months, we began to face the reality that my hearing would never return. I remembered the last voice I heard on the telephone while in the hospital and began to become frightened. It was as if I had cotton in my ears and felt like something I wanted to rip off or shake off. There was no shaking it off, this was part of me! I spent some time recalling all the sounds of the world that I had taken for granted and had even become annoyed with! I did see a plus, though, in sleeping – no snoring sounds would keep me awake. I contemplated on my latest interest in noise pollution and thought, "what irony." I thought about my job and my life in general and began to experience frustration and panic; how was I going to manage! At 47, this was not going to be an easy transition. It finally sank in that I was deaf and needed to do something!

Desperate to get started, I immersed myself into information about lipreading. I chose this form of interaction because it required only my effort in learning this communication form. My friends and family only needed to speak clearly so that I could read their lips. I was going to also pursue signing but knew that this decision would completely restrict my interactions to those who signed. While I wanted to learn signing, this communication technique was not going to solve my problem. It was very clear to me that I would be the one who needed to accommodate myself to the hearing world. All of my friends, business contacts, family, etc. were not going to sign to communicate with me. Continuing to read information about the deaf, each passing month brought with it new realizations of the challenges of the deaf and the unique niche that exists for this population of people.

My career came to a screeching halt because I could no longer hear. My position in project planning with a telecommunications company enabled me to deal with people all over the world via telephone. I was the liaison between the field and headquarters for new product information, software designs, problem resolution, and for payment to our representatives all over the world. I began to devise a system whereby I could continue in my position and communicate with the field via email. After all we are in the PC world and I thought this could work! Another learning curve – while we communicate via email to stay in touch, the really "hot" or important issues require immediate attention as well as the live voice of someone at headquarters to facilitate resolutions to concerns. Monthly meetings via conference calls with our affiliates worldwide were another of my responsibilities. It was frighteningly clear that I could no longer fill the project planner role. I was suddenly deaf with no plan on how I was going to overcome this communication challenge. The six-week leave provided in the Family Medical Leave Act (FMLA) passed and I was terminated.

Well, I finally realized the permanent impact of my condition and pursued answers from the medical profession. One of the specialists to whom I was referred confirmed that my natural hearing ability would not return. He also told me about the cochlear implant and the program at UCSF. Alleluia, hope! Until that moment, I had never heard about the program and neither had any of my friends or family. I was optimistic to learn of the cochlear implant device and process. I learned about the procedure and really began to believe that this could help me. I had perfectly normal hearing prior to the onslaught of meningitis and anything that could help me acquire some modicum of hearing ability was a very welcome option to me.

There's an old saying: "Absence makes the heart grow fonder" and while I believe that the adage refers to people, I certainly related it to the loss of my hearing ability. Before the meningitis, I never once thought about life without hearing or the challenges that non-hearing people face day to day. I tried to recall the sounds of birds, the sea crashing, or the sounds of kids shouting and laughing on the playground. I could bring back the memory of those events, but not how it sounded. My family and social life continued, but I observed that people were becoming annoyed or impatient with writing everything or repeating everything until my lipreading skills improved. Lipreading, one on one, is okay but in a group setting you cannot see everyone at once and I would quickly lose track of what the conversation was about. I remember thinking that I was only a beginner, maybe it would get better. I recalled the easy banter back and forth, in which my friends or family and I engaged and really reflected on how all these interactions help shape who I am as a person.

I began to lose comfort in speaking because I could no longer hear myself and felt I was forgetting sounds of words and became easily tongue-tied. You know, the constant reinforcement of the sound of language keeps us on track and without it, the speaking skill begins to slip, I believe. My confidence started to dwindle. Eventually, I began to withdraw socially, choosing to stay home vs. attend the various functions that were a part of my everyday life. I suspected that as time went on, my experience would become more unpleasant and I was feeling that this was only the tip of the iceberg. The telephone was actually a good experience for me. The TTY arrangement enabled me to converse with friends and family, and I commend that program and everyone engaged in it.

Finally my appointment time at UCSF arrived and I was diagnosed with profound hearing loss, in other words, NO hearing ability at all. I could not register hearing any sound. I was a good candidate for the implant procedure and was scheduled for surgery to implant the Clarion in December 1998. Learning about the process for the implant had me wondering about the surgery and I was apprehensive because I would be in the hospital only for one night. I wondered how something so intricate required only an overnight stay? Well, that's all it took for me and I was quite comfortable after the implant procedure was completed. The morning after the surgery, my doctor and audiologist came in to conduct the "tone test." They hooked me up to a device and tested to discern if I could hear any or all of eight tones.

After the appropriate recovery time, my processor was programmed

242

and I was "turned on" in January 1999 after having been deaf for 15 months. What a miracle! The day that the program was enabled, two of my friends and I went to UCSF, and the first voices I heard after 15 long months of silence were the voices of these dear friends. Their voices sounded exactly as I remembered them, and the little room in which we worked was the ideal place to experience this blessing. When we left that environment, I was shocked to experience all the sounds of everyday life; it was very noisy! I began to work with the program to adjust the sound levels and to discover what worked best for me. I went into the ladie's room to hear the sound of running water and to hear the toilet flush. Yes, it sounded exactly as I had remembered these sounds to be, but I would not have known that without the sense of sight or knowledge of what I was listening for. Hearing my son's voice and hearing my mother's laugh are sounds that I took for granted every day and now I was blessed to be able to experience these sounds again.

So, I began to immerse myself in the sounds of the world and took walks to experience as many sounds as I could. Initially, there is the stage of learning what the sound was, i.e., planes flying. I knew there was an overhead sound but I had to learn that it was the sound of an airplane. I worked with a very talented and patient therapist who systematically brought me through the stages of sound in language. "Mmm" sounds, "s" sounds, and all the subtle sounds with their unique attributes were the focus of our sessions. We began work on the telephone, using it as normal hearing people do. WOW! It's not perfect but it beats where I had been. Eventually, I met several people who were candidates for the implant and also met people who had been implanted.

A whole new world was opening up to me. The UCSF visits were always productive, and slowly we identified programs that worked increasingly better. I used the local library to check out books on tape as well as the accompanying book in order to read along with the tape. This helped me adjust to the new sounds. It is still surprising that when you can read along with the sound, you think, of course, that's the word. But when listening to the sound alone it was difficult to understand the word, because of the speaker's inflection or softness. All in all, this was a good process and I listened to books I would not normally have read. Now I felt I was ready to experiment with different environments, and the first "public" place was a café that my lovely therapist and I attended. OOPS...I had to read her lips because the environmental sounds, cacophony of voices, overhead fans, etc., dominated my hearing experience. I needed to learn to adjust the program or concentrate on her voice and block out the surrounding noise. I love movies, and a person whom I met through the UCSF program, who was implanted one month after me, also likes movies. We saw our first movie together after being implanted and found that we could hear most of it! What a thrill!

Over time, my comfort level with the programs increased. I have changed my career path because I could not adjust quickly enough to the demands of my position. I speak and hear on the telephone without peripheral devices but will attest to the fact that different equipment affects the quality of sound. European, Asian, and Australian callers create a challenge because of the distance. Some accents add to the challenge, and different cultures have softer presentation styles than those to which I am accustomed.

Meetings continue to challenge my ability to hear each person, and meetings in noisy places are not my preference. I believe that my comfort level in even these challenging environments will develop. I plan to continue to immerse myself in different situations in order to continue to develop my listening skills. My next focus is listening to music. Prior to losing my hearing, listening to music was total bliss for me and I lost myself in hours of listening magic. At a recent convention we learned techniques to develop our hearing skills and heard testimony from people who are in the process of mastering this joyous activity. I look forward to discovering the wonderful world of music. While my work in developing my hearing skills continues, I delight in the ability to "turn off" or decrease sound when in very noisy situations or at night when I go to sleep. It's the best of both worlds!

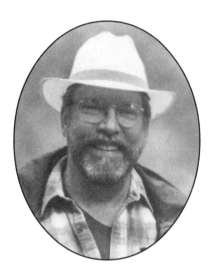

My Bionic Ear...By Greg Heller

I guess the easiest way to describe what a cochlear implant (CI) does is call it by a name that most everyone can understand. It, for all intents and purposes, is a "bionic ear". My hearing is 100% electronic. I lost my hearing due to a rare allergic reaction to what nowadays is a very common drug. I was prescribed this medication two different times, five years apart. The first time, I lost half of my hearing. The doctors could never make a determination as to why. In 1997, I was given the same prescription again. Two days and three doses later, I awoke to silence. I had normal hearing for 38 years, half of it for five years and then nothing... This was devastating.

The biggest problem with hearing loss is it affects not only the person with it, but everyone they come in contact with. My family slowly slipped away...my friends...my job was even threatened. My wife and I switched roles in our marriage. I had been the "social" person of the team and Debbie was the "wallflower." Previously, I used to make the arrangements for a backyard bar-b-que or dinner with friends at the local eatery, now it fell upon my wife to take care of the social planning. That is if she could talk me into attending any functions. At that point I preferred sitting at home with a book because it was easier than trying to carry on a conversation. Debbie also became my social secretary and took care of all the phone calls. She would carry on 30-minute conversations and then I would get the "Reader's Digest" version. I felt alienated in my own home but it wasn't my family's fault. My inability to hear affected all of us. After a lot of research, and talking with others who have a CI, I opted to have one implanted in February of 1999.

I have the Clarion, manufactured by Advanced Bionics Corporation in Valencia, CA. The surgery and all the follow-up programming of the processor were done at Virginia Mason Hospital in Seattle. Here's how it works...A microphone in the headpiece picks up the sound and the signal is sent down the wire to the processor. The processor turns the "sounds" into a digital code and sends it back up the wire to be sent across the skin, via radio waves, to the implant chip. The microchip in the implant, takes the data and breaks it down then sends it down the electrode array to the individual electrodes. They in turn, fire the nerve cluster in the center of the cochlea and the nerves send the signal to the brain to be interpreted as "sound." This all happens in "real time" so that sound is heard as it occurs. It sounds complicated...but it's like wearing glasses...I joke with my wife that I put on my "eyes" (glasses) so I can find my "ear".

Since regaining functional hearing with my CI my relationship with my family has improved considerably. My son was only seven years old when I lost my hearing and had just turned fourteen when I received my implant. The best gift the implant has given me is our renewed relationship as we are able to converse freely and have became much closer. Unfortunantly, I am one of only about 70,000 people in the world with one of these wonders. The sad part is that there are approximately 2 million people in this country alone with a profound/severe hearing loss. Thousands of people could benefit from this technology, but most don't even know that it exists. Control of my life was given back to me when I got my implant. I feel like a "torch" was passed to me to help educate and let people know of this wonderful technology. In close...I'm going to quote you some numbers that might help you understand where I was and where I am now. Before the implant, I only understood about 4% of what was said to me. The rest of it was picked up through my eyes...by lipreading. The rewards of gaining control over my life again far outweigh the fears and anxieties I went through to get the implant. Is it a magic cure? No, but it is a miracle to regain enough of my hearing to function in the hearing world again. I am, and always will be hard of hearing, but it sure beats the alternative of being deaf from my point of view.

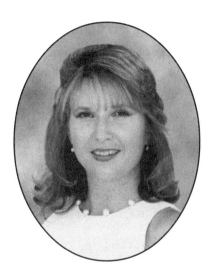

A New Lease On Life...By Cynthia Farley

Hello! My name is Cynthia. This is a narrative of my personal experience with hearing impairment, which was discovered initially by my preschool teachers. It was later determined that my hearing loss was caused by exposure to otoxic medication that I had received as a infant. I was first tested for hearing loss at the University of Kansas in 1969, where they discovered that I had a profound sensorineural loss in both ears with some residual hearing in my left ear. Subsequently, I was outfitted with a hearing aid at five years of age.

I adapted very well with my hearing aid. In public school I was placed in a special education class of about eight students with hearing impairments. All of us spoke and did not practice sign language. In the sixth grade I was mainstreamed half days to see how I would adapt to regular classrooms without special services. As long as I sat up front, watched the teacher, etc., I did just fine. There were, of course, adjustments on my part as well as the part of others, but overall it was a very positive step forward. Therefore in the seventh grade I was totally mainstreamed, and it was a very liberating experience after having been sequestered in a small class for so long. At that point not only had I adjusted, I excelled with honors, hence I was offered a transfer to a magnet school for the gifted. However, I choose to remain at my high school, as I wanted to go to the same school with my neighbors. High school was pretty typical. When I was 16 I landed my first "real" job as a sales-clerk at a retail store. (I had always been able to use the conventional phone with my hearing aid.)

After some college I was employed at a variety of positions including retail sales and management, the postal service, real estate ownership/development, and as an outside sales representative for Pitney Bowes. During my tenure at Pitney Bowes, my life changed drastically and very suddenly. That workday, I was returning from lunch in an instant it seemed like the volume just cut out with lots of static on my hearing aid. My reaction was to assume that my hearing aid was on the blink, so I went to my hearing aid center to get a loaner aid. When none of the hearing aids there worked either, even the brand-new ones, I started to become unnerved. I began to face the realization that the problem was with my ear.

I consulted with an ENT surgeon, Dr. Charles Luetje. I was in acute turmoil emotionally and physically. Dr. Luetje was very sympathetic and a real life line to me during this extremely rough patch. He pre-scribed a course of antibiotics along with prednisone to try and correct the loss that had robbed me of my remaining hearing. After that failed to produce the desired result, he stated to me, " I can restore your hearing with a cochlear implant, Cynthia." A bold statement to make, but he was that confident that it would work for me. And I, doubting Thomas that I was, had serious doubts as to whether an implant could really do the trick. So I consulted with other doctors for a second opin-ion. It was reinforced that I had suffered an irreversible deafness and that a cochlear implant was my only option if I wanted to regain any hearing.

During my 'deaf' period (eight months) I had to make many adjust-ments, so I truly have an insider's view of what it's like to be deaf. For instance, I had always been so independent to survive/thrive. Now I had to learn interdependence. In other words I had to accept help from others, whether I wanted it or not, a hard lesson for me. I could not hear, therefore my ability to communicate was severely impaired. My lifesaver was my ability to lipread, which served me well, as without the auditory information, I was totally dependent on lipreading and writing notes. This was not only tough for me but for those around me as well. My son was four years old at that time, and, having recently becoming a single parent it was quite a struggle, as you might imagine. My par-ents suffered as well by seeing their only child experience the helpless-ness of sudden deafness and its impact. It was a terrible strain. Daily life was very stressful at times without the hearing we have a tendency to take for granted. I couldn't hear the doorbell, the phone, music, voices, smoke detector, cars, etc. I was truly in a prison of silence, and it isolated me from people. I suffered much depression and grief for my loss of hearing. I remember trying to 'grasp' and retain the precious sound of my son's sweet voice as my hearing faltered even more. It was a nightmare from which I thought I would never awake from. I absolutely hated the looks of pity that I would receive from people. I didn't feel like I had changed all that much, yes, I was deaf, but I could still function and think for myself, thank you very much!

After the initial shock wore off I had to get a grip. I had to adjust because I'm not a quitter. I could no longer fulfill the requirements of my position at Pitney Bowes, therefore I opted to take disability as I could not communicate fluently and did not want to impose on others. I was given a TTY for telephone communication, which restored a measure of my independence, as I no longer had to rely on "mom" to make calls for me. However, it was very time-consuming (even with VCO) to use, and that was frustrating. I loved my alphanumeric pager because it would vibrate when I had a message, so it became my answering machine/outside communication tool for my hearing friends. I still drove, socialized, and participated in most of my previous activities. I had severe tinnitus with my deafness that was enough to drive most people over the edge. (Think of screaming elephants and insects— that's what it was like—a constant buzzing in the head day and night.) I had this the entire time and so had to learn to block it out mentally. I went through the period of adapting to deafness and see how it went; however, it was hard. Much harder than I would have ever thought. So, while I had tried to stay open-minded about it, the memories were too strong and I knew I had to get my life back.

I had finally come to the moment of truth and the truth was that I wanted to hear. I made the decision to have the Clarion cochlear implant. At that point I reasoned that anything was better than nothing, as it would just give me more information to work with. Something people with hearing loss do is put pieces of information together like what we heard, or thought we heard, or we read (lips), and other visual cues to formulate in seconds our response. My expectations at that point were to accept whatever benefit I would receive and maximize it to my best advantage. (Although it was my secret desire to get back on the conventional phone and donate that TTY!) My insurance company finally gave the authorization for my implant after much ado. The person responsible for making my life-changing operation decision was not very well informed about cochlear implants, and her attitude was "This device makes a deaf person hear? Yea right!" A common assumption in many people's minds, I'm afraid. However, she was convinced of its viability after working with Joanne Syrja of Advanced Bionics. Joann was in charge of insurance reimbursement at that time. During a conversation on the phone between Joanne and Barbara, when Barbara expressed her doubts about the implants effectiveness Joanne dropped the bomb. "Guess what, I'm deaf...I'm talking to you on the phone... and I wear the implant." That did it, and my approval to proceed was granted. Harrah for Joanne! She changes lives and in doing so is a true champion indeed!

At that point another hurdle was presented to me by my insurance company. They would only reimburse 100% if it were in-network vs. 20% I would have to pay for an out-of-network procedure. I reluctantly had to have my surgery elsewhere than with Dr. Charles Luetje who had fought the insurance companies so hard for me as I could not afford to pay the 20% that I would have incurred through his hospital. The surgery would have to be performed at a network hospital, since Kansas University had no experience with implanting a Clarion device (in clinical trials at that time), I chose to have my procedure performed at the University of California in San Francisco by Dr. Robert Schindler, whom I had seen before at the age of 12. I resided at my cousin's home in San Leandro for several months to be in close proximity to UCSF before and after the operation.

The surgery itself on December 5, 1995 was pretty typical, I had some apprehension, which is normal. I didn't have any problems, other than being a little weak for a few days. Everything went according to plan and I was released in less than 24 hours with no complications. At that point it was time to hurry up and wait till after the holidays for activation of my new "ear."

"Hook-up" day was on Jan. 5, 1996, at the University of California with my audiologist, Jan Larky. I wasn't sure what was going to happen, and it was a little scary not knowing what to expect. When the mapping session (programming of the electrodes in my implant) was complete, then came the moment of truth, would this work? Jan flipped a switch on my speech processor and I was on! Back in the hearing world again! Just like that! It was a miracle! Liberty! I could hear again! And it sounded natural to me. I was ecstatic to be back in the hearing world and released from the isolation imposed by my deafness.

Now I could really appreciate all that life had to offer, even more so because of where I had been. My memory of that day will always be with me, as I felt like a prisoner who was given her freedom, and it was such a profound experience. After leaving the UCSF that day my mother and I walked the streets of downtown San Francisco and celebrated my rebirth as a hearing person. We encountered a local street band on one of the sidewalks and we proceeded to dance in our excitement!!! It was truly a day to remember.

In retrospect I would like to add a few things. I've worn my Clarion CI for about six years now. Although I can use the conventional telephone fluently now with anyone (as long as they speak English!), I had to work to get to that point. It was not instantaneous. The day I was hooked up I tried it and failed to comprehend very many words. But I just kept trying. I practiced with voice messages and friends. I had several re-mappings (part of the program as a map will change as your ear becomes accustomed to sound). Within a month I was able to use the phone without any adaptive equipment. (I would just hold the phone up to my headpiece /ear level.) At that point I would still have to say "what" on more than one occasion! Since then I've had much practice and it's not really an issue anymore. My point is that I was very determined to regain this aspect of lifestyle and that I had to consciously work toward achieving this objective. As for listening 'rehab,' it was all 'self-directed.' I would check out children's books with tapes and read them with my son. (I would practice following the voice while reading the text on the page.) I have many fond memories of my son and I enjoying 'therapy' sessions. The '*Three Billy Goats Gruff*' was our favorite book!

Since regaining my hearing I've moved in new directions. In 1996-1997 I was busy supervising the historical renovation of an 1895 house that I owned. Within a year after implantation I met my husband Doug in Kansas City (he was in town on business). We dated across the miles for over a year prior to our marriage and relocation to Minnesota. My son Zachary has adjusted very well to all of the transitions and continues to grow up too fast! Currently, I'm in the process of starting a nonprofit venture which, I will hopefully have time for now that I've finished compiling this book. Last but not least, I would like to take this opportunity to thank all of those of who have spearheaded and supported the cochlear implant technology, for without them we would not enjoy the hearing we have today.

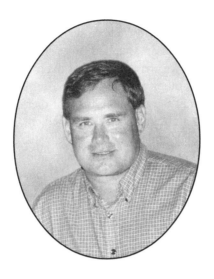

Here's the Deal…By Glen and Laurie Hommy

It is truly remarkable to think that Glen's cochlear implant surgery has been so successful that I actually had to review notes and resources to refresh my memory as to what it was like for our family to live with the hearing impaired. Doing so, however, has once again humbled me and left me in awe of the advances that have been made technologically in research and medicine. I am very thankful for the opportunity to have received one of them. We first sought help with Glen's subtle hearing loss in 1986, and gradually he became completely deaf in his right ear and totally dependant on a high-powered hearing aid in his left, prior to having surgery January 31, 2000. Considering that we procrastinated about going to seek help initially, we had a total of about 15 years living with a slight to severe disability. It was thought that Glen's hearing loss was due to an autoimmune disorder. In case you've never heard of these types of diseases, they are a group where the immune system is altered and the body produces antibodies against its own cells. Diseases like rheumatoid arthritis or lupus fall into this category, and it was felt that perhaps there was something of this nature going on in Glen's inner ear. During that time our three children, Breanne, Landon, and Parker, grew from infancy into young teenagers and dealt with their difficulty communicating in a number of evolving ways.

Glen was involved in business, having a passion for being an entrepreneur, and those years took us from Medicine Hat to Grande Prairie and on up to Fort McMurray where we have lived for the past six years. A gas station with an attached carwash and lube bay beckoned us up there, and since we arrived Glen has overseen their management, as well as taken on other projects. I am a registered nurse and am presently employed at the regional hospital there, where I work on a casual basis in their ambulatory care and medical units. We both came from rural backgrounds and believe in working hard, solving problems, and not being a quitter. Most of the time this allows a person to have a certain degree of control over their lives, but I must say that getting sick or dealing with a disability often takes away that sense of power or security. In dealing with Glen's deteriorating hearing, I think that that was one of the most frustrating feelings – the lack of control...but there were others that I'm sure that some of you will identify with.

Our world is very dynamic, and people have incredible demands on our time. We have become a society that has little patience with anyone or any circumstance that slows us down. Our frustration with the elderly, the disabled, or anyone who does not quickly execute day-to-day activities is very obvious in our facial expressions and mannerisms (or lack of them). Whether it be at the supermarket checkout, airline ticket counter, or with the local bank teller, speed is paramount and everyone is preoccupied with what we still have left to do. I include myself here because I still have to check myself to "slow down," listen, and actually offer assistance to those less efficient without being condescending. During Glen's disability I know that my body language often said far more than I spoke, and I did feel impatient as well. Then I would feel guilty for feeling impatient.

Because Glen could not hear, people would often talk to me so that I could explain things to him. Even though the topic may have been directly related to business or to him, they would not even make eye contact with Glen. I knew that this hurt and isolated him, and I would find myself looking at him while someone was speaking so that they would do the same. Sometimes it worked. Sometimes it didn't. I found that most people just do not know how to deal with a disability. We're not very good at saying that, and when Glen or I would tell them that they could help by just speaking clearly and a little slower and let him see them speak, it helped out everyone. Most people (again like myself prior to this experience) see someone with a hearing aid and immediately begin to shout. I remember the tension.

Over the years going out in crowds or to large social functions became more difficult. I would strain to listen carefully to the conversation so I could relay a condensed version back to Glen, but he is a very quick-witted, social person and it was so frustrating for him to always be that sentence or laugh behind. It was especially sad to see him miss the one-liners because they were a big part of his personality and somehow they're not the same if they are repeated. Occasionally he would jump into the conversation quickly with animation only to find out that someone had already said that, or he had misheard the previous speaker and he was off the topic. He would laugh but of course he was also embarrassed and it made him hesitant to take part again. Both of us would come home feeling exhausted. I missed the dancing. Glen was a great dancer and we tried to dance, but it was becoming difficult and occasionally embarrassing. We tried to have me lead, he tried to feel the beat in the floor, and we kept to the safe dances, but after a few humiliating moments we just quit trying. Then I felt guilty for missing it. I don't need to tell any of you about the feelings of isolation.

As Glen's hearing deteriorated and we were using sign language more and more to communicate, we did less and less socially as a couple and a family. We would go to where we felt the most comfortable…with established friends and relatives. We watched a lot of movies at home with closed captioning because it was something that we could all enjoy without straining to talk or to hear. Glen's balance was also affected, and he could no longer take part in the sports that he used to love – racquetball, hockey, volleyball – even swimming and golfing made him dizzy at times. This was a big change, as he was a phys-ed major and as a couple before we used to play a lot of sports or jog or hike together. I don't know if any of you have been on steroids, but the mood swings that one experiences, the change in metabolism, the weight gain, the change in body image – all of this contributed to a change in lifestyle. He tried so hard to continue with everything and to provide us with everything, but it took its toll. In the back of our minds we did not know how much longer Glen had left to hear, so our efforts became concentrated on making the most of business opportunities and getting things in order before he totally lost his hearing. Life became serious and focused on work.

I mentioned the children earlier, and their reaction to the decrease in hearing. It was very heart-warming at times watching them with their father, as they would help him in a crowd or protect him in a conversation. At other times you could sense their embarrassment or detachment. We all took sign language classes together, and before the implant we were relying on that a lot. I think that it was a big relief for Glen to have us in his world for a while and when everything clicked it was wonderful to be able to use just one sign to say so many words, but it was also frustrating because we were not all at the same level and sometimes, rather than talk or sign, there was silence. Again, this was very isolating for Glen. My experience as a nurse has shown me that often when there is a sickness or disability in the family, so much attention goes to the sick one that the development of the rest of the family is hampered or put on hold. Glen and I tried very hard to make sure that the children continued to take part in extracurricular activities and led as normal a life as possible. Were there occasional periods of anger, bitterness, depression, and self-pity? Of course! When you take your family's life and alter it midstream, lose your ability to pursue goals that you'd imagined you would, change your lifestyle or social activities and make some huge adjustments for the future, you're definitely going to feel the impact.

Sometimes I was angry at Glen because I thought that in some instances he could actually hear more than he let on and that sometimes his disability was a convenient excuse (similar to the men that you may know who pretend not to hear you hounding them to take out the garbage). Sometimes you just get tired of trying to be positive!

Fear comes into play as well, as you keep hoping that the hearing loss will stop or level off, but in the back of your mind you're wondering "What if it doesn't?" And you begin making plans for your life in case your partner is completely deaf. Looking back over those years the most predominant feeling I have is a sense of rising responsibility. By nature, like most women, I am a caregiver and used to try to take on the problems of all those around me. As Glen's hearing dropped I found that I was doing more and more to make it easier for him, making phone calls, setting up appointments, dealing with children's issues myself, encouraging them with sign language, doing more at home, and accompanying Glen to functions that he would normally have gone to alone. Because of my nursing background, of course, I was trying to solve the hearing problem and "play doctor." The autoimmune component was a big concern, and it was very frustrating at times to experience the health care system on the other side of the bed. Wellmeaning friends and relatives always had a new cure or herbal remedy as well and would often tell me instead of Glen or expect me to promote it.

When we moved to Fort McMurray I was planning on occasionally going into the convenience store to help out. As it turned out I ended up managing it. Glen managed the whole complex as I mentioned earlier and with his hearing decreasing, I took on more and more responsibility to try and take messages, relay information, make decisions, or even fill in for him. No one asked me to do it – I just decided that because that would be our main source of income if Glen were to go deaf, I would try to be a liaison between him and those he dealt with. The task, of course, was overwhelming. I was not really wired to be a manager. Glen and I really don't work that well together, and I couldn't devote all my energy to work because there were still three children at home. I finally reached a point where I said "God, I can't do this anymore." I say that in a sentence but it was something that built up over a three-year period during which I was exhausted, totally burnt out, and not really doing anything well.

Glen fired me, I went back to nursing, and our family doctor got us into the cochlear implant program. It took just seven months from his referral to the time that Glen could have his surgery and the rest is history. The difference has been amazing! Glen is now able to be totally independent and productive. I am in the profession that I should be, the children are maturing, Breanne graduates this spring and everything happens with such comparable ease. This is not to say that the same thing wouldn't have happened if we had become proficient at sign language and involved in the signing community. We are well aware of the fact that this has helped countless people around the world and if something should happen to Glen's implant we may be submerged in that culture again. Nor does it mean that we have only survived tough times – the whole experience has hopefully opened our eyes to the needs of others, made us more willing to help them, and challenged us as individuals to grow. We have also developed many strong friendships and become a close family unit as a result. In addition, there are many things to look back and laugh about. For now though – at the age that we are and with the mindset that we have – we are thoroughly enjoying this opportunity to continue in a hearing world again.

It is not very often that one gets a chance to get a sense back, and with something like hearing or eyesight, it has such far-reaching benefits. Our extended family, business partners, friends, and employees are sincerely grateful for the tremendous care, professionalism, knowledge, surgery and follow-ups offered to us by the whole implant team. You truly have made a difference! If there is one thing that you can take away from what we've said today it's 'DON'T GIVE UP HOPE!"

Keep trying new things. Keep asking for help, look for solutions, and do what you can to support each other and be healthy!

DEAFNESS MAY NOT BE A LIABILITY

Hello, everyone! My name is Glen Hommy and I am deaf (quickly attaches cochlear implant). Hello, my name is Glen Hommy and I can hear. Yes, it is that simple and it is beautiful!

Everyone should have the opportunity to experience deafness, only then can one experience the profound exhilaration of being able to hear, which hearing people only take for granted. There is an old saying that it is only when one experiences darkness that one can truly identify and appreciate daylight! Of course, this would only apply if you were as fortunate as I, who have experienced both deafness and hearing!

When I was asked to speak at this symposium I really didn't know what I could genuinely offer, other than a feel-fuzzy, feel-warm story about a middle-aging man who had gradually lost his hearing and through a series of trials and tribulations had miraculously recovered his hearing again with a cochlear implant.

Don't get me wrong, I am not undermining a feel-good story; indeed I am mighty thankful a thousand times over for my good fortune, but I want each of you to understand what it would be like not to hear, then just one day be able to hear again. It would sort of be like losing a loved one in an accident this afternoon and then having them return unexpectedly next week at your front door! Just imagine the rush that would be! Well, join me now, won't you, because that is how I had felt during that time when I was without hearin; I suffered my fair share of grief and despair. For those who hear…. Imagine ….the world of deafness…. Is it that bad, you wonder?….Not at all….And, I am sure, quite acceptable to those who have never been able to hear, but to us who have heard and then lost the ability, it can border on devastating, to say the least. It was to this world that I had traveled to, one of which brought along with it a feeling of hopelessness in my life.

But, it was also the best thing that ever happened to me on a personal basis. Let me explain. Deafness, inadvertently, made me a much, much better person. It has dramatically changed my life for the better!

The world of deafness…. What did it in actually do for me? First, it humbled me! I could count the ways, but it would take too long. Just trust me when I say, "Humility wasn't one of my strong suits prior to my deafness." Without humility, no one would be able to grow and flourish to one's fullest potential. In retrospect, I am sure one of the

258

factors that had helped bring on this humility was simply shear exhaustion....for, you see, lipreading, I would venture to say, has to be up there with the eco-challenges and the marathons. I would rather go for a swim in my winter parka than to try and communicate continually all day – every day by lipreading and writing notes back and forth. Being a businessman and working at getting through a day communicating from my deaf world was incredibly exhausting for me and, as well, by the people on the other side trying to communicate back to me.

Secondly, it taught me to listen. That's right. To listen...even though I could barely hear diddly squat. Out of desperation, I was forced and enticed to learn the art of listening to people....without my ears! If you really desperately want to communicate with someone and when you don't have much to work with, you use what resources you do have to help you out.

To begin with, I made time for people and I gave them my undivided attention. That was a good start in learning how to listen. Heck, all those years when I could hear I realized that I wasn't really listening to them at all. I had heard them, but I hadn't really listened to them.

While I was deaf the few words that I could pick up in a conversation I was now supplementing with my newly learned reading-people skills. Prior to this time, I had never quite appreciated the importance of learning to recognize and identify the body language which is so important in communication, and now I could practically communicate without hearing. For once in my lifetime, I was finally listening to what other people had to say to me. Needless to say, my wife is very thankful for this newly learned skill.

Last, but definitely not least, I got one heck of a lot closer to God. And this rekindled the strength that was required to conquer the fear, for it is fear that stymies healing and the feeling of hope!

Now, wouldn't you agree that all of these could be considered some very important intrinsic values that otherwise would not have been realized if one had not experienced deafness? These new-found values could be more appropriately considered "people" values but nonetheless hidden values gained from going deaf.

Now, how about other types of values, such as a financial value? Is there an intrinsic monetary value from going deaf, or would it simply be considered a liability? Warren Buffet, the famous stock investor, (who is worth some 40 or 50 billion dollars depending on where the market is on any given day), insists that one should never invest in a stock if there isn't an intrinsic value component. He claims a stock is only valuable if for some reason its intrinsic value is hidden, simply disguised, or has not yet metamorphosed into maturity and still unrecognized by the buying public. When this intrinsic value is identifiable and not properly accounted for in the stock price, one should buy and buy lots – for it only stands to reason that this intrinsic value is already the built-in profit. He has redefined the art of value investing.

What if I told you that there is a huge hidden financial value in cochlear implants and in the results that it can produce? That is right – profits. I have already told you about the intrinsic personal values that had made me a better person. Now, for the hidden financial value that needs to be identified, listen up now. I am talking real money and investments. Some of this money is yours. I'll tell you why in a second. As most of you already know, it is extremely difficult to make any profits if one doesn't invest and invest in the right things. I am not talking stocks and bonds....I am talking about investing in people, in my case "yours truly."

My cochlear implant, I understand, cost in the neighborhood of $50,000 so, how in the heck can one determine that this would be a financial investment instead of what looks like an obvious medical expense? This expense has been inherited by the government, consequently each and every one of us have participated to some degree in paying for this cost.

Let's examine where this financial value is....

Thankfully, I was chosen to be the recipient for this particular investment, which ultimately provided me with a cochlear implant and the opportunity to hear again. And I assure you that it was profitable!

For you see, after I was given the wonderful gift of a cochlear implant I was able to return to the world of hearing and I quickly regained a sense of hope! Remember the hopelessness I was referring to earlier? Well I was now making a 180 degree switchback turn and I surged with new business ideas and initiatives....."I was back!" I wanted to perform, and did I ever want to avenge the "deaf time" that I had spent in the business world! All those times when my lack of hearing had caused me to make many mistakes, ultimately causing a lot of unnecessary costs. I can honestly tell you that during many times in my initial stages of hearing loss, I would exit a business meeting not knowing any more than what I had before entering it. Can you believe it? I can laugh about it now, but on many occasions I bluffed my entire way through some of those meetings. You can imagine my idiocy. Hundreds of thousands of dollars at stake and I would just nod my head in approval of what someone was saying…..Yikes!!! As time progressed, I naturally came to realize that I needed allies to accompany me to these meetings. It was during these times when I was deaf that I came to depend on a lot of other people; many of them, very high priced. As well, many other people cared enough for me to go that extra mile knowing that I couldn't hear. Well, in many cases, they too had to be reimbursed for their extra time looking after my affairs. These "deaf times" cost my partners and me a lot of money.

Once my cochlear implant started hearing for me I became most interested again in my dreams and ambitions and I wanted to tackle the world again. My existing businesses grew, new ones were given a huge kick in the pants, and as a result economic productivity increased.

Any business depends on the people who run them. Businesses need people, and people need enthusiasm, direction, and the ongoing will to change. It takes leadership and leadership's energy…the very thing that fuels this initiative and ambition. These only coexist if there is even one person with a good dose of hope. This is what kick-starts the engines of any economy, large or small. The desire of individuals who have the dreams and ambitions to go forward!!!

I won….they won….It appears… everyone won!! Just because of the investment that was made in one person, that was me. Just think if we could keep making more investments in other deaf individuals, the government could have all kinds of surplus.

Money left to reinvest in more people who need cochlear implants. Consequently, more people would have hope and possibly our little personal manmade economies would prosper and contribute to the larger economies in our nation. Don't ever think that spending the money on a cochlear implant is a poor investment. I am living proof otherwise.

Before I conclude today, I want to take this personal opportunity to thank Dr. Oldring and his staff at the U of A for a splendid job performing my operation. Dr. Oldring had the foresight to proceed with my implant even though it may have been perceived to have an outside chance for success. Special thanks to Tracy Kruger and all of the people at the GlenRose Hospital for all their due diligence in making me a candidate for the program. They are a wonderful group of professionals! Of course, many thanks to Advanced Bionics for the fabulous technology that they have provided to the hearing industry. Also, I would like to thank Dr. O'Connor from Ft. McMurray for taking the extra personal time and demonstrating the persistence in opening the right doors for the implant program. As well, I would like to thank a special lady, Maryanne Banks from Calgary, who kept prodding my wife and me to push on with the cochlear implant initiative. And of course on the home front, my sincerest thanks to my beautiful, loving, and caring wife, without whom I wouldn't be where I am today. And naturally, I love and thank my kids as well, who were great…heck they actually were beginning to enjoy sign language. Also, many thanks to my extended family and friends who made special efforts to accommodate my deafness during some very difficult times for all of us….Thank you from the bottom of my heart! God bless you all, and I sincerely wish the best for each and every one of you in whatever role you may serve in life. Never, never lose hope, for it is the firepower one needs for tomorrow!

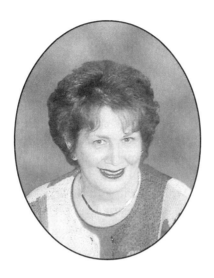

Yesterday and Today…By Carole Moravetz

Today I woke up with a feeling of anticipation. I have much to do today, and I am looking forward to it all. I teach school, and I am already planning my lessons in my head as I begin the morning routine of dressing for school. After school, I will need to stop by the printers and pick up the handouts I ordered for the private educational consulting business I own. I will barely have time to change into fresh clothes when I get home, as I am meeting a friend for dinner at a local restaurant. I make a mental note to call my friend and remind her to bring a book with her that I have wanted to read. I know I'll be pleasantly tired by the time I end my day with a quick chat with my daughter before I go to sleep. This sounds like a routine day to most people, but it never fails to excite me.

You see, I can have such a routine day because I can hear again. I have a cochlear implant, and it has re-opened the world to me. I lived in a world of silence for two years, when disease proved to be a thief that took my hearing from me. After living my life as a hearing person for all of my 43 years, I found myself lost in a world of silence. Each day was a challenge filled with loneliness and frustration. After having taught school for 20 years, I found myself unable to do so any longer. Along with my job went a lot of other essentials of my life, which I had previously taken for granted. The everyday activities, which had once kept me so busy quickly disappeared from my life, as I found myself unable to communicate effectively with those around me. Trying to constantly read lips well enough to understand the gist of a conversation left me so tired and frustrated that I quickly became something of a recluse. Watching my family suffer with me and because of me proved to be perhaps my heaviest burden. I have two lovely daughters who were used to a mom who was a carpool driver, a socializer, an organizer of fun and happy events. The limitations of my silent world made it difficult for me to organize much of anything. As days passed, and my world of silence seemed to be a permanent state, I found myself awakening each day with a feeling of dread. I tried my best to find things to do to keep myself constructively busy, but there were many days when the dark hole of depression grabbed me the moment I awoke and held me in its grasp all day.

Thankfully, I found a doctor at Emory University who believed that he could help me. He suggested to me that a cochlear implant would at least provide me with some improvement in my condition. After much thought and prayer, I decided to try it. I awoke this morning with a feeling of joy. Just thinking of all the routine activities waiting on me filled me with excitement. I reached, as I do every morning, for my speech processor, which will turn the world "on" for me. Over my ear. Attach the magnet. Click. *Sound!* Isn't it great?

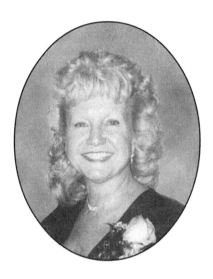

I've Got News for You...By Denise Kerns

"Go home. Write the 'Great American Novel.' And forget about trying to be a newspaper reporter." That was the "career advice" given me by an audiologist shortly after I was diagnosed with cochlear otosclerosis as a 21-year-old in 1970. I'd just graduated from college with degrees in English and journalism, and completed two summers as a newspaper intern, so news ink already was flowing in my blood. Needless to say, I was shocked for two reasons. My hearing loss had developed so gradually that no one suspected it until a chance test revealed its existence. And, for years, all I'd wanted to be was a reporter. I'd worked on my high school newspaper and served as editor of my college's newspaper for the past two years. Suddenly, my life seemed out of control.

Luckily, I also had a stubborn streak that my father always said I'd inherited from his parents, who were immigrants to this country from Germany. So, I decided, I *would* find some help for my hearing loss, and I *would* become a newspaper reporter. The latter turned out to be the easier of the two "jobs." I'd already proved my abilities through my summer internships at a local daily. My good luck returned strongly when the paper had an opening shortly after my graduation, and I was hired on a full-time basis.

Numerous visits to different doctors concerning my hearing loss, however, didn't offer me much hope. I was told I needed to start wearing a hearing aid, and to become reconciled to the fact that I'd probably lose even more of my hearing as the years went by. On the flip side, I found out, in a funny way, that I'd become an expert lip (speech) reader without being aware of that. One day, I was in the soundproof booth, working with an audiologist on the other side of the glass. My reactions to the "beeps" of the test were almost nonexistent. However, when he began to test my speech comprehension, I started doing pretty well. His expression grew more and more puzzled, until he suddenly snapped his fingers and left his side of the booth. He came back with a large square of cardboard to cover the window between us and began repeating the sentence comprehension tests. At that point, I became "lost" again, and my scores plummeted. When the audiologist asked if I knew I was reading his lips, I thought, at first, that he was accusing me of cheating! He laughingly explained that knowing how to read lips was a skill that would help me immensely in coping with my hearing loss.

His words and encouragement were prophetic. As my hearing loss progressed into my 30s, I began relying primarily on speechreading. By then, I was wearing two of the most powerful hearing aids available. However, they were of limited value, since I was medically classified as deaf in both ears by that time, with only residual hearing remaining. As my situation got worse, I learned of a wonderful organization, Self Help for Hard of Hearing People. A chapter had just been started in my hometown, and I eagerly contacted the founder to see if she or other group members could offer advice. My biggest problem at that time was getting up in the morning. (And I don't just mean not wanting to do that!) I couldn't find an alarm clock with a buzz or radio loud enough that I could hear. My husband traveled frequently, and my daughter was too small to realize the significance of the alarm clock sounding. And I worked for a newspaper, where every minute was vital in meeting that day's deadline.

The SHHH founder introduced me to the wonders of the bed shaker. The quality of my life – and my alertness during the day! – improved immediately. Who would have thought that such a small device could make such a difference? But that was my introduction to assistive devices and hearing technology outside hearing aids alone. Appreciative of the help of SHHH members, I became an active participant in the group myself and schooled myself on the devices and technology that were available for hearing impaired people. Therefore, I wasn't surprised when my doctor suggested, nearly 15 years ago, that I be evaluated as a candidate for a cochlear implant. The fact that I had residual hearing, however, and that my functional level was high with hearing aids disqualified me. That testing was repeated over the years, but I was turned down as a candidate twice more, the last time in 1997.

Meanwhile, my job and personal life continued to get harder as I struggled more and more with the stress of constant speechreading. I was fortunate to develop a love of computers that led me into editing jobs with the newspaper, so my hearing wasn't as critical any longer. However, I missed the interaction with other people that just wasn't possible for me in many situations. Some people were impossible to lip-read because of their facial hair, mannerisms that obscured their mouths, or just their failure to articulate well when they spoke. One of my favorite co-workers, for example, stuttered. We worked hard to understand each other, but trying to "read" his confusing speech took me months of efforts to accomplish.

Underlying everything during that period, too, was the fear that some-day I'd lose the last little bit of residual hearing I had and be relegated to silence for the rest of my life. Still, I was determined to do my best to prepare for and learn to accept the inevitable. When I was about to turn 50, my sister and I enrolled in a sign language class, so that I could learn another method of communication for my "silent years." Before the class started, however, I was in for another shock.

What happened next was one of the wonders of my life. On a routine visit to my hearing specialist, Dr. Brad Thediner, in Kansas City – an appointment I almost put off, but didn't, at the urging of my sister – he again suggested that I be evaluated as a cochlear implant candidate. Because I had so much respect for Dr. Thedinger, I went in for a consultation, as he'd suggested, but I told my sister, "This will be a waste of time. I've been turned down before, and my hearing hasn't changed." Both my sister and I were shocked when we were told I was a borderline candidate for an implant then, in 1999, not because my hearing had changed, but because the technology was improving by mountainous leaps. We wound up spending four hours with an audiologist at Midwest Ear Institute in Kansas City, asking her so many questions that she said we were "keeping her on her toes" with all our queries. The devices made by the three implant companies were shown to us, and the various features of each were explained. Then, I was sent home to start my insurance process and to make the decision of whether or not I wanted a cochlear implant and, if so, which device I wanted to have implanted.

What followed was a period where I spent nearly every waking minute away from work exploring the Internet, writing letters, and e-mailing and meeting other implant users. The things they shared with me were exciting. They told me of being able to hear speech again without lipreading and being able to use the phone without assistive devices, for example. I figured they probably were luckier than I'd be. I just couldn't believe those things would be possible for me after all the years I'd been deaf. But I decided that I probably could hope to regain some environmental sounds I'd lost over the years, like the ringing of the phone, the chiming of the doorbell, and the blinking of car turn signals.

Because I was getting more and better information from Advanced Bionics about the Clarion device – and because I was impressed by the reports of the advanced technology it was providing – I began leaning toward that choice. Then, I was told I could participate in field trials for the HiFocus device that was just beginning to be used at that time, so my choice of Clarion was cemented. I told my doctor my decision and asked him to schedule my surgery.

October 18, 1999, was the beginning of my "great adventure." My surgery went without a problem, my doctor saved a "fringe of hair" in front of my surgical site, and I went home looking pretty much as I always did. It was almost disappointing that there weren't many outward signs of the big step I'd taken.

Since my expectations were pretty modest and the loss of the already poor hearing in my implanted ear didn't affect me much, I was able to get through the four-week wait for my surgical site to heal without much nervousness. I experienced a little dizziness the first few days after my surgery and a feeling of tightness in my scalp due to the swelling. Otherwise, it was basically "life as usual" during that time. Deadlines at work also kept me so busy that I didn't have time to anticipate or imagine what might be in store for me on my "hook-up" date.

The newspaper I worked for wrote an article about my cochlear implant, so the day I was to get my processor on November 17, 1999, I was accompanied not only by family and friends, but by a reporter and photographer, as well. We all crowded into the office where the audiologist, Barbara Luikhart, was to "turn on" my implant for the first time.

When I was given my processor and connected to the computer, I began hearing high-pitched, LOUD noises, but I didn't think I was making much sense of them. As I talked with Barbara, I saw her give me a "look" before she got up and stepped out of the room. With a sense of déjà vu, I saw her return with what looked like a big embroidery hoop covered with black felt. She held it in front of her face, and I thought all was lost, like my earlier failure when I couldn't see the audiologist and, therefore, couldn't read lips.

This time, however, I was getting every word! The photographer snapped a photo in that instant when my face lit up and my fingers curled into a fist of triumph. I REALLY COULD HEAR! The shock swept over me and continued to shake me in the days and weeks that followed. Not only could I hear the phone ring, the birds sing, and other environmental sounds, but I could initiate conversations with strangers in stores and make my own telephone calls to reach friends or make appointments. One day, I even gathered the courage to find out if I could get a cell phone. When I went to the store to explain my situation, I found the young staff there fascinated by *my own* technology. They were delighted to experiment with me to see if the phone and I were compatible, and we hit it right off! I was experiencing the many freedoms that "hearing" people take for granted. I could drive to nearby Kansas City and call my daughter with my cell phone to let her know I was in town and to arrange a quick get-together or more leisurely lunch or supper. I could let people expecting me know if I got tied up in heavy traffic or delayed for other reasons.

Perhaps the two biggest "gifts" I've received from my cochlear implant are the reduction of stress in my life and the realization that I no longer have to fear that my hearing will get worse as I get older. In fact, I'm experiencing improved hearing each day, as I learn to work with implant equipment and re-learn to hear and understand speech and other sounds.

I'm reminded of a story about Helen Keller, who once was asked whether she considered her blindness or deafness her greatest handicap. Without hesitation, the story goes, she cited her deafness. Blindness divides you from things, she's reported to have said, but deafness divides you from people.

Restored hearing isn't just about recognizing sounds again and being able to function better. It's about becoming a full member of society, which is geared toward hearing. I find myself driving out of my way now to listen to the announcer talk on my car's radio. And I had to chuckle when one of the first commercials I could hear was promoting Viagra. Every morning on my way to work, it seemed to be repeated.

"Hearing" people, no doubt, would consider that a nuisance message, but it made me laugh each morning that I was able to get that "vital news" at last!

And I had to learn the etiquette of not eavesdropping on other conversations. At first I was so intent on "practicing" my new hearing skills that I realized that might be interpreted as just being nosey. (Well, maybe it *was* some of both.) Most of all, I've met wonderful people who also have cochlear implants. They all seem to have a delicious sense of humor (developed as a necessity from years of dealing with hearing loss?) and a wondrous and child-like joy in being able to hear, something taken for granted by most people on the planet. Their appreciation of the day-to-day miracles of life is infectious.

Since my own implant, I've retired from my job and begun working as a volunteer mentor for other implant candidates and giving talks to the general public about implants. None of my friends or family members believed that I could walk away from my obsession with newspapers, but I've found a new love in working to educate the public that cochlear implants are available – and that they're bringing daily miracles to deaf and hearing impaired people.

Often, one of the first things I'll say to a new acquaintance is, "I have a cochlear implant. Do you know what that is?" The answer, too often, is "No." But volunteers like me are working to help change that situation. The doctors, audiologists and other medical professionals can perform the miracles, but we 'implantees' can help them by telling people our own success stories. That's now my "calling," now as I've begun life all over again as someone who enjoys the symphony of sounds that is everyday existence. "Amazing grace! How sweet the sound...."

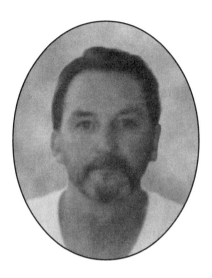

The Last Call...By Jerry May

My name is Jerry May and I used to be a firefighter for the State of Mississippi. My job as a firefighter related mostly to aircraft emergencies along with some structural firefighting. On the morning of June 1, 1996, I was riding as captain on the rescue truck when we were alerted to an in-flight emergency on a KC-135 aircraft used by the military. My job as captain was to gain access to the aircraft along with two other firefighters. We were to remove all personnel as quickly as possible to safety. We placed a 20-foot extension ladder on the wing and entered the door hatch of the plane. Upon entering the aircraft, we went to the cockpit to help remove the pilot, copilot, and flight navigator to safety. We assisted each one out the door and over the wing. By this time, other fire personnel had entered the aircraft and determined there was no fire hazard to be found. The "emergency" was actually a timed egress to see how we performed our duties in a certain time frame.

As captain, I was the last person to leave the aircraft. I had to make sure all power, doors, and anything else were shut down. I exited the aircraft onto the top of the wing and closed the door hatch. I then asked one of the other firemen to foot the ladder, as the top of the wing is approximately 20 feet high. I was headed toward the ladder to get

271

off the wing when it happened. I still can't remember what, or how, but I fell face first onto the concrete ramp. I was wearing full turnout gear with an air-pack on my back. The turnout gear along with the air-pack weighs an additional 50 pounds. This happened on a Saturday morning. I didn't remember anything until the next week when I woke up in the hospital intensive care unit. It was the strangest feeling I have ever experienced, because of the deep silence from lack of sound. My wife, Virginia, wrote several notes saying that I had been in a serious accident and that I had had surgery on my wrists and my face. She wrote that my injuries included fractures to the temporal bones inside my head. I had spinal fluid leaking out my ear that the doctor thought would go away in a few days and then I would regain my hearing. But the nerves that controlled my hearing and balance were damaged so badly that it never came back. In addition to these injuries, I had shattered the bones in both wrists. Obviously I had tried to use my wrists to break my fall before I hit the concrete. I had facial injuries to both eyes and my jaw. I dislocated my right hip, which has caused a lot of lower back pain since the accident.

As for my hearing loss, the doctors in the hospital in Meridian said it would probably only be temporary and for me not to worry about it. But after several days when it did not come back, and the spinal fluid leak did not stop, the doctor felt that I should be sent to a specialist in Jackson, MS. I was in so much pain that I did not realize the fluid leaking was spinal fluid. I was told that if they could not stop the leaking, I could get an infection and could die from spinal meningitis.

I was soon introduced to Dr. James House who would be handling my case. He explained to my wife that he would do some tests to determine what type of surgery was needed. He decided to do surgery the following morning, which was on Saturday. He was going to remove tissue from my stomach and use it to completely close off my left ear canal. This would stop the spinal fluid leak and reduce the risk of infection. He left the right ear canal open. He later stated that most people with temporal bone fractures do not live to get better. But God had other plans for me, the surgery was successful and the leaking stopped. He had told me that I would lose the hearing in my left ear and might retain about twenty percent in my right ear. Imagine how I felt when I learned that my world had gone from a normal lifestyle with a good career to losing so much in such a short time.

While in the hospital in Jackson, I also had to have additional surgery on both wrists due to complications from the first surgery in Meridian. I saw a doctor who specialized in wrists and he installed metal plates with external fixators to mobilize my hands and wrists. After all of these surgeries, the reality of being deaf began to set in. I was worried what the future held for me. After two long weeks, I was released from the hospital to go home. My wife, friends, and co-workers communicated with me through written notes. It was very frustrating for me to try to communicate with the outside world. I tried several different hearing aids but none seemed to help very much. Over the next few months, what little hearing I had left got worse and worse. I became very depressed about my life. I had lost a job I dearly loved. My two youngest children, David and Rachel, were age three years and one year at the time, and were beginning to do a lot of talking. They could not understand why I could no longer hear what they said. I never heard Rachel say her first words. My oldest son, Brian, was about to get married, and, even though I was able to attend his wedding, I was unable to hear any of the ceremony. I have always believed in God and had faith in him, but I was overwhelmed by my circumstances.

On one of my follow-up visits to Dr. House in Jackson, he mentioned that maybe I would be a good candidate for a cochlear implant on my right ear. The mention of an implant to me was surprising because I never figured on having some type of medical equipment implanted inside my body. After further discussing this with my wife, I concluded that if there was the slightest chance that I could hear again then I wanted to be a part of the hearing world again. Even though Dr. House could do the implant surgery and follow-up visits in Jackson, I wanted to go somewhere that was well known for that type of operation; I wanted a second opinion as well. My nurse/case manager, Lynn Love, put us in touch with the Shea Clinic in Memphis, TN. We contacted the clinic and set up an appointment with Dr. John Shea II to consult with him about the implant. He examined me and determined that I was indeed a candidate for the cochlear implant. He recommended the Med-El implant. I decided to go ahead with the procedure.

On February 1997 at Baptist Memorial Hospital in Memphis, TN, Dr. Shea performed the surgery. The surgery went very well although the incision was more than I anticipated. After the five-week waiting period had passed, my implant was "turned on" at the clinic. My audiologist in Memphis, Elizabeth Domico, was excellent at her job of programming the implant. When the moment of truth came, I could actually hear some sounds. It was a great step toward improving my life back to a way I had lived with for 44 years. At first, when it was turned on, I could only make out a few sounds. It took some time for me to get used to the implant. Elizabeth told me that as time went by I would gain more and more understanding through the implant.

I have now been wearing the implant for almost five years and it really has enhanced my way of life. I can understand a lot of different sounds and can make out some speech when I am in a good environment for hearing such as a one-on-one conversation. I am blessed to have been able to receive the implant. The wearing of the implant helps to mask the loud ringing in my ears, which I have had since my accident. I have to be honest, though- the implant is nothing close to normal hearing. The nerve damage was so severe that I don't get as much sound as other implant patients. I have had some classes in lipreading. This along with the implant helps me to make out some sound and conversation if there is not a lot of background noise. To me it is much better than the constant ringing in my ears.

I have been fortunate to have a family who has been very supportive of me throughout this ordeal. My wife, Virginia, and my three children, David, Rachel, and Brian, along with his wife Susan, have all learned to speak slowly and clearly so that I can understand them better. Last spring, I was blessed to become a grandparent to twins, Bonnie and Joey, who were born to my son and daughter-in-law, Brian and Susan. With the help of this implant, I hope to soon be able to hear them say, "I love you Papa." I am now wearing the behind-the-ear device, and it is so simple and easy to handle that I can hardly tell I am wearing anything. If you are profoundly hearing-impaired you should find out whether you may be a candidate for the cochlear implant. I have lived on both sides, the hearing world and the world of silence, and the hearing world has so many more advantages. I want to thank the people at the Med-El Corporation for their work on this device. The implant has helped me recover a part of my life that I had once known.

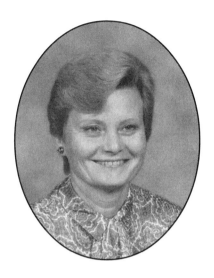

I'm Back!…By Elinore Bullock

"You won't be needing this anymore, " said the nurse as she wheeled the television set from my hospital room. She was angry with me for having turned up the volume too much and disturbing other patients. These words concluded a long scolding about my lack of consideration for others. During this scolding, she let it be known that "You won't be able to hear at all very soon, so get used to it." This nurse was not the norm, of course, but I had been unlucky enough to draw a mean-spirited one that day.

I was 14 years old and had been in the hospital for about three months fighting meningitis. Although I had watched my six-year-old roommate, Patty, change from a sunny, talkative child into a silent, sullen shadow of herself, and should have recognized the symptoms of oncoming deafness, I didn't think such a thing could happen to me. The nurse's cold announcement was the first I'd heard that deafness was a part of my prognosis, and everybody knew it but me.

When I couldn't hear the television as well as I had the day before, I assumed the volume control had been turned back somehow. I turned it up a little, but it didn't help. I turned it up a little more, and brought the wrath of this nurse upon my unsuspecting shoulders. Her parting words were numbing. She had flung them over her shoulder in anger, leaving me to cope with them alone and afraid. I felt I had turned to stone! The horror of her announcement was numbing. What could I do? There was no choice in the matter; I cried. I never felt so helpless and alone in my life before or since. Her words were painfully accurate. The scene with the television set happened in early August 1951, and by the end of that month I was profoundly deaf. I didn't have a clue about lip-reading or sign language, and I didn't want to. I just wanted this mistake, as I thought of it, to right itself.

Upon my discharge from the hospital, I asked the doctor, "When will I get my hearing back?" Very slowly he told this naïve 14-year-old, "Elinore, you will never hear again." "I'm not supposed to be deaf," I kept thinking. "This is a nightmare and I just need to wake up." It took me 42 years, and lots of help from Advanced Bionics, to awaken from that nightmare. During that time I did not use hearing aids except for a few short trial periods that usually ended with frustration. Everyone but me would hear the feedback from the hearing aid, and the ear mold caused discomfort.

When the implant re-introduced me to sound, it came as quite a jolt to my brain. It had become complacent and lazy during its long years of sound deprivation and it was reluctant to wake up and smell the coffee. "Go away!" it said to sound. "Don't expect ME to help you!" Although I could hear sounds, it was a whole other thing to learn to make sense of them.

My awakening began the day my cochlear implant was hooked up in December 1993. It happened at the exact moment I realized that the strange "buzzing" in my ear coincided exactly with my audiologist's lip movements. "It's you!" I said, pointing at her. "That sound is coming from you!" My husband of 34 years smiled, too. And he said those three little words that I had never heard him say before.

I had been implanted with the Clarion 1.0, but later I was able to upgrade my processor to the Clarion 1.2, which I still have. Although better implants have developed since then, I am content with all the 1.2 does for me. I feel as though I have lived three different lives: the one I enjoyed as a child with perfect hearing, the years of profound silence and isolation, and, best of all, the life I'm living now: the adventurous years of recovery, re-learning the fine art of hearing and understanding.

It's an exciting, ongoing process with a new audiological delight every day, even after eight years. Each day brings the thrill of a new sound, or the sudden recognition of a sound that I'd been unable to identify. This business of learning to hear again, after 42 years of sound

276

deprivation, is hard work, but it's also more rewarding than hard work has any right to be. I'm filled with anticipation each morning. What will the sound be today?

Today's new sound turned out to be a rhythmic knocking noise. Since I was sitting outside, I knew it wasn't someone at the door. I couldn't imagine what that sound could be, and had to ask my husband. "It's a woodpecker! A block away woodpecker! My thrill for the day! To think that not so long ago I wouldn't have heard a fire engine bearing down on me and now I'm hearing block-away woodpeckers!

Deafness, for me, was a total, cottony, empty-headed feeling, a feeling of isolation, of being almost invisible to the hearing people I lived with, of being an alien. I felt my intellect had shriveled, along with my personality and my ability to be the person I was meant to be. For me, the worst thing about being deaf was the loneliness, and the second worst thing was being mistaken for someone of limited ability and intelligence. Overshadowing those things was that ever-present, nagging feeling that I must wake up from this!

Six years after I lost my hearing, I met the man who would become my husband. He had normal hearing and was just finishing up his college studies. A very fine fellow, Jack was! For some reason he took an interest in me. Shortly after we met, as we were sitting together in my family home, Jack took my hand, faced me squarely, and said, "If ever, if at any time, ever, you do not understand me, I want you to tell me, and I will repeat it." Those were his exact words, just as I lipread them, just, as I will remember them for the rest of my life. The sincerity on his face was unmistakable as he made me promise to do this. No one had ever said this to me before! That's when I knew he was special. He understood.

Of course I had that guilty feeling that I shouldn't let myself into this man's life, to subject him to all those everyday limitations, irritations, and struggles that can so easily dampen a person's spirit. He had normal hearing, and he shouldn't have to put up with this pain and I should butt out of his life and be quick about it. That's hard to do when you love someone, though, especially when you're 20 years old. It didn't help that he kept turning up on my doorstep, either. And so we were married in September 1959. We're about to celebrate our 42 anniversary.

It was hard being the only deaf person in the family, but Jack's love and patience, my own stoicism and cheerful nature, our children's quick grasp and adaptation to the situation all worked together to provide a stable and happy life for us all. The children answered the phone for me, helped me out with store clerks when necessary, all with matter-of-factness and cheerfulness, an acceptance that "this is how it is, is all!" Jack overheard one remark by our four-year-old son who answered the phone for me one day. "My mommy can't come to the phone," said little Johnny, "she's death!"

There were less funny times though, those times when deafness could be a real pain for both of us. We had a sailboat that we raced on Sunday afternoons for many years. It was necessary for Jack, as skipper, to bark out commands to me, the mate. "Tighten the jib!" he would yell, or maybe "Lower the board!" Or, worst of all, "Coming about!" (Which means "duck!") I never heard any of these commands, and they needed absolute immediate compliance. Failure to act quickly could result in the boat capsizing or a painful whack on the head from the boom, not to mention coming in last over the finish line. Imagine how hard it was for me to understand unheard commands, to lipread from the heaving bow, where I might be, while he was manning the tiller at the stern! The boat would also be listing to one side, and forging its way through a surging sea. He had to bang on the boat's side to get my attention first, and then hope to heaven I would understand his orders. There was no time to say "What?" After a while, of course, I learned to anticipate what he would say, but there were always surprises I wasn't expecting. We rarely won these sailing races, but we never came in last either, usually crossing the finish line in the middle of the pack. We learned to be content with that, but it took time.

Being surrounded by hearing people meant I was always the odd one out. Attending dinners and other functions were painful and sometimes even humiliating. Holiday dinners at home with extended family were not the occasions of joy for me that they were for the others. I felt rather like the waitress, the invisible one most of the time. I didn't want my problem to affect the pleasure of others, so just quietly shrank into the background. Not the best attitude, I know, but then that's me.

Having known normal hearing, I never considered that I belonged to the deaf world and should seek it out. I thought, spoke, and acted like a hearing person in my own mind. Blessedly, a loving family surrounded me. And there was Caroline, next door, who was always there for me to make emergency phone calls, to field calls that came from the children's school when they were sick, to let me know there was a hurricane coming! I found ways to enjoy myself in my isolation. When the family watched television, I would read. Captions were still a long way off during those early family years, not appearing until about 30 years after I lost my hearing. Although living in silence was hard for me, I had my loving family to be grateful for. Jack and I raised two fine people, and we are proud of them. Both grew up to become respected in their chosen fields. Linda is an audiologist/speech pathologist working with mainstreaming hearing-impaired children in her local school system. (Where was she when I needed her?) John is a college chemistry professor, who now grasps the difference between death and deaf.

As I look back on those years of deafness, I sometimes feel immeasurably sad for the lost years. I feel as though those years went down the drain. But I find solace in the realization that I have so very much to be grateful for. I cannot remain sad for long. With the implant, gratitude is the theme of each day. Maybe without those long years of silence, I would take the sounds of life for granted and be unable to fully feel the joy of my husband's voice, our grandchildren's chatter, the cardinal's trill, the industrious woodpecker. After 42 years of silence, my brain is slowly accepting and understanding sounds that are new to me. It's almost like being a baby and learning what life is all about. It is such an exciting process!

I'm making up for lost time, joining committees that I never would have before, even becoming a chair. I get such a big kick of knowing when there is an opening in the conversation and being able to inject my thoughts into a discussion in my own natural way, feeling confident that I'm not interrupting, that my comments have not just been said by someone else, getting that look of respect and acceptance that I missed for so long. Each step of growth, or reaching out, leads to another. I can actually feel the self-esteem growing! It squares my shoulders and makes me feel tall!

The telephone presents a challenge. I am a bit afraid of it because it denies me the lipreading option that my stubborn brain still seems to need. I find the phone a bit intimidating, and I know I must get over that. I can hear the other person clearly, but just can't understand what is being said. I'm sure I will one day if I keep trying. I know this because it feels so close to happening now.

In the meantime, I've begun to listen to audio books over the phone. Jack will set the mouthpiece by the tape player, then ring me up on the other phone. When I answer my phone, he starts the tape, and I plug in my processor to the phone and just read along with the tape. I feel that this is a good way to acclimate my brain to phone sound. Although I still feel the need to lipread, I strongly suspect that I have an unconscious fear of letting go of my lifelong habit of "listening" visually, and that if

I could overcome this I could understand speech by sound alone. I'm working on that, but in the meantime, I have no difficulty keeping up with conversation in quiet situations. In restaurants, I rely on the auxiliary microphone, passing the mike end to my husband under the table. He attaches it to his collar and forgets about it. It enables me to hear his every word despite the noise around us. My audiologist has given me a "noisy situation program," and it works with the mike like a charm. I can even hear the waitress and speak for myself, thank you! I attend large conferences, another thing I never would have considered before the implant. FM or infrared systems plugged into the processor with a patch cord enable me to keep up with the proceedings nicely.

Music makes me so happy! Usually. I love the piano, especially George Winston's album, *The Forest.* The golden oldies from the late 40s sound good, because my memory fills in the gaps and distortions without thinking about it. You should see me light up at the sound of *Oklahoma*! I can hardly sit still!

I have a little Sony device, a gadget intended for use with video cameras. On Sunday morning I arrive at church a little early and place the transmitter on the pulpit. When I plug the receiver into my processor, it allows the pastor's words to come directly to my ear, eliminating the echoes that normally make hearing in church so difficult. When it comes time for music, I just unplug my end of the device and listen with the head microphone. I'll be honest with you and confess that I can do without the organ, but my gratitude still swells to a peak on Sundays!

I'm reaching out in many directions both to enrich my own life and to be of service to others. For the past two years, I served as president of the Association of Late-Deafened Adults-Garden State, and am almost as busy now serving as Past President. I attend state council meetings dealing with matters of concern to deaf and hard of hearing people, and I'm on a committee seeking new ways to make life for deaf people better in New Jersey, such as increased theater access and hospital sensitivity training. At church, I not only join committees now, and attend meetings with pleasure, but I have also become the head deacon! For fun, I have just joined a quilting group, a group where everyone else can hear! I feel so alive, so free, so capable, so whole, and so grateful!

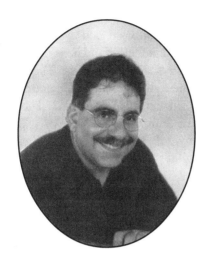

Back from the Silence…By Jay Bernstein

At 1:00 pm on April 24, 2001, after almost 40 years I removed my hearing aid for the last time. About 59 minutes later, after my audiologist, Betsy Bromberg, mapped and programmed my new processor, she turned it on. If I am blessed to live another 40 years, I *will* never forget what came next.

A sensation of sounds roared into my brain and rose into a rather high-pitched Donald Duck-like sound of "Jay, can you hear me?" For those of you old enough to remember, I thought of the Rock opera *Tommy,* performed by the Who and the line "Tommy, can you hear me?" Yes, I heard her and with clarity I never knew existed. After walking back to the train station, I was overwhelmed by the amount of sounds in the world that had come alive all around me. It was impossible to sort them out and I realized the doctor's words had become true. The surgery is the easy part. The real work begins as your brain has to relearn all the sounds. I sat in the train wondering how I was going to do this, everybody talking so loud into their cell phones, the loud speaker blaring, the guy in the next car with a boom box playing something funky, the train engine. Through all this noise, I unzip my briefcase to get to my laptop and I hear, crystal clearly, "zziiiippp." The zipper zips! It actually makes a zipping noise! So there I was sitting on the train, going back and forth with the zipper, zip-zip, zip-zip, zip-zip, zip-zip. How is that possible? The train is moving, and I hear the conductor enter the car from opposite end. 'Tickets, please." The conductor works his way through the car and he is now up to me. "Tickets please." I smile and he says "Fairfield, right?" he recognizes me as a regular as I have rode the train for eight years and never understood a word he said. I reply, " Do you always say this?" The conductor smiles, "Not if you're going to Stamford."

When I got home my wife and children were anxious to have their voices heard. All the voices were very odd yet I understood the words. My youngest, Laura, led me on a discovery of new sounds throughout the house. "Daddy, this is the doorbell, Daddy this is the refrigerator motor, this is my ducky, quack, quack." She gets her older sister "Katie, burp for Dad.".... One of her rare and many talents. The best moment was when Laura turned around with her back to me and said, "Daddy you can't read my lips. What am I saying? Daddy, you are the best daddy a kid could ever have." I heard every word, she then turned around and pronounced, "Dad, everything is fine now," and ran off to find her sister.

I have a special adaptor for the telephone. It's a wire that plugs the phone into the speech processor. I called my Mom and had a five-minute telephone conversation with her for the first time in nearly 10 years. It was not the best sound quality, there was still so much to learn, but it was great just the same. The TV was too much, as it was a long first day.

The second day, I returned to the audiologist and had more programming done. The voices were still very strange but I got a noise reduction program that cut out a lot of the unnecessary background. It also reduced the pitch of the voices. I was anxious to try this out, so I stopped by my office to see everyone. The elevator dinged between floors. "Ding." "Ding." This is wondrous for about 10 floors, after 15 it could be annoying. Everyone was talking at once. I heard the "whoosh" of the air conditioner vent in the hallway, too loud; I had to shut my door, then made another discovery. My computer mouse went "click." I never knew that. I felt the click before, but I never knew it produced a "clicking" sound. Awesome!

I took my family out to dinner Thursday night. I listened to a conversation between my wife and Katie all the way over, something I had never been able to do while driving. During dinner, the waitress mumbled something my wife did not understand. I said, "She wants to know what kind of dressing you want on your salad." The next morning I was up early at the crack of dawn, as I have a 9 a.m. meeting in New York. We live out in the country next to protected wetlands filled with birds. That morning I could hear them all calling. It was like a symphony. I almost missed the train as I could not get over the beauty of the birdcalls. I listened to the AM radio in my car on the way home. The announcer was talking about the weather, and I couldn't believe I understood every word and number.

It was an amazing first few days. I no longer consider myself deaf. I like that I have enjoyed a successful career as a sales executive, overcoming all the odds and rising to the top of my field. People are constantly amazed that I have accomplished so much without really hearing. My CI has given me so many more options that it feels like I can start over. I do not have to sit quietly and fear a conversation. I intend to do great things. After all, I have received the gift of hearing and am silent no more.

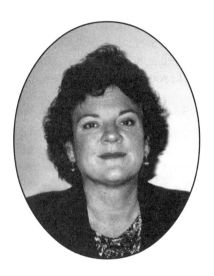

Life is Good…By Kim Afana

My hearing loss started at about the age of 18. I'm never quite sure exactly how old I was because I didn't commit the date to memory. I discovered I had a problem with my hearing, as I noticed I had been using the phone consistently with the left ear. In the past I had almost exclusively used the right ear to talk on the phone. When I held the phone up to my right ear, I could not even detect the dial tone. This was the beginning of a very long journey.

Later it was determined that my hearing loss was caused from exposure to loud noise after attending one rock concert. People always ask me what group was playing, but it doesn't really matter. I probably would have suffered the loss regardless of who was performing. And, yes, I was close to the speakers for half of the concert, but so were my friends who did not walk away with a hearing loss. My ears were ringing the next day and when I asked my doctor about this, he informed me that the ringing should subside within a month. The ringing did stop almost exactly 30 days after it began, but my hearing never returned to normal.

During my first visit to an ENT, I was told I had a 75% hearing loss in the right ear and a 25% hearing loss in the left ear. The diagnosis was Rock Concert Syndrome. I really don't know much about the diagnosis other than the doctor told me that Keith Moon, from the rock band The Who, suffered from the same type of loss. He told me nothing could be done to help me and sent me on my way. No mention was ever made of a follow-up appointment or hearing aids. Thinking back on this now, I realize I probably should have returned for an annual re-evaluation.

This initial loss happened at a time in my life when I was very busy with college and work. In all ways I functioned normally. I could participate in normal conversations and use the phone. I do remember paying close attention to the faces of persons speaking, such as college professors, so maybe I was coping with my loss on some level that I was not aware of.

In 1983, I graduated from college with honors and began working in my selected field of Information Management. Originally, I had planned to attend law school with dreams of someday serving in the U.S. Senate. At some point, I considered my hearing loss and how it would impact this type of future. I don't think my hearing loss was the deciding factor in whether to attend law school or not, though.

As a single professional, I spent many evenings going out with groups from work. I was always careful to wear earplugs if we went some place loud even though the earplugs were kind of embarrassing. Considering the alternative of my hearing being further damaged, I took precautions to protect myself.

At 24, I took a new job in my hometown and got married. Part of my employment required a physical. During the physical I told the doctor about my hearing loss, but since it was expected to remain stable, and because I was able to converse normally on the phone and in person, my hearing loss was not an issue.

When I was 28 and six months pregnant, my husband and I got into a terrible argument. The next day I noticed ringing in my ears which still persists today. My hearing began to deteriorate rapidly and I went to see another ENT. This time, the audiologist tried to fit me with hearing aids. By the time the aid on the right ear was loud enough to detect sensation but not sound, I nearly passed out from the dizziness. The left ear was more cooperative, so we decided on crossover aids that would at least let me detect sounds on my right side.

By the time my son was born, three months later, I couldn't comprehend very much even with the hearing aid. Additional tests were run and I was diagnosed with tinnitus and Meniere's disease. The ENT also suspected that I had something wrong with my autoimunune system and referred me to Dr. Brian McCabe at the University of Iowa in 1990. In Iowa, I learned about cochlear implants but was told I would not qualify to be implanted. I asked for literature about the devices anyway so I could learn more. I remember being upset about the fact that the surgery was restricted to one ear only. After all, I had a problem with both ears and I knew what it was like to have normal hearing. I wasn't willing to settle for anything less than having both ears fixed.

Hearing with only one ear was very bothersome. I found my life centering on the position my left ear was relative to every sound in my life. When walking with friends I would always shuffle around them to get my left ear facing them. Even while sleeping I somehow thought I could protect my remaining hearing by sleeping with my left ear in the pillow. I realize this seems silly now, but there are still times I find my neck twisted uncomfortably to the left in an effort to protect that ear.

The test results from Iowa were positive and I was diagnosed with autoimmune sensorineural hearing loss. This was determined by the results of a blood test called the Western Blot. Miscommunication between Iowa, my local ENT, and me resulted in my not knowing the results of this test for over two years. Dr. McCabe finally contacted me directly and asked why I had never started the recommended treatment. At the end of the one-year treatment Dr. McCabe wrote me to tell me I could halt the treatment since no changes were noted. I continued having my hearing tested regularly. Then one day a new audiologist in the ENT's office tested my hearing and told me my hearing had dropped dramatically. I had not noticed any changes and communicated this to Dr. McCabe. He told me that my hearing had been reported as being better than it had been in many years and he thought it was from the treatment. I was completely shocked. I told him if my hearing had taken such a dramatic nosedive, I would have noticed it.

Dr. McCabe contacted me again and recommended I switch ENTs and audiologists. He even provided me with names of ENTs in my city and their educational backgrounds. For this, I will be forever grateful. This was quite possibly the first step in the right direction. The new audiologist tested me and still did not think my hearing was poor enough for a cochlear implant. Once you've had several audiological examinations, you can pretty well guess the test ahead of time. Cowboy, airplane, and ice cream are all words the hearing impaired population is familiar with. I think we do ourselves a disservice by guessing at the words sometimes. It would probably be beneficial for the tests given in the soundproof booths to be changed frequently and for the audiologist to remain out of view. Still, I was able to convince both the audiologist and the ENT to refer me to Iowa for a cochlear implant evaluation.

I think it is important to point out that, for a period of about six years, I was extremely depressed. I wrote poetry that was very dark and probably bordered on suicidal. If there were one piece of advice that I could emphasize to every person in the medical profession, it would be this: Any type of loss requires a grieving period. It also requires acceptance and learning to cope. The patient may not necessarily recognize this. The best tools that a medical professional can provide to the patient include education on their affliction, what to expect in the future, and a referral to a good therapist.

I returned to the University of Iowa where I was evaluated for a cochlear implant. My test scores were 0% across the board. Because of the history of my hearing loss, I was asked if I would consider participating in a study for bilateral implantation. Participants in the study had to be 18 years of age or older, post-lingually deafened, and have a different type of hearing loss in each ear that occurred at different times.

My evaluation was in January of 1997. The hospital was just beginning the paperwork for the required FDA approval for the study. I contacted Iowa about once a month to see if they had received approval yet. Mary, my audiologist, and soon to be dear friend, wrote me to tell me I didn't have to wait. She suggested that I go ahead and have one ear implanted. But I wanted both ears done and opted to wait.

Eleven months after learning of the project, I was implanted. My sister traveled with me the 415 miles to Iowa. We arrived on December 10, 1997, and my surgery was scheduled for December 12. One piece of information I learned when we arrived was that my head was to be completely shaved. They thought this would be better than having a Mohawk hairdo. The idea of being bald bothered me a little bit at first, but I was not really offered an alternative. Now they usually just shave a portion above the ear that is hidden by longer hair.

The night before the surgery, my sister and I went to a local restaurant. As we were eating our dinners, my sister asked what I wanted her to bring to the hospital after the surgery. I can't tell you how happy I was that my sister is a nurse. I told her the usual items such as toothbrush and toothpaste, pajamas and bathrobe, and several other items. She kind of gave me a funny look and asked me if I didn't want my hairbrush too. I reminded her I would be bald after the surgery and the two of us laughed until we cried. Each time we would try to start

288

eating again, we would get the giggles and start all over again. Her comment was completely unplanned, but it certainly helped relieve the stress of the impending surgery.

The day of surgery I was doing pretty good before going in to the operating room until one of the residents reminded me my head was to be shaved. I still hadn't grown accustomed to that thought yet. The operating room was full of people. Since I was the first person to receive two implants in a single surgery, it seemed like everyone wanted to be present to see history take place. Even some of the persons from the marketing department of the manufacturer had requested special permission to be present during the surgery. Before being wheeled in, I had to give up my hearing aid and since I could not hear, and because the staff was required to wear masks, communication was nearly impossible. One very dear person removed her mask, held my hand, and told me what I needed to know.

My surgery was on a Friday and lasted about five hours. I woke up briefly on and off that evening. I remember Dr. Gantz and some of the residents coming in to my room about 4:00 p.m. to tell me the surgery went well and that my left ear tested slightly better than my right, although my right ear was responding. I slept most of the night except for begging to be fed. Jello and broth do not qualify as food. Then I took a walk with the nurse around 10:30 p.m. The next morning, I woke up when my sister came in with my things. My head was completely covered in bandages and the areas over my ears stuck out from the rest of the dressing. I later learned I had been dubbed Princess Leia after a character in the Star Wars movie that wore her hair in buns over her ears. I think it was a pretty fair comparison.

The resident came in and asked how I was doing. I told him my lip was a little bit numb and he had me pucker and release my lips to make sure they were okay. He also changed my dressing and I got my first glance at my bald head. I kind of liked the new hairdo.

Seven weeks after the surgery, I was hooked up to the external speech processors. That day, I heard and comprehended speech for the first time in a very long time. I spoke to my mother and then six-year old son on the phone. I danced to music on the TV, I heard squeaky tennis shoes, and I prayed.

The goals of the bilateral implant project were to try to determine if there was a way to know which is the better ear to implant by implanting 10 persons meeting the project criteria. The results of the Iowa project were that they would have been right 50% of the time, which also means they would have been wrong 50% of the time. In my own situation, the ear that had never been aided performs marginally better than the ear that had the slower loss and that had been aided. The differences measured in the lab, though, don't measure my own experience. And that is I hear more clearly with my right, or pre-implant bad, ear.

Other benefits I am receiving from having bilateral implants include the ability to hear better in noisy environments and to detect the direction of sound. There is still some question whether or not all persons with bilateral implants have or will receive these same benefits, and more studies are being conducted. I'm just glad that I was given an opportunity to participate in research that will hopefully answer a lot of questions for the researchers.

Having hearing and losing it can cut a person off socially and emotionally. For many of us, it is a living hell. The first day of having the implants activated, I was able to realize there was again hope for me. It didn't really sound very good but the potential was there. My cochlear implants brought me back into a world I forgot existed. Where people really are kind and caring. My self-confidence took a big hit during those years of deafness. It's not back 100% yet and I'm not sure if it ever will be. My only goals with the implants were to be able to hear my son say the "Pledge of Allegiance," hopefully a valedictorian speech, his wedding vows, and "I love you, Mommy." I have gotten so very much more than I ever dreamed. I hear everything now. I may not necessarily comprehend everything I hear 100%, but I do hear. When I heard the click-click sound of my little poodle's toenails going across the linoleum floor, I knew I could hear anything.

Having the implants and being socialized back into my world again is not enough. There are too many professionals in the hearing field that are unaware of the advances in cochlear implant technology. There are too many hearing impaired persons in the world who don't realize hope exists for them. And there is too much misunderstanding by others in this world about how to treat persons with disabilities. Cochlear implant technology has only scratched the surface in dealing with hearing loss. It is my duty, and my great joy as a recipient of this technology, to join other implant recipients in educating the professionals, giving hope to the hearing impaired, and teaching our neighbors, one by one, to understand. Life is good, life is VERY good.

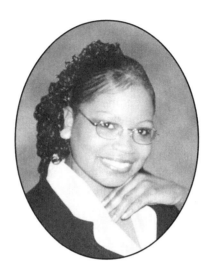

Overcoming Obstacles…By Donna Stephens

Born and raised in Washington, D.C., I was diagnosed as having bilateral hearing loss at the age of five or six years old. My grandfather was spending time with me when he noticed that I could not hear. He immediately went to my mother and stated that I might have a hearing problem because each time he said something to me I wouldn't respond. The only time he said I responded was when we were facing each other, because I could read his lips. He suggested that my mother take me to a doctor for a hearing test. After the hearing tests were performed, my grandfather's suspicion that I could not hear was confirmed. The results were that I was deaf in my left ear and had sensorineural hearing loss in my right ear that could be helped with the use of a hearing aid.

When my mother and I returned home from the doctor's office, I remembered her holding me closely, apologizing and crying. As I got older, I asked her about that day and her motive for being so upset. She stated that, before she found out that I was deaf, she had been punishing me for misbehaving. She said I never did what she asked me to do. She thought I was ignoring her. She also recalled a day that broke her heart. She stated that after disciplining me I was very tearful with an expression on my face as if I was asking her what I did wrong. She broke down and cried with me because, she said, she did not know how to handle me and had no idea during that time that I had a hearing disability. Ever since then and until the time of her death in 1996, she was always concerned about the things going on in my life. She needed to know if I was hearing okay and getting respect from people regarding my hearing.

After three months of attending Junior Primary, I began to dislike going to school every day. Children used to make fun of me and asked silly questions about my hearing aid. When I did not hear them, some would laugh at me and slowly pronounce words to me. Their behavior upset me a lot. My teachers were understanding of my problem and made sure I sat in the front row of the classroom. It wasn't long before I moved to the back of the classroom. While sitting in the front row of the classroom, some kid sitting behind me would deliberately say things to me behind my back knowing that I would not hear him. To keep myself from being bothered by him, I sat in the back of the classroom against my teacher's request to remain seated in front of the classroom. At the age of 13 years old, I got tired of being teased and quit wearing the hearing aid. I tried hearing without the hearing aid with difficulty and I learned to read lips very well.

As I got older and more mature, I realized that without sufficient hearing, my grades and the ability to socialize with people were very poor. I soon began wearing the hearing aid again. Whenever children or young adults asked me about my hearing aid, I would tell them that the hearing aid helped me hear better and if they didn't like the way it looked on me, not to worry because it was my problem, not theirs, and to mind their own business. I would encounter other problems. When I did not hear what a person said the first time or second time, I would ask them to repeat what they said. I noted that some folks just didn't have any patience and would practically scream what they said. I would get sarcastic by telling them that if it bothered them to repeat what they said to me it was okay because I didn't care to talk to them in the first place. Soon, I was getting respect from anyone who cared to get to know me and understand my hearing disability. I was asked by some students to have lunch with them. I was even invited to parties and to the movies. I also had a special group of friends who simply liked me for who I was. Whenever they heard of anyone they knew or did not know disrespect me, they would give the culprit a piece of their mind. When I entered high school, the harassment about my hearing problem ended. I received help from some of my classmates by sharing notes with them and confirming what the teacher asked us to do. My classmates' assistance helped increase my grades and self-esteem. I completed and graduated from high school in 1981.

After graduating from high school, I attended college and it was not successful. The classroom setting was not arranged to accommodate my needs, and the professor's lack of knowledge of how to deal with a hearing-impaired student was obvious. I think that was a large part of the reason I always got poor grades. I could not hear or understand most things that the professors said. My request for the professors to keep still and face me while speaking normally failed. I tried just going by the book but ended up failing anyway because I was reading and studying subjects the professors did not request. I quit college early until I found the resources I needed to succeed in my studies. I remember thinking that there had to be a way to overcome those barriers and achieve my goals.

In March 1985, I joined a program that helped young mothers get off of welfare by enrolling them in job-training programs to become independent working adults. I accepted a job-training offer at the U.S. Department of Labor as a Clerk-Typist trainee. My hours were from 9:00 a.m. to 5:00 p.m. I felt pride in the fact that I was making preparations to become a part of the workplace. Before I could start applying for jobs in the government, I had to pass a typing proficiency test. I was very determined to pass that test. I typed 55 words per minute with no errors and I was so excited about my success. In June 1985, I landed a job at the U. S. Environmental Protection Agency (USEPA) as a Clerk-Typist. I am currently with the agency as an Information Management Specialist.

In 1995 I lost total hearing in my only hearing ear (right ear) due to ear surgery. That was the most devastating moment of my life. I could not imagine living my life as a deaf person. I began the search of getting my hearing back and was referred to Dr. John Niparko, who is the Director of the Otolaryngology Head and Neck Surgery Department at Johns Hopkins University Hospital, in Baltimore, Maryland. Dr. Niparko took me through a battery of inner ear tests, which indicated that I was a good candidate for the Clarion cochlear implant.

In May 1996, my right ear was implanted with the device. For me, the healing process was long and miserable. When I finally healed from the surgery, I was able to have the speech processor programmed. The sounds received from the cochlear implant at first were awfully bad. Everyone sounded like Donald Duck speaking. I could not clearly understand what people were saying since I never understood his language. For that reason, it took a while for me to understand speech again. Despite the aggravation of the sound quality from the cochlear implant, I was satisfied that I was hearing *something* rather than nothing at all. Over time, I have been receiving sounds from the cochlear implant better. As time went on I was amazed that I was able to hear conversation on a regular telephone. I am also using a cell phone. However, I can hear what men are saying better than what women are saying over the telephone. Before that, my only means of communicating on the telephone was through the TTY. I disliked the idea that a third party was listening in on my telephone conversations.

Today, I am hearing so well with the cochlear implant that I forget that I am using one. I sometimes even forget to bring extra batteries with me when leaving my house! I find it so inviting to be able to engage in social conversations, hear the voices of children playing, cars and trucks passing by, listening and dancing to my favorite songs. At bedtime, I continue to use my implant for hearing; I do not like sleeping without being woken by sounds in my environment. The only time I cannot use the implant for hearing is when I shower or go swimming.

I recently attended the University of the District of Columbia (UDC) to study Business Administration. Before attending classes, I had to explain my hearing situation and needs to the school, and request that they assign a note taker for each of my two courses, Business Management and Business Communication. One student in my business management class volunteered to be my note taker. Because of her help, I was able to understand what was being said during classroom discussions and what the professor requested for homework. I've promised myself that in the future, I would choose a school that is better equipped to accommodate the hearing impaired and willing to provide me with reasonable accommodations. If possible, I plan to overcome the barriers of learning in a classroom setting, by considering the option of a college that would allow me to study on-line. Without my hearing I felt lonely and isolated from the rest of the world. I was very unhappy. It is so wonderful to have my hearing back. I highly respect and commend Dr. John Niparko for a job well done.

I would like to encourage the deaf population about the benefits of hearing with the use of a cochlear implant and see for themselves how beautiful the world sounds with hearing. My experience with losing my hearing and having it restored has made me a much stronger person and communicator.

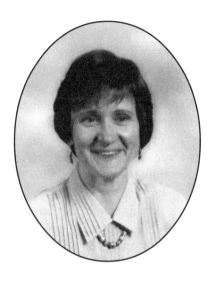

A Future and a Hope...By Sheila Adams

"For I know the plans I have for you, declares the Lord, plans for welfare and not for calamity to give you a future and a hope." Jeremiah 29:1 (NASV)

"What'd he say?" my husband asked absently. A young man, who was carrying his young daughter, had just exited the elevator at the Outpatient Center at Johns Hopkins University Hospital. The dangling, bare foot of this little one had captured our attention, because it was so peculiar for a cold December day. "She just got her cast off," I replied as we also made our way out of the elevator. We were at the hospital for a "mapping" appointment, scheduled after two months of sound generated by my cochlear implant. It took a few moments before we both realized that a very significant event had just occurred. Could it be that I had heard a passing comment that Gerry had not heard? This was definitely a new experience for both of us, something that had never happened in all our married life!

The Descent

My hearing problems had begun soon after beginning my career as a special education teacher and had progressed (or should I say regressed) in the pattern typical of a person plagued with sensorineural hearing loss. Bi-annual trips to the audiologist inevitably meant the sad but not surprising news of yet another drop in decibels and the need to invest in a better, more powerful hearing aid. My journey toward deafness was gradual and spanned over two decades, but that did not diminish the devastating effects on my life, professionally and personally. When it was time to speak to my employer about accommodations in the workplace, it felt like the beginning of the end of my professional competency. It was a fairly "tall order" for me to continue to teach phonics to elementary age children with any degree of effectiveness.

I knew that the occasional remark from a colleague or parent indicating that my hearing loss would serve to make me a better, more understanding teacher of children with disabilities was well meaning and sincere. Yet it simply was not true. I had always cared deeply for my young charges and had empathized with their struggles to achieve success in school. I had prided myself in my skills as a resource teacher, honed by nearly 25 years of experience with teaching students of all ages. I knew that what I was dealing with was a decline in teaching skills, not an enhancement, because of my hearing impairment.

My students, for the most part, had been eager to help and to serve as my "ears" whenever they could. My employer was also gracious and willing to act on my suggestions for equipment that might help, such as an amplified phone, a newer model window air conditioner designed for quiet running, a fire alarm with a strobe light, and an FM system to use in class and during faculty meetings. While these assistive devices were immensely helpful, I was still having a difficult time coping with the hearing demands of the job.

I guess there is a "line in the sand" when any additional loss in hearing capacity, however small, puts you over the edge in terms of speech comprehension. For me, it occurred sometime in 1999. My acquired lipreading skills, my ability to fill in the missing words through context clues, and my seasoned aptitude in "faking" it had kept me functional for many years. Now these compensatory strategies were no longer enough. It seemed that the addition of any background noise or any other voices beyond the one person speaking directly to me caused a significant breakdown in communication. I just couldn't grasp what people were saying! I think the private realization of my approaching deafness came when I began to understand that being deaf was not really defined as the total absence of sound but, rather, the inability to understand speech if your eyes are closed. You see, I could no longer understand anything people said when I could not see their faces. Using the telephone, even with a patch cord to transmit the sound to the FM boot on my hearing aid, was not satisfactory. There were the colossal headaches and the ever-present fatigue that come from the stress of always being on the alert for conversation that might be taking place around me. Many of the sounds amplified by my aid were not only distorted but also painful because of my recruitment problems. I began to dread the thought of another day of social encounters. I had long since removed myself from the daily lunchtime crowd in the teachers' lounge, choosing to close my classroom door and relish the silence. I prayed that somehow I could make it through the afternoon with some semblance of efficiency.

There were many humiliating incidences that I still recall with raw emotions during those dark days when my hearing aid was no longer adequate for the demands of my job. I had arrived early one morning and had hastily clamored into school with an armload of files and with a mind preoccupied with the myriad of things on my "to do" list. It was now several hours later when I happened by the side door as a colleague was entering the building. She asked, with finger pointing toward the parking lot, "Isn't that your car over there with the motor running?" I mumbled a feeble, "Yes, thank you" and dashed red-faced to the car. There had already been private embarrassments at home when I would return to the bathroom for a last-minute mirror check and discover, to my surprise, that I'd left the water running in the sink, but this event seemed to me to be a very public declaration of the magnitude of my hearing loss.

The social and psychological impact of a profound hearing loss on a person who grew up with normal hearing deserves greater attention than it's usually afforded. An enormous amount of emotional energy is expended in a desperate attempt to stay connected with friends and family, to continue to share in the spontaneous flow of ideas that maintains relationships. But you sense that you are losing the battle for equal access to communication with each passing day. No more listening to a cassette of relaxing music or keeping abreast of current events by listening to the daily news on the radio during the commute to work. No more picking up the phone to chat with a friend about trivia or about more substantial things that are vital in sustaining friendships. No more enjoyable social outings to restaurants, concerts, movies, or the mall. The burgeoning fears, anxieties, and apprehensions that are attached to new situations, chance encounters, or other social obligations can begin to transform you from a relaxed, confident, and spontaneous person to a withdrawn, tense, and intense observer of life. In short, the stress of my profound hearing impairment was exacting its emotional and physical toll.

The Decision

In March 2000, I was once again seated before my doctor to discuss my annual hearing tests. The additional decline in hearing capability was no surprise, but the news that I was now a possible candidate for a cochlear implant was unexpected. My otolaryngologist explained that his policy was to implant the better ear because there was a greater chance of success in the ear that had the most recent stimulation. He suggested that I give it serious consideration and that I pick up some literature at the front desk. My response to this recommendation would have been an immediate, "Let's schedule it!" if he had advised an implant for my left (deaf) ear. But I was not ready to sacrifice the only residual hearing I had left in my right ear. Driving home, Gerry and I discussed the idea of getting a second opinion. The next day he called our insurance company and then the Listening Center at Johns Hopkins and arranged a consultation for May 11, 2000, the first of six appointments in the candidacy process. I was encouraged by the knowledge that surgeons often implanted the "worse" ear and with great results.

By the time the verdict was in, I was more than ready to proceed with surgery. An implant in my left ear offered me a hope for the future, the possibility of some restored hearing and the prospect of enough speech comprehension to resume some degree of independence and connection with people. The Listening Center was careful to emphasize that there were no guarantees, only the prediction that it was likely that I would hear more environmental sounds than what I was hearing with my hearing aid. Fine ... I had nothing to lose and everything to gain.

The Discoveries

I busied myself during the one-month recovery period between surgery and activation by learning Cued Speech. I reasoned that Gerry and I needed a means of communication that would help me with sounds that I might have trouble processing. Cued Speech is a system of hand placements used in conjunction with speech that corresponds with the

298

44 phonemes of English. Learning Cue has proven to be a wise and practical decision. Gerry uses it to "talk" to me late at night and early in the morning when the implant processor is not connected, or in noisy environments when I'm struggling to understand a word or sentence.

My parents joined us for the momentous day called "hook-up." I was blessed with being able to hear most of the words of all those in the room from the long-awaited moment when all channels are activated, but no one's speech possessed a human quality. Gerry's was sort of a Darth Vader clone, and Mom's voice did not even sound feminine. But I was thrilled! Let the adventure begin! Each subsequent "mapping" session at Johns Hopkins was both encouraging and challenging. Joy and amazement swept over me when we compared my pre-implant audiogram and my current post-implant audiogram. Scores on tests of repeating single words had risen from 6% to 84% in just six months! After auditory testing came the exhausting work of "re-mapping" as the audiologist attempted to make program adjustments to address my complaints. It was no easy task for me to accurately describe what I had been hearing that didn't sound quite right. Initially, both male and female voices sounded similar, like everyone was underwater, having a kind of a monotone "boink" attached to their words. As time passed, it changed to a muffled, fuzzy sound with a buzz like that produced by an oboe. With a later map, the words still seemed too resonant, like rever-beration in an overdriven stereo speaker. But I knew the changes were in the right direction, toward the goal of human-sounding speech, and my brain was working overtime.

"What's that sound?" was my perpetual question to anyone who chanced to be near me. I was like a toddler, alert to every sight and sound and curious about each new sound discovery. Inside my house, I discovered that my dog's toenails made a clicking sound as she traipsed across the kitchen floor. The microwave beeped, the refrigerator hummed, the water cooler gurgled, and the wall clock audibly ticked away the seconds. The computer was not the silent technology I had always known. From its musical announcement of start up, to its *thunk* when I click on the wrong thing, or its chattering as my fingers de-pressed the keys. Who would have thought? The companion printer was also a noisy machine, producing rumbling and chirping sounds in addition to the light and motion and, eventually, the printed page.

The outside world was an even greater wonder. Traffic noise and the roar of airplanes overhead became annoying noise pollutants that interrupted my investigation of more pleasant sounds. Last season's grasses in a nearby meadow made a crunching noise under my feet. There was a veritable serenade to experience when walking in the woods as twilight approaches: twigs snapping underfoot, leaves rustling with each gust of wind, and tree frogs and cicadas announcing their presence with a continual concert. There was something soothing and serene about listening to the sound of a tiny stream as its crystal clear water trickled over the stones and wound its way downstream. And the birds... oh, the birds! Had their songs had such sweetness and energy when I heard them in my youth?

Gerry's whistling and the tinkling sound of music boxes were a plea-sure within the first week of "CI" sound and especially when I began to recognize some of the melodies. I so longed to have music back in my life that I even made a trip to the local Costco store just to finger an electronic keyboard on display, holding my aux microphone next to the speaker. A strange phenomenon occurred at various times on the de-scending scales: a note would go up instead of down. No wonder Gerry, who is gifted with a beautiful baritone voice, was now singing off key! Patience and practice, I'd tell myself. The music of *Peter and the Wolf* was the first recording that sounded somewhat like I remem-bered it. It was a great CD to use as a kind of aural therapy since it begins with the identifying of single instruments with their melody "lines" and has narration throughout the score.

There was a longing during the first few months of CI sound for that promised return of more human-sounding voices. I had not expected to experience this yearning, a kind of grieving, I suppose, over the ab-sence of that "natural" sound of speech. Though acutely aware of the rich blessing of comprehending most of what people said when I could see their faces, I still wanted to hear people sounding like people! I was only vaguely conscious of a gradual evolution occurring in my brain's perception of speech, a subtle change from the Darth Vader men and the computerized women's voices to a sort of tunnel-like, public ad-dress system quality to everyone's speech. At about the time Gerry began to "sing well" again, I realized that people's voices had more intonation and inflection than in previous weeks. When we arrived home one evening from a visit next door, I recall telling Gerry, through tears of gratitude, "Angie sounds like Angie!"

The Delights

New delights and unexpected surprises defined the wonder of this ad-

300

justment time. These "CI moments" were awesome and created in me a deep sense of gratitude to God for this miraculous technology. Simple things like hearing someone call my name or understanding a private, whispered message brought a smile to my face and heart. I never realized how much more enjoyable television and films could be when you're able to process more than the visual images and the closed captioned words. "I heard that!" I exclaimed one night when the captioning indicated that the actor had emitted a soft sound. Many outdoor dialogues have a lovely background of chattering birds in the sound track. Watching a biography of the life of John Philip Sousa would have been an educational, engrossing experience in my hearing aid days, but now it was an emotional and moving one as my heart swelled to the sound of his rousing marches, like *The Washington Post* and *The Stars and Stripes Forever.*

I remember feeling triumphant one evening when, as a passenger in the front seat, I realized that I comprehended most of my brother's words as he chatted from the back seat! Then at a religious convention in March, just five months after activation, I sat with a silly smirk on my face after correctly answering the question asked by the woman seated next to me ("What was that hymn number?"). Even mundane chores became CI moments, like the time that I had a real shock when my headpiece crackled with static as I emptied the dryer of its "electrifying" contents.

The developers of our residential community sponsored a fireworks display recently that could be viewed from our upstairs bedroom. I positioned myself at the window and prepared to watch with minimal interest, my enthusiasm dampened by the unconscious expectation that I would need to turn off the sound of those painfully loud bangs and just experience the visual display in silence. But, wait... the explosions were loud but not uncomfortable. Were there some pleasant whistle sounds and a swishing noise as the spiraling colors lit up the landscape? I asked Gerry to describe what he was hearing, confirming that my CI was giving me those same sounds. Wow!

The Destination

Adjusting to CI sound is an amazing journey that has no pre-determined destination. With each small victory on the telephone or each independent trip to the store or doctor's office, I feel like I'm reclaiming the lost ground that was so reluctantly and painfully surrendered over

301

the years. It's as if the person of Sheila Adams is re-emerging after years of dormancy and despair. Those who knew me then and who know me now speak of the subtle changes in my speech and my demeanor. That blank expression that was often pasted on my face does re-surface from time to time, but the stress from not hearing and the fear of appearing rude or foolish are no longer my constant companion. The future is no longer bleak and limited, but now filled with promise and potential. That sense of being lonely-in-a-crowd is slowly fading as the confidence in my ability to hear is gaining strength. So many of my professional skills are also returning, such as being able to write down what one of my learning disabled students is dictating to me without having to stare intently at his face and then to frantically scribe as much as my short-term memory would retrieve. Maybe one day I will be able to follow one of the many pockets of conversations that go on in the teacher's workroom at lunchtime. Perhaps soon I will operate the copy machine, collate pages, label files, and talk to a colleague at the same time or perhaps not.

It always shocks me when my battery dies and the world becomes so suddenly and starkly silent, but with a quick change of the battery, the wonderful sounds of life come flooding back. This routine experience is not without purpose, because it is a healthy reminder that I am still deaf and that I dare not take my hearing for granted. The gift of a cochlear implant "keeps on giving" and, in the process, keeps on affecting all aspects of my life in monumental ways. And tomorrow ... who knows what "CI moment" is awaiting me around the next corner! Thanks to God!

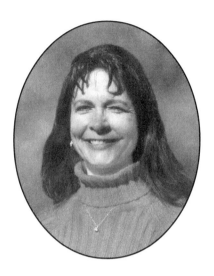

What Are You? Deaf? Hard of Hearing? Hearing?...By Sharaine Rawlinson

In the summer of 1974, I was spending my usual 12 weeks up north in Duluth, Minnesota, with my father and his new wife and her three daughters from a previous marriage. My brother, Scott, and I would fly up to Minnesota each summer and for a week at Christmas, so this year was no different than the others. Or so I thought.

Ever since I was five years old, I longed to be a pediatrician. I knew with every cell in my body that medicine was my calling. So, it was only natural that, when I became bored with my routine of watching soap operas with my stepsisters, I decided to telephone every hospital in Duluth to see if I could find one that would allow me to volunteer. I was able to locate one and quickly settled into five of the most satisfying weeks of the summer.

I volunteered as a candystriper 40 hours a week. I saw every inch of that hospital, with the exception of the operating room and even then, I saw the waiting room where patients are prepped before being wheeled into the OR. I loved what I did, and it only served to confirm my conviction to become a doctor.

In no time at all, the five weeks flew by in a blur. The next thing I knew, I was flying home to Albuquerque to get ready to start my sophomore year in high school on September 3rd. While I did eventually make it to high school, a detour to the hospital was next on my calendar even though I didn't plan on it. I spent 10 days in quarantine with spinal meningitis, barely holding on to my life. I had a fever of 105 and was paralyzed from the waist down. When I awoke from the coma, I didn't realize I'd lost my hearing, all of it. "It's only fluid build-up in her ear canals. Give it a month or so and her hearing should return," the doctors told my mom. A hearing aid, the big bulky kind, was of no help. It just gave off feedback when I turned it up to 10 in an effort to hear something. Three weeks after discharge, I was back in high school and trying to learn a new way of learning. School was always easy for me, I had to study, but I loved to do so and always did well in my studies. Without hearing, learning was presenting me with totally new challenges.

My parents bought carbon paper that I would give to classmates in each class who had volunteered to take notes and give me a copy. Using an interpreter was of no assistance and never attempted during my sophomore year. My friends taught me the manual alphabet and my speech teacher taught me beginning sign language. Regardless of the struggles, I somehow managed to graduate number 106 in a class of 610. Not bad for a girl who couldn't hear a darn thing and was assimilating to a new way of life.

I had a scholarship offer to the University of Arizona, but turned it down because it was too far away from Albuquerque. Then my parents heard of the National Technical Institute for the Deaf at Rochester Institute of Technology in Rochester, New York. When the bulletin catalog arrived in the mail, I took one look at the cover photo replete with green trees, green grass, and open spaces. In no time at all, I said that was where I would be going to college. So much for "too far from home"!

My four years at NTID were wonderful. I learned American Sign Language fluently and utilized the services of interpreters and notetakers to the maximum. College was definitely harder than high school, but the environment was good for me. NTID was at RIT and there were some 12,000 students, of which 1,000 were deaf. I was in both of my worlds, the deaf and the hearing. I started out a biology major, intent on going to medical school. That only lasted one quarter, when I switched to social work. I reasoned that to become a doctor I would have to depend on hearing people to tell me what was going on inside my patients. Independent as I was, that didn't sit well with me. Of course, pathology was an option, but the last thing I wanted to do was work on cadavers. So, off to social work I went. The years flew by and before long I was graduating with honors from NTID/RIT. Graduation was a wonderful time of pomp and circumstance. The staff of the NTID Social Work Support Team had thought to get inflated balloons for each of the graduates who were deaf so that we could feel the music vibrations.

Over the years, my life went through many ups and downs. I married young, a year after graduating college. Three years into the marriage, *Newsweek* magazine carried a story on cochlear implants. Of course, I knew of them, but they were purely experimental. And besides, it was against the beliefs of the Deaf Community to get a cochlear implant. My career was in its infant stages and I was fighting to gain acceptance in the Community. The fact that I was born hearing was already a strike against me. To get a cochlear implant would be a double whammy, one I didn't want to risk. Time went on and I continued my work with the Deaf Community. I went to church where there was an interpreter and I had friends, deaf and hearing. I was still inundated with people suggesting that I get a cochlear implant (CI) and I finally gave in to being evaluated for one. My rationale was that I didn't expect to benefit from one and this would put all of the prompting to an end, once and for all. I was tested and heard sound for the first time in 11 years. It wasn't normal sound, but it was sound.

I went home and discussed this with my husband. Yes, there were risks like facial paralysis, not to mention the normal risks associated with surgery of any kind. Plus, if it was a success, would I spend all of my time listening and put aside my graduate studies at the University of Kansas? In the end, I opted not to be implanted. I would complete my master's degree in the coming year, and then would re-evaluate my decision.

Time flew by and before long one year became 11. Divorced and doing very well in my career, I still missed music. That had been the one thing that hit me and stayed with me when I became deaf. My love of music would never go away. Still, I was happy being deaf. I'd met so many wonderful people as a result of it; Jehanel Sadat, the widow of Egypt's president Answar Sadat, for example. I'd danced for Mikhail Baryshnikov at NTID. I was considered a "one-woman army" by Governor John Ashcroft of Missouri, for the work I did on behalf of deaf and hard of hearing Missourians with mental health problems. The list was endless; among those big famous names were the lesser known that meant more to me than anyone. My friends, Gerry and

Judy, had stood by me through thick and thin. Family and friends across the nation urged me on when I wanted to give up. Truly, becoming deaf had been the best thing to happen to me. Instead of being an obscure pediatrician, I was enjoying traveling, building my career, and making a name for myself.

In 1996, I took a leap of faith (another one!) and decided to get a cochlear implant. I was implanted on March 27, 1997 at the Mayo Clinic in Rochester, Minnesota. After four weeks of healing, I was "hooked up" and mapped on April 22nd. It was unbelievable. I now heard sound, although it was nothing like what I remembered hearing to be. The decision to get a CI had not been an easy one. My desire to hear music was still there inside of me. At the same time, I'd had so many close calls with death as a result of not hearing snow plows and ambulances behind me, that I figured access to even a little bit of sound would be of benefit to me. Surely, I wouldn't ever hear again like I had previously, but this was something I wanted to do. It was a tremendous risk career-wise. Yet, I had accomplished so much in my work and established a name for myself, I figured that if folks wanted to fire me, I would find another job rather easily. I was finally able to say, "This is for me, it's my decision and no one else's, so back off."

It's been almost five years since I was implanted and the benefits I have derived from my implant are far beyond anything I dared to hope for. I use the telephone with some difficulty, I hear music although it's not perfect, and I know when my cats are mewing at me. I've heard the birds sing, the wind in the tree branches (I thought it was water in a river!), and water trickling through gutters after a night's rainfall. As expected, I took and continue to take criticism for getting an implant. Yet, I've been able to stand my ground and prove that, though I can hear some when I have my CI on, I am still deaf and will always cherish that part of me. I'll always use sign language, even when I'm speaking. People challenge me at the talks I give across the nation: "What are you? Deaf? Hard of Hearing? Hearing?" I struggled with that one at first, but finally came up with the right answer, "I'm Sharaine. Take me or leave me. This is the way I am."

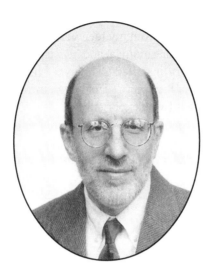

It's Really About The Music…By Robert Beck

When you come right down to it, music's return to my life was the most overwhelming outcome of the cochlear implant. My implant surgery took place on September 15, 2000, about 25 years after my hearing took a substantial nosedive. My musical knowledge and appreciation were arrested about the same time. I had been a decent folk musician, mostly playing the guitar, a bit of the banjo and, rudimentarily, a few other stringed instruments. My hearing loss and the subsequent loss of ability to take in the higher frequencies pretty much did me in musically.

One memory of the slow but steady decline in my musical world has me sitting in our music room, surrounded by a great speaker system. I was frantically attempting to absorb as much as I could before the loss became more substantial. I feverishly pursued classical music, having previously neglected learning more about the classics. But the hearing went, music became nothing more than noise, my instruments played not a note, I bought no more LPs, and never learned how to open a CD package.

Along came the implant, a Nucleus 24 Contour. I rapidly adapted, my audiologist made the adjustments, and I was on my way into the world of hearing. Not wanting to get my hopes up, I was too fearful to ask about whether I would be able to hear music. One morning on the way to work I took a CD from my wife's cache. I went for the music that had been my favorite from my teen years. It was early Bob Dylan with acoustic guitar and harmonica, and his raspy but familiar voice. In a new car with a factory-installed CD player I never thought I'd use, I figured out how to get it going. Tears began to flow from my eyes. I could not believe what I was experiencing.

Each morning on my short ride to work and return at the end of the day, I have to be pried from my car. I don't want to let go of the indescribable pleasure I experience with my growing CD collection. In many ways, the return of music to my life transcends the equally, if not more, important changes which have taken place with family and friends, at work and on the phone.

The answer, my friends, was "Blowing in the Wind."

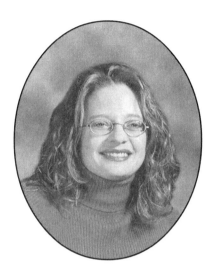

My Story…By Linda Cecutti

It was just over a year ago that my husband came rushing into the kitchen and pulled me by the arm to the front step. I stood there looking at him, expecting some sort of explanation for the commotion. Then I heard them. "Birds," I said in a state of amazement. "Yes, birds," he confirmed, a smile broadening across his face as tears welled in our eyes. It was the most beautiful thing I have ever heard. For 12 years I never dared to even dream that I would ever hear birds again.

Shortly after I started kindergarten the teacher called my parents to tell them I was mentally retarded. This lead to the discovery that I had a mild to moderate hearing loss. I was fitted with two hearing aids and managed well with them.

A few weeks after my fifteenth birthday this all changed. I awoke to find my mother at my bedside gently nudging me. "You don't want to get up this morning?" she teased as she reached down and flicked the switch on my alarm clock. Her comment confused me, and I was wondering why she was turning my alarm clock off. But it was six o'clock in the morning and I was not quite fully awake, so I just went about my usual morning routine. When I turned on the hairdryer I noticed there was no sound coming from it though the air was blowing out. I turned it off, then on again, hoping to discover some mechanical failure, still no sound. With panic beginning to build within me, I started banging on my desk, praying to hear something. Nothing. I put my hearing aids on, but to no avail. In desperation I even changed the batteries. Surely that must be the answer. But of course, it was not. The only answer was that I had suddenly lost more hearing. I now had a moderate to severe loss.

This was a huge adjustment for me. Being 15, I just wanted to fit in and be like everyone else. I was the only one in our small town high school who had a hearing loss significant enough to warrant hearing aids. So I continued to hide it and told only my closest friends. I refused any type of extra support in school and relied on my friends' notes to get me through high school.

At this point in my life people started saying I could teach deaf children when I finished school. I resented this, only because I felt they thought it was the only thing I could do. Reluctantly, I went to visit a class of deaf children as arranged through friends of my parents. I enjoyed the visit but was not prepared to give in. As we were leaving the class, one of the students ran up to me and grabbed my arm. With her teacher interpreting, she asked me if I would come back and teach them some day. At that moment I chose my career.

With the support of an electronic notetaker, I graduated on the Dean's Honor List with an Honor's Bachelor of Arts in Psychology from Laurentian University in Sudbury. I then moved to Toronto to pursue a Bachelor of Education and a specialization in Deaf Education. I returned to Sudbury and was hired by the local public school board a week later. That fall, I was teaching the same class I had visited seven years earlier.

It was two years later, ten weeks before my wedding, when I gradually lost more hearing over a period of five days. I was now profoundly deaf. Up until this point I had never considered a cochlear implant. With my wedding only a few weeks away, I desperately wanted one and I wanted it now. However, that was not possible. My wedding went on to be everything I had dreamed it would be and more. My only regret was, and still is, that I could not hear the music.

A few weeks later I was at Sunnybrook and Women's College Health Sciences Centre in Toronto, undergoing tests to determine my candidacy for an implant. I was successful at getting on the waiting list and was told it would be at least April and probably the following summer before I would be implanted. My husband and I went home and did our research. We asked questions and read everything we could find on cochlear implants. Meanwhile, I had learned to adjust to my new level of hearing. I was no longer desperate but ready to make an informed decision. Finally, during the Christmas holidays when I had time to really think about all we knew, I decided to go for it. The risks were deemed small compared to the potential benefits.

On January 31, I received a letter from the hospital informing me that my surgery date was at the end of the following month. My first reaction was "I can't do this. It's too soon!" It was all becoming a reality sooner than I had expected. Though I was scared that I was making the wrong decision, I was excited, too. In the weeks to come I cried every time the surgery was mentioned. I could only think of the "what ifs." Never once did I allow myself to think of what it would be like to hear the birds again.

On February 29, 1999 I was implanted with a Clarion S-Series co-chlear implant. I was discharged from the hospital the following after-noon. However, I became very nauseous from the anesthetic and had to be re-admitted to the hospital for three days. Once that problem passed, I became stronger each day.

My "hook up" was on April 5th. I remember it being everything they said it would be. It was not a feeling of "Oh my God, it's a miracle! I can hear!" The audiologist's voice reminded me of a news broadcaster's. It was mechanical and sounded far off. But I felt a wave of relief that at least I was hearing something. The surgery was a success after all. My husband and I left the hospital to go back to my brother's house where we were staying. I was constantly listening to hear sounds that I had forgotten existed. The brushing of my pant legs rubbing against one another as I walked to the car, the sound of our feet scraping against the pavement, the money crackling as it passed to and from the parking lot attendant. I was excited! I spent the entire dinner looking around as the silverware tinkled against plates and lids clinked against bowls. How amazing! It was the noisiest dinner of my life!

The next morning when we went out to the car to return to the hospital for my second mapping, my husband asked me if I could hear something. I could hear something, but it was not at all clear. He pointed out that it was a bird. I felt a wave of disappointment wash over me because it sounded nothing like a bird. However, after the second mapping I felt more confident that things would get better with time, as I had been promised from the beginning. I distinctly remember hearing the keys jingle in my husband's hand. I could not hear that the day before.

I was especially excited to return home to see what discoveries I could make in my familiar environment. The first was the beeping of the house alarm as we entered our home. I sat on the bed that night counting how many beeps there were before the alarm went into the armed mode after I pushed the button- there were 49 beeps and 11 warning tones. The microwave beeps five times when it is finished. The timer on the oven is one long beep. The breadmaker beeps five times when the bread is finished. And I never knew the dishwasher beeps when you push the buttons. Suddenly I felt so connected and so "at home" again. I could hear the house alarm beep when someone came in. I did not have to constantly look over my shoulder to see if the microwave had shut off or glance at my watch every five minutes to see if it was time to take the cake out of the oven. I cannot describe what a feeling of empowerment and freedom that is. You do not realize how much you rely on something until it is gone.

After about a week I noticed myself counting everything I heard. That is when I realized my fear. Without knowing it, I was afraid I was going to lose this hearing. I had never gained hearing before, only lost it. And now I was afraid of losing it again. A year has come and gone. I don't count the beeps as much anymore. As I sit here writing, birds twitter in the trees outside my open window. They sound like birds now and they don't all sound the same. Every chirp fills me with gratitude. I continued to be amazed on those occasions when I am able to understand what someone has said even though I am not lipreading. I often initiate conversations instead of turning away. After every phone conversation I am grateful for the chance to do this again. I feel more connected with my family and friends when I can pick up the phone and talk to them any time. I feel safer when I am alone in my home because I can hear when someone comes to the door or when someone comes in. I feel more confident in my ability to follow along in meetings and social interactions. I feel more at ease no matter where I am. Above all, I feel blessed to have been given the chance to hear again.

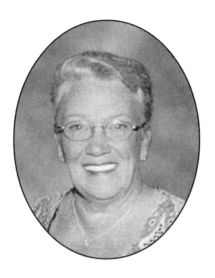

My Journey to Hearing...By Judith Hansberry

My journey to hearing began in June 1997 while my husband was hospitalized for kidney surgery at the University of Pennsylvania, in Philadelphia. On the day he was to be released from the hospital, a nurse came in to give me instructions on how to care for him. When she began, I told her that I would need to see her lips to aid my understanding because I was deaf. When she was finished, she asked me to accompany her to the nurses' station, where she wrote down a name and phone number. Little did I know that the name, Dr. Douglas Bigelow, and audiologist, Kris Rafter, would have a profound effect on the rest of my life. The floor for kidney patients was also the floor for cochlear implants. Had my husband not been so ill, I would probably still be deaf. A true case of divine intervention if ever there was one.

After being evaluated as a viable candidate, my surgery was set for October 22. I was implanted and hooked up for the hearing world on November 14, 1997. I respectfully call November 14th my birthday now because I have a whole new life.

I began losing my hearing at 30, and by 35 hearing aids were no longer helping me to hear. When I decided to have the implant, I only wanted to hear conversations again. It has given me so much more. It has given me music and laughter and all the environmental sounds that we take for granted when we can hear. It has given me confidence and a great feeling of independence. I have re-entered the working world as a teacher's aide in the public school system. Before my implant, I would never have dreamed that was even a possibility.

The time between surgery and hookup is an emotional roller coaster ride. I questioned whether I did the right thing. Did it work? Will I be able to hear? I would count the days until I was to be hooked up. I would dream of hearing my grandchildren's voices, then I would wake up deaf again. Each person implanted will go through this time differently. The benefit from this turmoil during this time is that you will never take your implant for granted! You can't! Each night before you go to bed, you unhook and become that deaf person again. Then when morning comes, you hook up and begin a new adventure. I have the rest of my life to enjoy the sounds of the world. It's the simple things that bring the most joy – the rain on the porch roof, the dog snoring at your feet. These sounds make me feel part of the human race again.

After my initial hookup, the sounds I heard were monitone-ish. I couldn't tell the difference between male and female voices. I did hear and understand most words in a quiet room. The sounds were very mellow, not at all like the harshness of my hearing aids. The environmental sounds were fascinating. Many of those sounds did not exist when I last heard. The microwave dinging, the phone ringing were all so exciting. I wanted to hear it all! Now after three years, I still hear new sounds everyday. Sometimes I'm not sure what I'm hearing – so I ask or I file it away for later – then I just smile, because I did hear something. That's more than I could say before the adventure began.

Which brings me to my next point! There comes a time as your hearing improves that you must learn to tune out some sounds so that you can understand what you want to hear! Basically, you have been given the opportunity to hear, now you must learn to LISTEN.

I think it is extremely important for all potential candidates to meet an implanted person. The smile on our faces says volumes more than technical data ever could. I have already met with the 82-year-old grandmother of one of our cafeteria workers. She was implanted and is doing extremely well. Her one wish was to speak to her brother in Oregon on the phone. He has Alzheimer's and it was important for her to be able to speak to him while he could still remember who she was. Only a week after hookup, she was practicing on the phone with her daughter. Ruth got her wish and spoke to her brother just two months after her hookup. Determination, desire, and a special need are three of the intangibles that go with a successful implant.

My life wasn't always this rosy! Before my implant, I was becoming more isolated and alone daily. I no longer went to any social gatherings. Even when I went to the grocery store, I couldn't hear, but most people didn't believe me. They would just talk louder or speak to me like I was mentally disabled – none of which helped my understanding. A few minutes into our attempt at conversation, we would both be uncomfortable and just make our excuse to get out of the situation. To eliminate this trauma from my life, I just stayed home. Since two of my sons were grown and on their own and my youngest was away at college, there was no one to speak to but my husband (God bless him) and my dogs. Since my husband is a policeman and works 12-hour shifts at a time, I was alone a lot. My dogs became my friends that I talked to. I didn't need to hear them talk back to me. From the hermit that talked to dogs to the person that I am today is the difference a cochlear implant has made in my life.

Only three weeks after my implant, my youngest son was involved in a musical production at college. To sit in the audience and hear him sing brought tears to my eyes. While in high school he was involved in drama and the musicals. Each year the cast would give me a copy of the script in an attempt to help me enjoy the play. I would memorize the play along with the students. To actually hear my son sing was so overwhelming and made me realize what I had missed through the years.

My husband has always been a Doo-Wop music fan. Unfortunately, I could not appreciate his love for the music. Now we put the top down on his convertible, pop in a CD, and sing all the way to our destination. Yes, even with the top down, I can pick out the music and sing along. I never realized how much I missed the music until I heard again. It can be relaxing, or uplifting, or happy. Emotions – that's what hearing comes down to – emotions.

As I mentioned earlier, only four months after my implant, I took a job at our local high school as an inclusion specialist. An inclusion specialist goes into a classroom to assist mainstreamed Special Ed students in a normal classroom atmosphere. Most of my students are not mentally or physically handicapped but emotionally disabled or behavior management students. On my very first day, the teacher I was working with introduced me to the students and told them of my implant. One young man asked me if I was like the Bionic Woman! I answered with a resounding, "YES"! During the first few weeks they pulled a few fast ones on me. The PA system was difficult for me to understand. They would tell me that I was needed at the office, but then they would laugh, and I would know. Then we would have a good laugh together! At the end of the year, the students wrote me little notes thanking me for all the help—I know my life is great!

The one problem having an implant gave me was the loss of a dear friend. For years we had shopped and lunched together. My newfound confidence and independence intimidated her. She told my husband I changed after my implant. He told her, "No, my old Jude is back. This is the Jude I married." While we are still friends, our relationship can never be the same.

My only other problem was the telephone, I was so afraid to try to hear someone without the benefit of lipreading. I had used a TTY for years and hated it. It made me feel even more handicapped! My audiologist, Kris Rafter, assured me that it was a conquerable task. Through tears of fear and unending patience by Kris, the telephone has become my friend. I do use the phone adapter that came with my implant kit, most of the time—mostly because I was left-eared and right-handed. My implant is on the right side, so the adapter makes me left-eared again and allows me to be able to write things down. The adapter also filters out background noise, which helps with my confidence.

This wonderful little piece of technology is not perfect. It never will be, but it allows me to be part of the world around me. I've learned to adjust to its flaws and my own. I've learned it is OK to say, "Sorry, I didn't get that." I've learned to be patient. I've learned to enjoy what I am hearing and not dwell on what I have missed. The most important thing that my implant FIXED is the loneliness. When you cannot hear, you are so alone. I am no longer the woman who hides in the grocery store or looks at her feet in the elevator. I welcome the questions about "that button on your head" and I can't wait for my next adventure to begin!

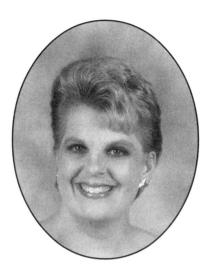

The Wonders of Sound...By Denise Pieper

As a white middle-class female in a small town in Iowa you might not think that I had experienced discrimination. The primary discrimination I have faced would probably be because I am female. But...I have faced another kind because I am deaf. When you cannot hear, many people assume that you cannot think, or maybe that you cannot feel. Being hearing impaired is a strange thing because even a person with the most profound hearing loss has some residual hearing and uses it as much as possible. This means that there are times that you totally miss what was said and other times that you catch at least part of the message. It seemed I always understood when someone said, "She can't hear, you know" or "Just forget it, you can't hear me!" It always made me feel as if it was my fault, and I felt ashamed. Worst of all was when someone threw up their hands, slumped their shoulders, and walked away. I could understand body language.

My being deaf had a profound effect on my whole family. My son would literally bounce off the walls trying to tell me something. My daughter learned from infancy to take my face and turn it toward her if she wanted to talk to me. I got into the habit of bringing her into our bed in case she woke up at night because I'd never hear her cry. People whom I thought were friends quit dropping by. If someone said, "I'll call you" I felt fear. My husband had to make phone calls for me, and I had my son taking messages from any callers, telling them I was busy or in the shower.

In 1988, after our daughter was born, I didn't work. During this time I lost more hearing. By 1990, my hearing loss was profound in both ears. At last I decided to get a hearing aid from what I now know was a dishonest dealer. This person was not an audiologist, but a certified hearing aid dispenser. When he found out I had health insurance coverage, he appealed to my sense of vanity and sold me the most expensive in-the-canal model. It was completely inappropriate for the degree of loss I had. The hearing aid amplified everything, but it was very distorted. After a couple of months it was in the drawer more than it was in my ear.

When my children were six and one, my husband's factory began massive layoffs and we feared he would be next. We had been through this before, the company where he had previously worked before closed their doors. It was time for me to find a job. I was terrified. When you cannot hear, your self-confidence is at a low, and I needed to find a job! I finally summoned all my courage and went to apply at a factory to work as a seamstress, where I had worked in 1980 and 1981, before I was married and before any noticeable hearing loss had occurred. I knew the woman who was the personnel director, and I knew she had a hearing impaired sister. She said, "Denise, you do not have to hear to do this job." Maybe not, but it sure would have helped. My supervisors had to write notes to me. Plant meetings were a joke, as I couldn't hear a thing. I did not know I had a right to ask for special treatment and I would have been embarrassed to ask. So I went to work everyday and didn't make waves.

In 1991, my (now ex) husband was still working at a factory that was 35 miles away, the 3 p.m. to 11 p.m. shift. He often stayed up after getting home at midnight and watched TV. He liked *Hard Copy*, one of the original tabloid TV shows. Late one night they had a report on something called the cochlear implant. The show featured a woman who was profoundly deaf. She turned her implant off and they read to her from a book, she understood one or two words facing the person reading. She turned the implant on, the reader stood out of her sight, and she missed only one or two words! How could that be? She could really hear, without lipreading! My husband said what struck him the most was the look on her face when she couldn't hear them. It was the same look I always had.

318

This was a real turning point in my life. I began the quest to find out about this invention. It sounded too good to be true. I went to an audiologist in Mason City; he in turn made an appointment in Iowa City at the University of Iowa Hospitals and Clinics. Following this I had more hearing tests than I had ever had in my life. The very first day that I met Mary Lowder, the audiologist at UIHC, she said, "You have nothing to lose and everything to gain." She was so right!

I was accepted for the new grant program to be a part of the clinical trials for a new device called the Clarion cochlear implant. They couldn't guarantee the results- they were optimistic, but no promises. I wanted to know if I would use the phone again all they said was "maybe." That was good enough for me. They didn't want to get my hopes up. None of us knew my hopes would all be surpassed, as a miracle was going to take place.

My surgery was on July 8, 1992. A doctor from California was there to assist and there were 15 people in the operating theater. I was the eighth person in the USA to receive the Clarion. During the surgery the electrodes are activated to see how much the surviving nerves will respond to the stimulus. Mine looked very good. When I woke up Dr. Gantz was there and gave me the thumbs up. Then came six weeks of healing before the electrodes would be activated. Those were the longest six weeks of my life.

August 20, 1992, the day I will never forget. Next to the birth of my children this was the biggest turning point of my life. Now it was time for more exhausting tests. I had to listen to what seemed like endless beeping, telling Mary when I could hear it, when it got loud, and on and on. Then it was time to turn on the "live voice" microphone.

I have been listening ever since. The birds singing, the water dripping, the wind blowing, people laughing. I had a test of my own to try when I got home. My husband went next door and called me, I could hear him. I could repeat everything he said. I jumped on the phone whenever it rang. People who called that knew me would stop and ask, "Who is this?" They didn't think I would be answering the phone! It was (is) wonderful!

Without the implant I really don't know where I'd be, maybe in a grave, or institution, or maybe I would have accepted my fate and turned myself around and made the most of my life as a deaf person. As a hearing person with this wonderful miracle, my life has changed so much. I ended my marriage, a difficult thing to do, but it was the right thing. I then decided to return to college and take the nursing program.

I graduated as an LPN in spring of 2000. I am taking classes toward my RN and working 24-32 hours a week. My life is very busy and I like it that way. It will take me awhile to get to where I want to go but it feels good to have a goal and to work toward it, and I really love my job in a long-term care facility.

The experience of living as a deaf person has taught me to not discriminate against anyone no matter what his or her handicap or disability. To walk though this world with a disability is a challenge. It can be hard to remember that if someone treats you unfairly it's their problem, not yours. I can now use the lessons I learned as a deaf person, and remember them everyday as I meet all the fellow humans in this journey of life. I also believe in miracles. The best is yet to come.

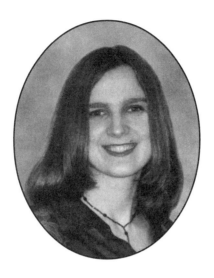

The Best Day of My Life…By Svetlana Kouznetsova

August 6, 1998, was one of the best days of my life—it was when I heard for the first time with a wonderful technology called a cochlear implant. It has changed my life so greatly. In fact, it's impossible for me to imagine what my life would be like now without this advanced technology available today for people with severe to profound sensorineural hearing loss.

I was born with normal hearing, but became profoundly deaf in both ears at the age of two due to meningitis. Before getting the implant, I wore hearing aids. They were not very helpful to me. Although I could hear some sounds that were loud enough for me, I couldn't recognize them all, let alone the complex sounds of speech. That was the main reason I decided to get a cochlear implant.

As for communication skills, I'm bilingual. My languages are Russian and English. I use voice and speechreading and/or sign language depending on the situation and whom I talk with. Since I am the only deaf member in my family, I learned to speak and lipread because my parents wanted me to be able to communicate not only with them, but also with other hearing people. It is easier for me to understand people if they speak clearly and don't talk too fast. I use sign language mainly to communicate with deaf signers. I came with my parents and sister to the US from Russia, so our native language is Russian. We still use it to communicate with each other and with other Russian-speaking people.

I started to learn English at age 11 in a Russian school after I was transferred from a school for the deaf to a regular public school. I had spent the first four years with deaf students and hearing teachers whom I could easily understand through sign language. Therefore, it was quite a challenge for me to be in a new school where I was the only deaf individual and had to rely on lipreading to communicate with hearing students and teachers whom I couldn't always understand. I had to do more work than my hearing classmates to replace the missed information in class by reading more materials and asking more questions. However, thanks to support from my family, school teachers, and some classmates, I learned to adjust to this environment and made it to high school graduation. A good secondary education and knowledge of English as a foreign language helped me get into the Rochester Institute of Technology (RIT). I graduated in 2000 with a bachelor's degree in Graphic Design. Now I work in a graphic design firm in New York City.

I am also fortunate to live in this country, where the conditions for people with hearing loss are much better than in Russia, since there are laws to protect their rights, as well as technology and services to make their lives easier. I've been taking advantage of these opportunities, such as watching TV and movies with captions, talking on the text phone, and using sign language interpreters for group events as well as for classes I attended at RIT. However, I wanted to broaden and improve my communication skills and saw the cochlear implant as the opportunity to enrich my life with sounds and to become more confident and independent in the hearing world.

My family and I had been interested in cochlear implants and impressed by their performance since the time we first heard about them. However, it wasn't easy for us to decide to get one for me, mainly because of surgical intervention. We hadn't known much about this technology, and therefore we weren't sure how effective it was in comparison to hearing aids that I wore then. Besides, we were so confused with opposite opinions of proponents and opponents of cochlear implants. Only when we met CI users, were we convinced of its effectiveness. Most of them were happy with their CIs. They turned out to be the best people to explain what it was like to hear with a cochlear implant, and therefore we received more credible information from them. I was fortunate to be able to contact more CI users and to go to CI support group meetings at the League for Hard of Hearing (LHH) in

New York City and at RIT (while I was a student there). This helped me become more confident about my decision to get a CI and be better prepared to enter the world of sound.

After having taken different tests and talking with a surgeon and audiologist who were CI specialists, I was told that I could receive benefits from this technology. I was warned, however, not to have unrealistic expectations. I had been deaf for a long time and it would therefore take longer for me to learn to understand sounds, especially speech, than for those who had become deaf later in their lives or those who had been deaf for a shorter period of time.

Finally, I had to decide which company's cochlear implant to select, as well as which ear to choose for implantation. As for choosing the ear for implantation, the CT scan and MRI showed that my left ear's cochlea had some ossification as a result of meningitis, while my right ear's cochlea was clear. Also, my right ear had more response to amplification than the left ear, meaning that it should have more surviving ganglion nerve cells. So my surgeon suggested that it would be best to operate on my right ear, but he also told me that it was up to me to decide. The problem was that at first I didn't want to risk my better ear. However, having talked with some other CI users who had their good ears operated, I realized that my hearing loss was so profound, that even with a hearing aid in my right ear I could not hear that much anyway and couldn't understand speech without lipreading. So I decided to follow my surgeon's advice and to have my better ear implanted to maximize the results.

My surgery was performed on July 7, 1998, and went well, without complications. A month later, during CI activation, I heard sounds for the first time in 18 years and was very surprised by their quantity and quality! Cochlear implants outperform the conventional hearing aids that just amplify some sounds, without helping me to hear and understand them. I liked the cochlear implant right away! With it, I hear many sounds of different volume and frequencies at different distances. I can hear, for example, the sounds of a computer's keyboard, my sister playing the piano one floor above, the phone ringing in another room, the doorbell, people talking, music, water running from a faucet, a whisper, the rustle of leaves under my feet, sounds of animals, and various musical instruments. Of course, it was unusual for me to hear so many sounds in the beginning, but with time I became used to them and started to understand them. I'm better at identifying common environmental sounds that I hear many times. This is due to the fact that they are easier to remember and recognize than the complex sounds of speech. I can't understand all words by only hearing them yet, but the cochlear implant facilitates my lipreading, especially if there are no loud environmental sounds around that make it hard for me to hear speech. I can also hear my voice and control its volume, although for the time being, I can't fully eradicate the so-called deaf speech.

The cochlear implant changed my concept of sounds and helped me better understand how hearing people perceive them. One of the most important changes that the cochlear implant has brought into my life is my ability to use a regular phone. So far I can talk on the phone only with my family members who know what words I can understand. But the important difference is that before the surgery I couldn't use a regular phone at all. Now, I can recognize the ring, dial tone, and the busy signal of the phone without difficulty, and can tell if it's someone in my family answering the phone or the answering machine picking up. I can hear when someone answers my call and start a conversation, or get an answering machine and leave a message after the beep.

Cochlear implants have some limitations. For example, I can't use a speech processor during the night (it's not comfortable to sleep with it on); I have to take it off before swimming and cover it during heavy rain (water can damage the external component). As for the sound quality, a cochlear implant can't replace all the damaged hair cells of the ear's cochlea and therefore can't produce all the sounds that can be heard by a person with normal hearing. Besides, it's not enough to just hear with a cochlear implant, it takes time, hard work, and patience to learn to understand sounds. Therefore, the success of a CI user depends not only on his/her deafness history, the cause and duration of hearing loss, but also on himself/herself, on his/her family's support, and on how he/she is using the device. That's why people shouldn't assume that cochlear implants cure deaf people and make them hearing and that new CI users can understand everything right away.

Some people ask me why I decided to get a CI back then and not wait until the technology becomes more advanced. It's true that there may be some better solutions for hearing loss in the future, but cochlear implants have already improved so much over the past several decades that I didn't want to wait another few years to take advantage of hearing sounds. I think it was the right time for me, because the earlier I got the CI, the more years of hearing I would have. My hearing and speech comprehension is still improving every day.

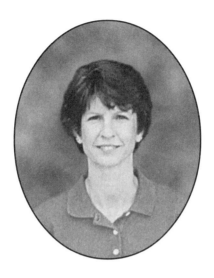

I Hear This Wild, Wonderful World Now…By Teresa Jackson Jones

I began my journey into a world of silence 40 years ago. I was diagnosed with profound hearing loss around the age of two. I contracted the measles when I was three weeks old and had very painful ear abscesses until I reached school age. Hearing loss runs in my mother's family even though she wasn't affected, nor was my younger brother. It was really never determined exactly what caused my hearing loss, but over the years the silence became total. I like to think I was the one with hearing loss because I could handle it best.

I was raised as a normal hearing child, I was never told I couldn't do something because I couldn't hear. My mom and dad always encouraged me to try. I grew up to be a very hard-headed, determined little girl, which has served me well over the years. It was so very important to me to be considered "normal." Back in the 60s hearing aids were boxes with wires that you wore on your shirt. I hated the thought of having to wear those things and was determined to manage without them. I was 'mainstreamed' into regular schools. Over the years, school became increasingly difficult, but I managed with my self-taught lipreading skills and was fortunate to have very caring and understanding teachers. But there were lots of things that I missed out on because of my hearing loss. I lived out in the country so most of my playmates were cousins, people who knew me well and knew to look at me when they were speaking.

Our son Jon was born just before my 20th birthday. It was soon after his birth that I had to accept the fact that I was going to need help, because I couldn't hear him cry. Being deaf and raising a child was difficult I was totally dependent on my husband Garry to wake me at night and during the day, and I had to keep Jon in sight. I got my first hearing aid at age 20 and another one seven years later when Jamie, our daughter, was born. Even with the help of two powerful hearing aids, all I could hear were loud, unintelligent sounds. I have been blessed with two normal hearing children, both of whom are excellent lipreaders and were making doctor and dentist appointments when they were just over two years old.

I first became aware of the cochlear implant in 1995. My Department of Vocational Rehab counselor mentioned it to me while we were working on my case. I was looking for more help than the hearing aids were giving me. After getting a voice-carry over phone, a lighted doorbell and alarm clock from Vocational Rehab., I experienced my first real taste of independence. Two years later, Jane once again brought up the cochlear implant and the improvements that had been made since we last talked about it. I had become pretty comfortable with my life, I could communicate over the phone with the VCO and awake on my own with the lighted alarm clock, but I promised I would think about it. It took me three years to decide to look into the CI further. After a lot of praying and soul searching, I decided that I had so much to gain and so little to lose and if this didn't work out…well, I had better things to do than feel sorry for myself.

My first appointment with Dr. Raleigh Jones at the University of Kentucky Medical Center in Lexington, Kentucky was in December 1999. I guess I was hoping he would say, "Teresa, I cannot help you, go home and get on with your life" and I wouldn't have to make this decision. I was surprised when he looked me straight in the eye and said "Teresa, I think you would be an excellent candidate for the cochlear implant."

I was wired March 30, 2000. This was the beginning of a remarkable, scary, overwhelming, and wonderful adventure. Not only could I actually hear voices, I could make out the different tones of the sounds. Some sounds were easily identified because they sounded like I thought they would, others sounded nothing like I had imagined, and there were things that I never dreamed made any sound at all. The first voices I heard were squeaky and muffled. Mr. Shelton, my audiologist, told me that this was the way Mickey Mouse sounded, but I had never heard Mickey Mouse. Over time, the squeakiness disappeared and sounds became more defined and clearer.

People would ask me after my surgery, "Can you hear me?" Oh yes, I could hear them very well, but I cannot understand them without reading their lips. This is so hard for people to understand. Speech sounded like I imagine a foreign language would sound. But with time and patience, I have learned to pick out a word here and there. Imagine hearing your children's voices for the first time when they were 14 and 20 years old.

It was a thrilling experience to hear my mother's voice over the regular phone and actually understand her simple sentences. Even after 17 months, I am still learning. I still rely on my lipreading skills but am slowly learning to trust what I am hearing. I did experience some emotional spells after receiving my implant. My kind CI surgeon, with whom I still keep in contact via e-mail, assured me that this was a normal reaction to such a major life-changing event. He compared the feelings I was having to those associated with childbirth, marriage, major relocation, etc. It was helpful, too, that I could talk freely of my fears with my new audiologist, Jinger.

I took speech therapy for a while, even though the therapist told me that I spoke very well considering my hearing loss. I learned to say the 's' and 'f' sounds and actually understood my first sentence during therapy. Learning to understand what I was hearing had become an "effortless effort." The harder I tried to understand, the more difficult it was. I learned to just sit back and let it come as it would, and it has. It is important to realize that with a cochlear implant learning to hear and understand, is a slow, gradual process, especially for someone who has never been able to understand speech and hearing for the first time.

The support of family and friends play a big part of the success with the CI. Having someone who has experienced what you are going through both physically and emotionally can make a big difference. I have been fortunate to meet some wonderful people over the Internet, who have made my journey into the hearing world so much easier. As much as I had come to love my silent world, as safe as I felt in it…. I love this wild, wonderful, noisy world more….much more.

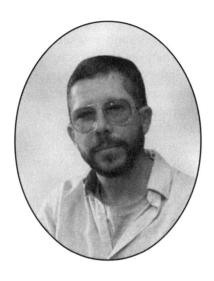

My Hearing Odyssey...By Paul Thompson

I was born on September 3, 1957, in East London, a small town on the southeast coast of South Africa. I had the good fortune to be born hearing and had learnt the rudiments of speech, when around the age of one and a half I came down with a simultaneous infection of Rubella (German measles) and whooping cough. It is conjectured that the fever damaged the hearing nerve and since then my hearing has slowly but steadily declined.

My parents discovered that I was deaf when I started school. My teacher noticed that I did not appear to hear unless I was looking at her and that my speech was not always as clear as it should be (I had a tendency to swallow my words which I sometimes still do). When she queried my parents concerning this, they said, yes, they had noticed but just thought I being stubborn and maybe a little slow with speech! I had taught myself to lipread.

Much to my disgust, I was then sent to Collage Street, a normal school with a hard-of-hearing department. While there, I had a speech therapist named Miss Vice. This remarkable woman took me under her wing and spent many hours improving my speech and lipreading. I

329

have her to thank that today I speak as clearly as I do and for my excellent lipreading skills. She also taught me that you could get anything you want, if you will but apply yourself with single-minded determination in pursuit of whatever it may be that you want. I remained in Collage Street until Grade 5. Then, as there was no facility in East London and I was losing more of my hearing, I was sent to St. Vincent's School for the deaf in Johannesburg, where I was a boarder. I remained with them until Grade 8.

As I was the only person going on to matric that year and the school felt that it was not viable for them to employ a teacher for just one pupil. It was decided that I should try a hearing school. This did not work, mainly because normal South African schools are bilingual and in the deaf school we were only taught in our home language, so I earned my matric via a Damlin correspondence course.

In 1977, my formal education having come to an end, I went out into the world to try my luck at earning a living. My first job was that of a draughtsman, but it did not work out. I was a cheeky little bugger and did not want to accept what I was told. The net result was that after six months, my long-suffering employer suggested that maybe I was not meant to be a draughtsman. This resulted in the two of us parting ways. Possibly a little wiser but not in any way sadder, I looked around for some other way of earning a living. Quite by chance I came across an advertisement offering a course in COBOL, a computer language. Knowing nothing about computers but thinking it was something a deaf guy could do (computers, at least in those days, do not talk) I enrolled and three months later I was the proud possessor of a COBOL diploma. Since then I have worked in the computer industry.

After being sidetracked many times (hiking in Europe and Africa, racing motor bikes and cars etc.) In 1989, I finally started to do something about achieving my dream of building a yacht and going sailing. It was to be one of those decisions that change one's life forever.

When growing up in East London, one of my favorite playgrounds was the harbor. I enjoyed watching the shipping being maneuvered by the tugs and would dream of the faraway places that they came from, wondering what it would be like to travel seas and be meeting people in foreign lands. One day when I was down at the docks I met another boy, who, too, was watching the shipping. It turned out that he lived on a yacht with his parents and they were sailing around the world. Their boat was in East London for an overhaul. Anyway he invited me to come and have a look at the boat. I spent the rest of the day exploring the boat with him. That day my dream was born. At the age of 11 I decided I would one day have my own boat and I would one day, sail the seas. I have never forgotten my dream. Today *La Chico* (the name means "My Girl") is not very different from that first boat which inspired my dream.

The building of *La Chico* was in many ways the most difficult and ambitious task that I had up to that time undertaken. To an outsider the prospects could not have looked good. I had a history of not finishing my projects, as I allowed myself to be to easily distracted and side-tracked into other things and despite having been draughtsman to Angelo Lavrano (South Africa's best known yacht designer) for two years, I still did not know anything about building boats, apart that is, from what I learnt from books. I must point out that almost everything that I know today, I taught myself, usually from reading the relevant book.

It took me from September 1989 till late 1992 to build *La Chico*. I had to learn the skills of a welder, electrician, plumber, carpenter, rigger, upholsterer, and mechanic. At the end of the day, as far as the building of *La Chico* is concerned, all I can say is that *La Chico* made me and I made *La Chico*. Without the trail of building her I would probably never have been able to sail single-handed. Building her, I learnt about perseverance, about sticking it out. Today they call me stubborn - maybe I am, but that is what it takes to do what I do. It is also what it takes to survive as a deaf person in a hearing world.

In the 1993 Cape to Rio, I skippered *Acid Rain* (I took on the job, after the original skipper defected) a boat with two blind people (Neel's and Hein). It was the first time I was in command of a crewed yacht. It was also the first time I crossed an ocean. Today I am still proud of that voyage. I turned what was threatening to turn into a disaster into a successful voyage, and I earned the affection and esteem of my crew. After the race I delivered a St Francis 43-ft. catamaran from Rio back to Cape Town (with two crew and owner onboard).

In May 1994, I was finally ready to leave Cape Town in my own yacht, *La Chico*. I sailed alone and was thus the first deaf person to cross the South Atlantic single-handed. I then spent the next seven and a half years sailing in Brazil, Venezuela, the Caribbean islands, and the Eastern Seaboard of the USA. I had many interesting and (mostly) enjoyable adventures, amoung the highlights being Hurricane Luis (St. Martin, Sept. 1995) during which I nearly lost *La Chico* as she went ashore just after the hurricane peaked. Fortunately, she is built of steel and is nearly unbreakable and I was able to pull off the shore and get her sailing again within a week. Other highlights were being a paid skipper of an 85-ft. ferry in St. Martin and cruising America's inland waterway. I also met many interesting and wonderful people, many of whom went out of their way to be kind and helpful.

Suddenly, during April 2000 in the midst of preparing for a solo circumnavigation effort, my hearing went from a severe hearing loss to a profound one. Two weeks later my hearing started to fluctuate between profound and a complete loss, and I was relying almost exclusively on lipreading, as my hearing aid was no longer of any use. I gave up the solo effort on being advised that the sooner I get an implant, the more likely it was that it would be successful and so, after the American Navy offered to let me store the boat in their yard, I left for Cape Town, South Africa.

I was implanted by Dr. Wagenfeld on Dec. 11, 2000 (becoming his 167th implantee), with Cochlear's Nucleus Contour 24 electrode and use the Esprite 24 BTE processor with the SPEAK strategy. Switch-on was three days later, on Dec.14th. This was rather unusual, as it is normal to wait at least two weeks. However, with hospital and audiological staff going on leave for the Christmas period, my surgeon thought it would be worth the experiment. So I was able to hear for Christmas.

The other wonderful thing that happened during 2000 is that I got married and promptly acquired not only a wonderful wife, Elmarie (whose uncle is Prof. Johannes Swart, Dr. Wagenfeld's compatriot in Pretoria), but also two very energetic boys!

For me the cochlear implant has mostly been a success. Immediately after switch-on, I was able to understand voices. At first they did not sound very normal, having a very hollow and insubstantial sort of sound. Also the clarity was poor and music did not sound good at all. After my second mapping things improved and speech began to sound much more normal.

The first six months, the improvement after each mapping was significant. Thereafter the differences were subtler. Nonetheless, each mapping brings out details that I did not hear before. The above not withstanding, I still need to lipread to a lesser or greater degree, depending on the environmental (background) noise and how well the person I am communicating with enunciates their words.

The telephone, which in the days when I still wore a hearing aid, I could handle with possibly a 50% chance of success, I can now only claim about a 20% success rate. Mostly I am only really successful with people I know well. Knowing what the subject is about beforehand or being able to catch on to what the person on the other end is trying to say is half the battle.

Music has proved to be another story entirely; so far it is not a success. I used to be a great borough and classical music fan so this has perhaps been the greatest disappointment of the implant. A short while ago I was able to borrow a Sprint body-worn processor. The Sprint, unlike the Esprit is not just restricted to the SPEAK mapping strategy but can run ACE and CIS as well. It is also possible to control the rate of electrode simulation more finely. Anyway, I found that with both ACE and CIS, music sounds a thousand times more like music should sound. Of the two strategies CIS seems to hold the most promise. Other implantees have confirmed this as well.

At my one-year check-up, my audiogram showed that with the implant my response curve is now a near flat line, with a threshold at 250 Hz of 28 dB continuing to 6000 Hz also at 28 dB. This is better hearing than I have any memory of in my life. Single-word recognition is still poor at about 15%, but in sentences I am doing much better with about 60% recognition. In reality I am able to follow a conversation at 100%, as my lipreading makes up for any hearing deficiency. Of course that does not help on the phone, and likewise I do poorly when trying to follow TV or the radio.

In conclusion an implant does not make a deaf person a hearing person, but it most certainly makes life a lot easier and also enables one to be more independent of others for assistance in hearing matters. If anyone were to ask me "Was it worth it?" my answer would be a resounding YES.

Seniors' Stories

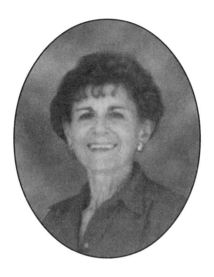

Prelude to a Song…By Rosalie Orinson

Bells were ringing. No, not the Bells of St. Mary, but the high school hand bells during the holiday music program. I strained to hear the melodic resonance and prayed for a miracle. In a few moments I would gaze proudly upon my son, who was first clarinet in the HS band and symphony orchestras. But I would not hear the Mozart magic, the Christmas carols, or the Chanukah songs. Two weeks earlier, a sudden, total, and irrevocable hearing loss destroyed my life's momentum and trapped me in a world of silence.

Both my daughter and my son were seniors that year and during their entire HS career I had never missed a performance. In the spring, before graduation, both would star in *My Fair Lady*. It took steel nerves to attend the show, to conjure up memories of the libretto and the sparkling score and behave, as I now perceived myself to be a hearing person who happened to be deaf. Nothing outwardly defined my difference. I did not grow horns. I cheered and applauded with the others, but I was totally dependent upon lipreading, stage direction, and visual cues on that soundless stage. Formerly a blithe spirit, a dancer, a casework supervisor in a children's home with several college degrees, I was now dependent for the simplest of life's needs even for an ordinary phone call. My change of life started before menopause, in one life-shattering and isolating blow. I was no stranger to hearing loss. My odyssey with difference began at the age of three when scarlet fever moderately impacted on my hearing acuity. I was already involved in singing elocution, tap and toe dancing. My mother's love of music and the performing arts became a treasured legacy that sustained me throughout my life, especially when I was struck by deafness. Whereas my mother sang like an angel, my brother played the violin, and my father could whistle, I chose dance and never stopped tripping the light fantastic.

"Bluff and Anxiety" was the name of the game I played during my growing-up years. Being petite I had the good fortune in school to be seated up front, but keeping up with teacher tactics and class discussion was a tremendous drain on my energies. I was a good student, made class honors, and experienced a boost to my ego by being awarded the art medal at graduation. I had many friends, but still... I was different.

Dance remained my most precious outlet. During my teen years I was a member of a club of 14 girls from my neighborhood. We grew up in a beach community well typified by *The Brighton Beach Memoirs*. Art, swing, modern dance, and boys rounded out my social existence. My first experience with a hearing aid, (artfully concealed) was at NYU, but every lecture was a challenge. Many post-war professors grew mustaches and beards. Although I informed them of my problem, they strutted around the classroom, turned their backs while speaking, and much depended upon my ability to surreptitiously copy a fellow student's notes. I worked hard at concealing my problem. I had aspirations of becoming a doctor, but realities tempered that dream. What chance would a Jewish, hard of hearing young woman have of being admitted to medical school when top priority was given to the returning war veterans? I worked in the Occupational Therapy department of the Hospital for Special Surgery one summer, but, despite my good performance, my hearing loss was a deterrent. Would it always be the monkey on my back?

Armed with a useless bachelor's degree in Psychology, I tried my wings in a vast variety of services. Among them I led a journalism group in a lower East side community center, taught art for the Police Athletic League in Hell's Kitchen in NYC and upper Manhattan, was a camp counselor, learned to type in a local high school and finally applied and was accepted in the University of Pennsylvania School of Social Work social group work program. Life was definitely not beautiful. It was hard, demanding, and for the first time I had to deal with the effect of my hearing loss on others. I was capable, creative, and challenged and knew graduation was incumbent upon change! Two years later I was armed with a MSW degree but vestiges of a lifetime of bluffing and non-acceptance of my hearing loss accompanied me to my first job in Denver, Colorado. I was director of the children's program in a Jewish community center with a dwindling membership and endless phone responsibilities. Hearing loss always added to my anxiety. This became a frustrating and unfulfilling experience, and I finally made the change to become director of a recreation center in a culturally mixed lower income neighborhood with large family groups. Along with children's activities I developed women's self-enhancement and fund raising programs. It was creative, challenging, and I felt competent.

A new love interest in my life followed me to Colorado where he completed his Ph.D. in Psychology at Denver University. We were married that year, and after two years of completing course work we left the majesty of the mountains for his internship in St Elizabeth's Hospital in Washington DC. Our son was born during those trying times. We had few amenities to ease the boredom.... no TV; little money for entertainment and walking around the grounds of a mental institution was not my idea of amusement. Listening to the radio was difficult. My love of reading was a blessing and an escape to the outside world. Special friends made the difference as they still do today.

Our daughter was born 15 months later, adding to the pressures of parenting. My hearing loss, primarily in the low frequencies, had increased over the years as a result of ear infections, and in retrospect I now realize that I had been blessed to be able to hear the babies crying, the violins, the clarinets, and even the infernal shriek of the teakettle.

After several moves in the east, we developed roots in Rockland County in NY where for seven years I worked as a casework supervisor and director of volunteers in a children's home. Over the years I became aware of more deaf children needing appropriate placement and in the fall of 1974 I decided to take a graduate course on the Psychology of Deafness in NYU. I wanted to learn about the field, not become a statistic.

The following events changed my life forever. Just before Thanksgiving there was an economic cutback at the home. One-third of the staff was given notice and my job was taken over by a member of the convent. A week later at a group home meeting with one of my clients, who had a voice like an angel, the last I ever heard naturally, there was a shrieking sound and then silence. The whole way to NYU that night I figured my hearing aids had broken. By the next morning I knew the truth. I could not hear myself screaming. I was deaf.

THE DEAF YEARS

What had happened? Medical authorities could only say, "The Lord only knows." Many diagnostic tests followed but nothing changed. My world remained silent and joyless ... until an eternal spring of resilience took hold. I found my lipreading skills had not abandoned me. I continued my studies in deafness and worked toward a degree. I negotiated with Rockland Community College to present a full-day conference on "The Psychiatric Dilemma of Deafness" in the spring and engaged the deaf community in the planning process. For the first time I became aware of deaf culture, deaf pride, and deaf humor. I still get a few chuckles showing how a few minute differences in hand movement can inadvertently change "hungry" into "horny."

The conference was a huge success. It became the springboard for new programs at the college on hearing loss that followed: individual and group counseling, sign language, captioned movies, and conferences exploring the social and emotional impact of hearing loss. We brought in vocational experts, specialists in technology, the Little Theatre for the Deaf, the Gallaudet Dancers, and groups acting and singing with signs.

The phone remained my biggest obstacle during the dependency decades. The relay was not a full-time service. With necessity being the mother of invention, I developed a device, "The Extra Ear" which enabled a third person to listen to a phone conversation via an ear piece and interpret orally (or with sign). The deaf person held the receiver and could respond verbally. At last my children could not hang up until I was ready to sign off. The Extra Ear was marketable for a brief period until the relay service was established 24 hours a day and portable phones enabled ease of third-party listening.

Desirous of more therapeutic involvement, I wrote proposals for special school and hospital services and worked as a counselor for the hearing impaired in mainstream schools in New Jersey and New York. I developed a private practice specializing in deafness and spoke at conferences and seminars. I gave courses for first persons responding to the scene of an accident: EMT, police, and fire Departments and became an adjunct professor at Ramapo College in New Jersey teaching "The World of the Deaf and the Hard of Hearing."

Dance and theater were my passion throughout those 15 soundless years. I performed in folk and ballroom programs while conjuring up the music in my mind's ear. I attended theatrical performance where the script was available or I knew the interpretation would not be solely ASL. Wherever needed I used oral interpreters for conventions and important events.

In spite of many loving, rewarding years, my marriage crashed on a rocky road. Deafness exacerbated the problem. However, by the time I presented the workshop, "Deaf, Divorced and Daring to be Different" at the SHHH convention in Colorado, I had become an "independent woman." I began to train in professional ballroom studios, I taught teenagers swing and Latin dancing in the New York School for the Deaf, and became increasingly involved in conference development in college hearing-impaired programs. Life was manageable and predictable until the MIRACLE!

THE COCHLEAR IMPLANT

In 1990 a friend suggested I consider the cochlear implant. She had been my audiologist in better days and knew I had nothing to lose. I was intrigued. I made an appointment with Dr. Parisier at the Lenox Hill Hospital in NY, followed through with all the audiological tests and was declared a candidate. Where would the money come from? My insurance company at work would only commit themselves to a fraction of the cost. I was ready to consider utilizing my son's colleague, a surgeon who had trained in this procedure but had not yet performed the operation. He would do it without cost as a professional courtesy. I soon learned that a major requirement for success was a trained and knowledgeable audiology team. He was not prepared for that. For a short period of time I felt a wave of disappointment then shelved the idea. I knew I would have to return to Lenox Hill ... but when?

A few weeks later a chance meeting with a psychologist who had recently been implanted renewed my determination. I would explore every opportunity to establish funding. I met with the CI hospital staff with my congressman, and I offered to provide counseling services at the hospital for the balance of the funding not provided by my insurance company. My request was accepted but in the final stage. My company came through with flying colors.

My stay in the hospital was more primitive in those days. The nursing staff was less informed, special needs such as TTYs, and TV captions were delayed, and I was detained for three days because of fluid drainage. Once hooked up six weeks later, life became fuller and more exciting. I knew I would have some clarity and worked diligently at training my auditory word recognition through reading books, records, radio, and human speech. My perceptions of music blossomed. I could now dance to the rhythms of reality. Symphonic, big band and modern rock mixed with memory became increasingly pleasurable. Voice telephone became my instrument of choice soon to dominate all phone contacts. I joined Toastmasters and became more proficient in delivering speeches and truly enjoyed my 10 minutes "on stage." Dance and theatre continue to captivate me, and I am now involved with a team devoted to bringing captions to on-stage performances.

I am still hard of hearing. As magical as the cochlear implant is, friends and family require sensitivity, understanding, and patience in situations where my hearing loss still prevails. At times I receive substantial aid from assistive devices such as infrared systems, phone adapters, etc. My speech has become clearer and more precise. As my caseload increased to include hearing as well as hearing impaired students, I lectured as the "Bionic Woman" in every classroom about difference, hearing loss and the cochlear implant. I have encouraged many profoundly hearing impaired people to become implanted and hope to devote my post-retirement years to educating the public about hearing loss.

During my residence in Florida over the past two years, I have given seminars on deafness, family dynamics, coping with hearing loss and the cochlear implant at local colleges, libraries, senior centers, and adult communities with the hope that some will be inspired to live fuller, happier, and more productive lives.

I am no longer the "Bionic Woman." A behind-the-ear processor has eliminated the need for wires and has afforded me the renewed freedom of fashion and athletic comfort. I continue to view my experience as a miracle...a prelude to a song. Once past the surgery, the early discordance and the adaptation to unfamiliar sounds, the ultimate joy experienced from the voices of loved ones, from music, and from the delightfully diversified sounds of nature is incomparable. Once again the bells are ringing...and I can hear them!!!

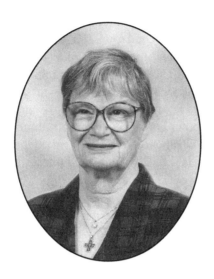

My Implant…By Virginia Anderson, Ph.D.

I haven't always been deaf. When I was thirty-something, during the winter of 1967-68, our chimney plugged, and carbon monoxide entered our home every time the gas furnace came on, and in North Dakota that's pretty often! By February, when we discovered the problem, we were all sick, but, luckily, not dead.

A few years later it was obvious I wasn't hearing well. A visit to the speech and hearing clinic confirmed it. After hearing my history of carbon monoxide poisoning (my blood CO level on a day I felt well was 23 – 18 is usually considered fatal!!), the audiologists suggested that my hearing loss was probably caused by oxygen deprivation atrophying the cilia in my inner ears. (Our four children also have hearing problems, which tends to confirm the theory.)

My next stop was the rehabilitation center, which fitted me with behind-the-ear hearing aids. I also received a lesson in lipreading from my audiologist there. I practiced a lot, especially on television newscasters. I also learned to do a lot of guessing from the context of the sounds I was hearing! But my husband learned to laugh pretty often when the answers I gave bore no relation to the questions he asked.…

By the early 80s I graduated to two in-the-ear aids, which were more advanced and gave me more help. In the 90s I was teaching large

343

lecture sections of Introduction to Computers at the University of North Dakota, and was really having trouble hearing questions from my students beyond the first or second row. The first digital hearing aids were coming on the market, and I tried them. I also tried Starkey aids with Manhattan switches. These were just as helpful as the digital, and cheaper, so we went with them. Needless to say, my students had lectures on how the ear and hearing aids work (or don't work)!

One of my computer books had an article about cochlear implants, with a reference to Cochlear in Denver. I called them, but was told I'd never qualify if I could talk to them on the telephone. They sent me some literature, however. I read through it, but was not thrilled with their "state of the air" technology at the time (early 90s).

I was really limited in hearing over the telephone – only the old AT&T phones with amplifiers worked for me. (I still use that old phone.) My daughter, who is a computer software engineer in Virginia, got so upset with my not being able to understand her on the phone that she got on the Internet and found Advanced Bionics. At her request they sent me some literature and a videotape. Their state of the art technology impressed and intrigued us. My husband called them, and they encouraged us to consider a Clarion implant. They thought I sounded like a good candidate. We found that an ear surgeon, Dr. James Frisk, and his audiologist son, Matt, in Fargo, ND, just 75 miles from our home, were in the process of getting implant surgery done there. They had both been certified by Advanced Bionics, but the hospital in Fargo was dragging its feet.

After consulting with the Frisks I was tested by Matt and passed the audiology criteria of Advanced Bionics and Medicare. I could understand vowels, but consonants were a guessing game. The Hi-focus electrode was in the final stages of getting FDA approval, and Matt suggested we go to Dr. Samuel Levine and his audiologist Sharon Smith at the University of Minnesota-Fairview Hospital in Minneapolis, MN., where the Hi-Focus trials were taking place. In fact, Matt set up the appointments for us. After spending a day at the clinic in Minneapolis, including psychological tests, CT scans, and interviews with Dr. Levine and Ms. Smith, I was given final approval, and surgery was scheduled for July 31, 2000. In the meantime, the Hi-Focus approval was finalized so I would not be part of the test group, meaning I could have all my mapping session done in Fargo, a savings of more than 500 miles per trip!

Since I had only about 10% hearing in each ear, with virtually no difference between them, I decided to have the right ear implanted, taking advantage of the fact that the right ear is tuned more to speech, leaving the left to music and environmental sounds. Dr. Levine concurred.

When the time came for my initial activation, August 24, Mary Barker, clinical specialist with Advanced Bionics who was instrumental in developing the mapping program for the Platinum Series, came from Denver to assist. I was to be one of the first to be hooked-up to the Hi-Focus electrode Platinum hardware. After a very quiet three weeks, I was hearing again. But understanding? Hardly.

So I practiced. It occurred to me that if I talked out loud to myself, I would know what words I said, and my brain might make the connection between the words and the sounds. Yes! That worked pretty well, and I still do it. Another trick I used was to listen to talking books over my Bose sound system. Book narrators enunciate very clearly, and again, I might make the connection between sound and meaning. And I went back to my trusty TV newscasters – this time with the sound on – they enunciate well, also, and since they usually face the camera, I could combine lipreading and meaning to find words to connect with the sounds I was hearing.

One of my resources was Beverly Biderman's book *Wired for Sound.* Another resource, which I found very useful, with lots of information about hearing, was the audiotape *Mozart as Healer* by Don Campbell. In fact, I collected Mozart CDs and a player and took them to the hospital with me. I had a monaural earphone and played Mozart most of the time I was there. I still listen to classical music and find I am hearing more and more of the high frequencies. I am also doing better with television, especially narrated programs like those on the History and Discovery channels. Sports events have too much intentional background noise for me to decipher what the commentators are saying, however.

I still have trouble hearing in crowds, as I hear (but do not understand) all the conversations within range (and the range is very wide!). I do best in the car, because it is an enclosed space and sound waves cannot escape. It also is very well insulated so there is little background noise.

An interesting and happy side effect of my implant is an alleviation of migraine headaches. I have had frequent migraines since I was a very young girl, sometimes lasting as long as a week to 10 days. Since my implant I've not had a single migraine! I also had a tendency toward sinus headaches. They, too, have diminished in frequency and intensity to almost nothing. Two daughters-in-law in the medical field have suggested that it might be the magnet, or just having my skull drilled, a la ancient Egyptian practices!

I had been warned prior to surgery that I would waken with "the worst headache you've ever had" – that also didn't happen. I was completely comfortable, without even my usual post-anesthesia nausea. I had requested lots of oxygen, which I was given, and that may have had its desired effect.

Overall, I'm glad I have the implant. I anticipate that my hearing will improve over time, although I realize it will never be complete. I will always give funny answers to some questions….

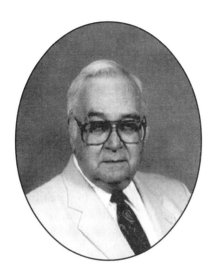

Do You Hear What I Hear?...By Dave Emerson

In the normal course of life we expect to be blessed with five senses: vision, hearing, taste, touch, and smell. Sometimes through accident, illness or genetics one or more of those senses may be lost or non-existent. That loss may occur at any age or, in some people, it may never have been there. The normal world takes all of these senses for granted. We usually don't give much thought to how we see, hear, feel, taste, or detect odors; and we give less thought to how we would react to a sudden loss of a sense.

In my case I lost my hearing suddenly over the space of one week some 20 years ago. On Monday morning my hearing was fine; by Friday I had no hearing. In addition to the loss of hearing I encountered extreme photosensitivity - I had to wear sunglasses inside at night. There was also intense vertigo, nausea, as well as loss of balance and equilibrium, and very annoying tinnitus. Looking back at the event there were clues that my hearing and balance were somehow being affected. Sharp noises were very uncomfortable and in playing golf I found that I had started to miss the ball on the tee. That in itself shouldn't have been a cause for concern; it happens from time to time, usually accompanied by laughter from ones playing partners. But it had started to happen with uncomfortable regularity.

The week of my severe hearing loss and other problems occurred while I was away from my home. I was working on a research project at a university in North Carolina, 1500 miles from my home. The project was one that was critical for my employer and was to be set up and conducted during a week's time. The facility was a multi-storied structure and directed by an individual who happened to be deaf. My work was going well in spite of the progressive hearing loss during the week. I was rushing to get it completed so that I could get back to my personal physician for diagnosis and treatment. That meant working after hours until late evening. One night the director was closing the facility and securing. He would turn lights off on one floor and then go the next. I couldn't yell at him to stop, so I tried to catch him and in the process would turn the lights back on. I think that finally he noticed that the lights weren't staying turned off and he looked to find the reason. That's when we discovered each other. I told him that I was almost through and was having problems. He was completely sympathetic and very understanding.

At that time, I was working for one of the major pharmaceutical companies. The FDA considered the early cochlear implants experimental devices, and as a result most insurers would not cover the cost of the device or surgery. My employing company had been established a number of years ago by a one very compassionate individual. At the time of my hearing loss this individual realized that our insurance would not cover the cost. He authorized the company to pay for it all, including the device, surgery and rehabilitation, out of company funds. The company took pains to help locate meaningful work for me elsewhere in the company. I become involved in medical writing and eventually was a team leader in developing the regulatory programs, strategies, and documentation leading to drug registration and continuing research. I have since retired following some 20 years with the company and its ever-changing departmental structures. I was fortunate to have been employed by that very understanding and supportive company. I was also very fortunate to have been the recipient of a few awards along the way.

During the course of the week I called my wife to explain my problems and ask her to set up appointments for me as soon as I got home. I had decided to call while I still had a little residual hearing. By Friday evening all hearing was gone. Early Saturday I drove as best I could to return a rental car and to catch a flight home. As luck would have it, the flight was not a direct flight but required a change in planes at

348

another airport. Through trial and error and a very helpful group of airline personnel I managed to catch the correct flight and got home where I went directly into a hospital on the advice of our family physician.

The cause of my hearing loss and other problems could not be diagnosed immediately. It didn't fit any of the known parameters. I was referred to Dr. Charles Luetje for further assessment and testing. Since my eyes were giving me so much trouble, Dr. Leutje suggested visiting with an ophthalmologist, Dr. K. C. Place, whose office was just across the hall. This fortunate referral and assessment led to the diagnosis of Cogan's Syndrome.

I continued under the care of both physicians for some time, but since there is no known cure for Cogan's Syndrome the conditions could not be reversed. My hearing loss was profound and permanent.

Dr. Luetje was one of the early workers in the field of cochlear implants and he suggested that we might wish to consider that device to restore at least a partial sense of hearing. That was indeed good news. However, there were problems with some of those early devices and so we had to wait for several months for the technical problems to be resolved. While waiting is always a difficult chore for some, it was especially nerve-wracking for me. It was a constant battle to avoid unreasonable expectations. It is a great temptation to expect the cochlear implant to restore hearing as we remember it. It does not. It can be devastating to sit on a peak of high expectations and then fall in a deep valley of depression when they are not met.

I was implanted early in 1982 with the House 3M Single Channel device. Surgery then was done early in the morning with an overnight stay in the hospital. There was a period of a few weeks before the final hook-up of the external device and programming. I recall very clearly that first time when the device was turned on. At first I thought, 'It isn't working.' I could hear nothing except my own tinnitus. Then I realized that no one was saying anything and there was only the slight sound of the ventilation system. That first voice startled me- "How does it feel?" I could only say "Great."

From that point onward it was a matter of training and practice with the speech pathologist and the audiologist. It cannot be emphasized too greatly that training and practice are a continual and ongoing effort. I have been at it some 20 years now and every day there is something new to learn and to identify by sound. One disadvantage of losing ones hearing later in life is that we try to force the things we hear now into the mold of how we remember things sounding long ago. It doesn't work that way. We have to take what things sound like now and try to store that information. It cannot be a conscious effort, since we have no direct control over how our brain works. It is more of an attitude than anything else. It's a matter of not saying 'that sounds like sounds like so-and-so; it's saying 'that is so-and-so.' A bird singing is a bird singing. A siren is a siren. They are not things that "sound like" birds singing or sirens warning.

Once one has a cochlear implant it opens up the world once more to our own individuality and a whole new set of experiences. I meet people who want to know what the implant is, what it does, and what it sounds like. I have found no way to explain what it sounds like because it sounds slightly different to everyone who has an implant. The only thing I have found to compare it with is to imagine a color you have never seen and then tell me what that color is.

I now have the 22-Channel cochlear implant. I use it exclusively but still have the single-channel internal coil in place. I consciously listen to everything at all times. It's a matter of identifying sounds, voices, and the sources of sound. I talk on the telephone using the relay system. Others I know are able to speak on the phone and carry on a near normal conversation. I cannot, but that is just my individual situation.

It would have been very easy to become depressed and discouraged very early on. It would have been tempting to ask "Why me?" But I have always considered that question to be meaningless. It serves absolutely no purpose except to try to place blame for an event for which there is nothing or no one at fault. It detracts from the effort needed to learn and grow in the use of the life-saving cochlear implant system. Changes are constantly being made in the equipment and strategies of implant technologies. The future may hold new and improved ways to do things. Still, the human being is the key to benefiting from any technology and methods. It is a long road but a thrilling ride, and each day is new with new things to hear and learn. It is one of my greatest joys now to be able to hear my new grandson laugh and say his first words. There are new worlds and new sounds to experience just around the bend.

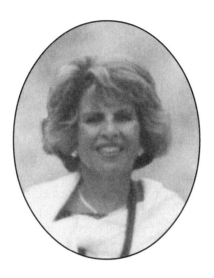

My Story... by Geri Young

In 1969 at age 30 and after giving birth to three children, I noticed one day that I was having a great deal of trouble hearing a friend of mine on the telephone. Upon asking my friend to repeat herself several times, I began to feel embarrassed and concerned about what was going on. This was the beginning of what turned out to be a very difficult and relentless series of episodes that were the cause of my deafness. I noticed that this problem seemed to fluctuate so that there were times during a month that I heard better or worse. As time went on, I chose to ignore this problem. However it continued to get worse, and so I decided to consult with a well-known otolaryngologist. He seemed confused and asked me to take a hearing test, as though that would, like magic, fix the problem. Each time I went back, he would again order a hearing test.

Years passed, and of course my hearing grew worse as well as my fluctuation. As my children were growing up and going to school, I wanted to work in my chosen field of Education. I substituted for a short while, but found that it was next to impossible to communicate with the children. Somehow choosing to ignore this difficult situation, I decided to go back to school and get a master's degree with a focus in Reading because there was such a need for this! I managed to get my master's in about four years, but I could only manage to see one or two students at a time in a tutoring situation because I knew that I would not be able to face a classroom of 30 children. Over the years, I did a great deal of tutoring in schools and in my home, but when my hearing began to worsen to the point that I couldn't hear parents on the phone who were calling to get their children to see me, then I had to stop tutoring. I did continue to want to work, somehow never really giving up that idea. For a while I owned my own discount clothing business until I moved to Florida. Coming back to my continued hearing loss, it was terrible because I never knew on what day or what week I would have an episode and my hearing would became worse and worse to the point that I didn't feel comfortable socializing; especially parties where I'd spend a lot of time excusing myself and going to the restroom to recuperate from the strain of listening and trying to hear, and come up with an appropriate response.

About five years after I first noticed this problem occurring, I called my otolaryngologist and said that this is getting very bad in that the episodes were occurring more often and lasting longer. What I mean by episodes was buzzing, ringing, and fullness in the ear, as well as a sudden decrease in my hearing. These episodes could last as long as two weeks. He immediately said that he thought I had Meniere's Disease, which is an inner ear disorder that causes fluctuating hearing loss due to a pressure that occurs in the inner ear due to a buildup of fluids that are not draining. He suggested I see a doctor in a nearby city. This doctor thought I might be helped by a surgical procedure called inner sac decompression, which is supposed to alleviate the pressure in the inner ear by removing the bone around the sac and therefore lowering the inner pressure of the sac. He also told me that I didn't really have Meniere's but that I had Lymphatic Hydrops.

After having the sac decompression surgery, I waited for the fluctuations to stop but it never did, so my hearing loss continued to progress. At this time I was 39 years old and the problem became relentless and continued until I lost all my hearing.

As the years went by and the problem worsened and I wore two big hearing aids covered by medium length hair, I was still having a lot of trouble understanding speech, due to very poor discrimination as a result of this inner ear disease. My frustration and anxiety levels were very high as I realized that there was no end in sight! Upon returning to my ENT doctor, he suggested I see an otologist in Nashville, Tennessee. I saw him and he suggested I go on a low sodium diet and that if

352

my body absorbed little salt, maybe these fluids would decrease but that didn't work either!! After seeing several otologists in California and Colorado who each had a different slant on this subject, I began to realize that this problem wasn't going away and I had better make my adjustments. At this time my hearing loss was in the "profound" category around 75 to 80 decibels.

In 1989, someone told me about SHHH, (Self Help for the Hard of Hearing). First I must mention that I tried to start a support group in Ann Arbor, Michigan, but to no avail. However, when I heard about SHHH, I wrote to the national organization in Bethesda, Maryland. They wrote back and sent me a great deal of materials and encouraged me to start a chapter in my city! I was so turned on by this prospect that it seemed to take precedence over the misery of my hearing loss. It distracted me and gave me a purpose and managed to increase my self-esteem, which wasn't very good at this time. I was fortunate to get in touch with several people who were more than anxious to help me start a group and viola!!! We started a support group of people of all ages and stages of life and we laughed, ate, talked, used devices, and had a lot of fun!!!! This saved my life and my spirit. An article was written in our local newspaper about how I started this chapter. One of my former neighbors wrote to say that I had turned lemons into lemonade. After three years my husband and I decided to retire and move to Florida. The members of the SHHH chapter suggested that I might want to start a new chapter in Boca Ratan where we were moving.

I went to several national conventions (I found them to be very inspiring and informative), but one in particular in Cedar Rapids, Iowa, had a Florida meeting. I met a woman who is very responsible for the success of the Delray Beach chapter, Regina Rabinowitz, and she told me to contact her when I moved to Boca. My husband and I did contact her and she gave me a lot of support. She suggested that I come to a meeting in Delray and that she would let me stand up and introduce myself and announce that I wanted to start a chapter in Boca. When the meeting was over several people came up to me with their business cards and told me to contact them. One of the most wonderful people I have ever met in my life was one who started this chapter with me. His name was Walter Saks and he had been very active in SHHH nationally and locally in New York as well as in volunteering at service agencies for the deaf to help people find the appropriate assistive listening devices (ALDs). He lived in my development and we spent many hours deciding how to start a local group. We met at my house in

January 1993 it's now 2001 and we're going strong with over 60 members, a board of directors of 12 wonderful people, and a solid treasury.

Three years after starting the chapter, in 1995, Dr. Thomas Balkany, and his staff from Miami were asked to speak on cochlear implants at one of our meetings. I was aware of and knowledgeable about CI's and even consulted with an otolaryngologist in Ann Arbor a few years before and was told that I wasn't a candidate yet. It was our most well attended meeting due to wide publicity in Miami and Boca. They showed slides and discussed the procedure in its entirety, including possible candidacy. When I saw their slides, read their brochures, and listened (via audio loop) to what they were saying, I knew this procedure was for me and I cried!!!! When I was evaluated, Dr. Balkany told me that I was an "ideal candidate." I had the procedure performed in June of 1995. Immediately, I seemed to have good results, didn't require too much rehabilitation, and began using the telephone. The results were so great that I was asked to speak at a meeting of doctors and audiologists who were learning about cochlear implants. Gradually my hearing improved more and I began to use cordless, cell, and regular phones. I began to hear environmental sounds for the first time in fifteen years. I began to enjoy conversations mainly on a "one to one". I can enjoy music and if I train myself I can identify songs of the past. I can hear my grandchildren talk, which was one of my greatest concerns. Socializing has become much more enjoyable.

It's not perfect and at times I still struggle a little but the improvement is enormous and I realized that one must have realistic expectations with cochlear implants. They aren't perfect, but they can make an enormous improvement in one's ability to communicate and in the quality of one's life. Both SHHH and my CI have turned my life around. I have enjoyed the satisfaction of leading two groups and meeting so many wonderful people along the way who have been an inspiration to me in coping with my hearing loss. It's been wonderful to be part of a group where everyone has the same problem and is willing to share their concerns and approaches to coping with it. This has given me support and great joy! One person I roomed with in Denver at a convention was a single woman who felt that SHHH gave her somewhat of a family that she wouldn't have otherwise had. In her words, "I don't know what I would do without my hearing loss and SHHH!"

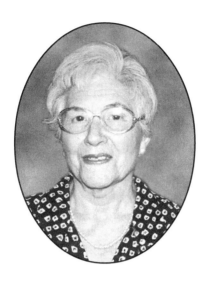

Irene's Story...By Irene Ellis

I was born in 1920 and received a new lease on life in 1999. Three months before my 79th birthday, I received a cochlear implant. I'll soon be 81 years old but my "hearing age" is two years. Just like a curious toddler, I'm discovering new things every day. Did you know that wind sounds different when it blows through different types of trees? If you've always had normal hearing you probably have never noticed. After being deaf for almost 15 years, I notice. I'm listening with new ears and I love it!

I was born with normal hearing but began to lose my hearing around age 50. My hearing loss was progressive. I tried to wear hearing aids, but after a time, did not receive much benefit. By the time I was 65 years old, I was profoundly deaf. I couldn't talk on the phone at all. Even in a face-to-face conversation, I couldn't make out what people were saying. Like most hearing impaired people, I learned to read lips to an extent. However this just enabled me to get bits and pieces of the conversation.

I have always been a very social, outgoing person. I've always been active and interested in everything. My hearing loss was slowly putting me into a prison. I stopped going to certain places because I knew I wouldn't be able to communicate. My family has always been very close, but even family gatherings became less enjoyable. I simply was not able to participate in the give and take of conversation. I was starting to become a loner. I started keeping to myself because I couldn't understand what most people were saying. I would give wrong answers, which was embarrassing, especially with new acquaintances. I was becoming miserable. I was totally out of things. Most of my communication was through the written word. I carried my notepad with me everywhere. People had to write things down for me. This was a tedious, time-consuming way to communicate! My daughter Jane lives in Florida and I couldn't talk to her on the phone at all. She and her family gave me a fax machine and we faxed letter back and forth every day. This was the only way we could stay in touch.

Those who have never experienced severe hearing loss have no idea how terrible, sad, and pathetic it is not to understand people talking to you. I was missing out on so much that normal hearing people take for granted. In December 1998, my son Glenn said that something had to be done. He made an appointment for me to see Dr. Gregory Tarasidis at Greenwood ENT Center. My examination showed profound hearing loss in each ear with no speech understanding ability even at intense levels (90dB). Due to my limited speech understanding ability, it was felt that I would not benefit from a hearing aid. Dr. Tarasidis recommended that I be evaluated for a cochlear implant. His audiologist talked to us about the implant and gave us literature on it and a videotape to review.

After reviewing my options (remaining deaf or trying to do something about it), I decided to be evaluated for the implant. Dr. Tarasidis arranged for me to go to the University of South Carolina Speech and Hearing Clinic for the implant evaluation.

From that point on, I never looked back. I had no reservations when I was told that I was an implant candidate, even though I would be the first senior citizen to be operated on by the University of South Carolina cochlear implant team. I decided to have the surgery and set my heart on success. From the first, I felt like it would be a complete success and that I would be able to hear.

I underwent cochlear implant surgery at Baptist Medical Center in Columbia, South Carolina, on May 5, 1999. I was dizzy for two weeks after the surgery but had no other complications. I didn't have any pain at all. I went home the day after surgery and began one of the longest waits of my life – the time between surgery and actually activating the implant.

356

I was told that it would be about four weeks before the implant could be hooked up. However, I healed so well, that I was hooked up just two weeks after my surgery. I had wondered what I would hear first. I couldn't have guessed if I had tried! When the implant was activated, Dr. Tami Bradham, the audiologist from the implant team was standing behind me. I heard her say, "I have two dogs." I said, "You have two dogs! What are their names?" It was wonderful!!! The doctors and nurses were amazed at the way I could respond.

When I got home, I could hear the phone ringing when we pulled into the carport. My son could not believe it when I told him I could hear the phone ringing. The phone stopped before we could get to it, but started ringing again in a few minutes. I picked up the phone and said, "Hello." When the caller answered "Hello," I said, "Hey, Eleanor." It was my sister from Simpsonville. I had recognized her voice over the phone! We talked for 5-10 minutes and it was absolutely wonderful. She immediately called my brother Fred in Greenville and told him, "Irene can hear! I talked to her on the phone and she heard every word I said." He couldn't believe it so he called me. I recognized his voice immediately and we had a wonderful conversation. I can't describe how happy and excited we all were. I hadn't talked on the phone for over 15 years.

It's been just over two years since my implant and I continue to be amazed at the changes in my life. The implant has done more for me than I ever really expected. I feel like I've come out of a dark prison into the sunlight. I am so active again! I visit neighbors, go out socially, go shopping with groups of friends and out to dinner. I have been given a new lease on life. Every sound is precious. I notice everything. It's hard to pinpoint the best thing, but I would have to say that it is a baby's cry. Shortly after my implant, my niece was down with her baby. He was fretting for his bottle and began to cry. It sounded so sweet. I asked to hold him and I know I must have driven the mother crazy because I kept pulling the bottle away so I could hear him cry. I don't know when I had last heard a baby's cry.

There are so many sounds. Sometimes I just sit and listen. My hearing is so keen now that I pick up so many things – sounds that I had forgotten even existed. Some sounds are a puzzle at first until I realize what the source is. At age 80, I am experiencing a brand new world. If I could tell people one thing about cochlear implants it would be that you are never too old to consider this as an option. I would do it again tomorrow. Don't let the notion that you are "too old" keep you from hearing again and taking part in life. Hearing helps you to stay alert and keeps you in the mainstream. I'm looking forward to what I'll be hearing and doing for the next 20 years! In hearing years, I'm still a child.

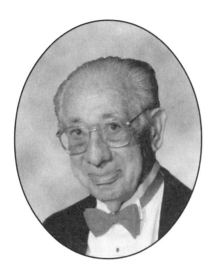

Rabbi Silver's Story...By Barbara Liss Chertok

In his lifetime, Rabbi Sam Silver has been the recipient of many awards. The Dovetail Institute for Interfaith Family Resources gave the rabbi its first Father Dan Montalbano Award for Promoting Interfaith Understanding. But Silver was the recipient of a more life-impacting award last August when he received a cochlear implant at the 'tender' age of 88, making him possibly one of the oldest if not the oldest person in the U.S. to have one.

Born in Wilmington, Delaware, Silver studied at the University of Delaware and was ordained a rabbi at Hebrew Union College in Cincinnati. During World War II he served as a U.S. Army chaplain for four years, performing services for everyone including Protestants and Catholics as well as Jews. After the war, he served as rabbi for 18 years at Temple Sinai in Stamford, Conn. It was there that a congregant whose daughter was about to marry a non-Jew asked Silver to perform the ceremony. Silver was reluctant at first but with his wife's encouragement he agreed. Thus began over four decades of performing interfaith marriages, now numbering over one thousand.

Rabbi Silver and his wife Elaine, an accomplished Julliard concert pianist, have been married 46 years and have five sons, 13 grandchildren and one great-grandchild. The Silvers travel throughout the country presenting a program: "Jewish Music Is Not Sad" at synagogues, churches, nursing homes, and schools. Sam lectures on the subject while Elaine demonstrates it on the piano.

After settling in southern Florida in 1977, Sam became rabbi at Temple Sinai in Delray Beach, a position he held for 18 years. For the past three years, he has been leading biweekly Sabbath services, with Elaine providing the piano and organ music, for the 75-member synagogue I: Dor Va-Dor - translating from Hebrew, it means From Generation To Generation -where most members are converts from other religions.

On August 17th, I visited Rabbi Silver in the hospital where he had just undergone cochlear implant surgery. Standing by his hospital bed as he came out of the anesthesia, the rabbi, in his typical joking style, quipped; "I needed this like I needed a hole in the head!" Two days after the surgery, using his hearing aid in his unimplanted ear, Rabbi Silver was back in the community officiating at weddings and funerals.

INTERVIEW

Q: You are father to five sons. Did you ever pray that you and Elaine might be blessed with a daughter?

A: It took me a long time to learn how to diaper a boy baby, and I understand that girl babies are diapered from the other end. I feared that I would never be able to learn how to do it right and the result would be that I would stab the poor thing - we used diaper pins in those days - so I was glad to have all sons.

Q: What led you to become a rabbi? Did any of your sons follow you and become a rabbi?

A: I was inspired by another rabbi when I was in High School. He was my mentor and a was a major influence in my life. My third son Barry, a lawyer and a Hebrew scholar, became a reform rabbi a few years ago and has officiated at many weddings. I will have the great pleasure of officiating at Barry and his fiancée Francine's wedding when they marry a few weeks from now.

Q: You have authored five books on religion. What are they about?

360

A: I'll mention two of them: *Explaining Judaism to Jews and Christians and Mixed Marriage* explains why I will perform a wedding ceremony to an interfaith couple. The reason is because more and more Christians are happy to be married by a rabbi to a Jewish person. I also explain to them that the ceremony that I offer them is exactly the same ceremony that united the parents of Jesus.

Q: Aside from the usual weddings and funerals, what else takes up your time?

A: I do baby blessings and I write a column on religion for the *Sun-Sentinel.* I also continue to lecture, as I have for the past 20 years, at Palm Beach Community College.

Q: Is there a spiritual leader whom you especially admire today?

A: Billy Graham because he's very eloquent and he very forcefully urges people to improve the quality of their daily life. He demonstrates great skill and the ability to lift the sprit of the people who are listening to him. He's a role model for me as a preacher. Even at my age, I'm still looking to role models.

Q: What can you tell us about your hearing loss?

A: The hearing in my right ear was destroyed due to a botched stapedectomy operation about 40 years ago. As I aged, the hearing in my left ear began to deteriorate. I used a hearing aid in that ear ever since I was about 50 years old, but my hearing got progressively worse. I was implanted last August, in my right "dead" ear, by Dr. Mark Widick, at the Cochlear Implant Center of South Florida in Boca Raton. I thank Dr. Widick for my swift and uncomplicated recovery.

Q: What made you decide to get a cochlear implant?

A: You did, you were my role model. I didn't know what a cochlear implant was until you came along, and I still don't know how to spell it.

Q: What was the most difficult part of dealing with your severe hearing loss all those years?

A: The hardest thing for me was the lack of personal contact with people. I felt so embarrassed I used to avoid meeting people even though I'm a gregarious person by nature.

Q: In what ways has the implant changed you or your life?

A: It has stimulated more contact with other people. At services where I officiate, people who talk to me now are more audible than before, making it easier for me to communicate. And people who normally would shy away from me are now communicating with me. An other way is that I can appreciate my wife's piano playing more because the music is sharper and clearer with my implant.

Q: Your audiologist recently said; "The last time Rabbi Silver was in our office we did some testing in the booth and he performed wonderfully with his implant." That's a very good report for someone whose implant was activated only last October. How do you feel about your implant?

A: I'm glad I got a cochlear implant, and, because of my experience with it, I'm now urging other people with impaired hearing to consider having one, too.

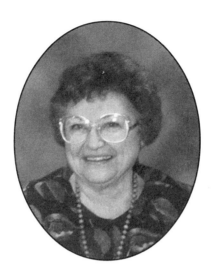

Back in the Hearing World...By Audrey Mueller

On a Sunday in July 1996, I woke up and realized that I had lost my hearing overnight. This is not quite as drastic as it may sound, since I had already lost about 90% of the hearing in my left ear. This happened to be a gradual loss over many years, and actually started after the replacement surgeries of both stapes bones during my late 20s and early 30s, due to otosclerosis.

Since I was only using my right ear to hear (with about 80% function left), this left me not able to hear anything except very loud noises. The Monday following, I went to my doctor's office to determine what happened. She said she didn't know, but gave me the basic hearing test and referred me to an ear, nose and throat doctor at my HMO. After having the audiologist confirm that I was now profoundly deaf, we sat down to talk about my options.

I was the one who suggested to this doctor that I was a candidate for a cochlear implant. Since I have had hearing problems for most of my adult life, any newspaper or magazine article, TV show, radio talk, etc. that concerned hearing problems was of immense interest to me. Lately I had been reading about cochlear implants and this was the first thing that came to my mind when my hearing left.

My doctor told me at that time that nothing should be done for at least

363

a year, because in cases of Sudden Hearing Loss, sometimes the hearing returns naturally. Well, knowing my history I was pretty skeptical about that. My mother had very good hearing, but there was some deafness in her family. My father was hard of hearing from the time I can remember, and by the time he died at the age of 92, I'm sure he would have been diagnosed as profoundly deaf. With only one brother who has normal hearing, I figured that I got all the "bad genes."

Weeks and months went by with my husband and I trying to lead a "normal" life. In meetings and for speeches, he would sit by my side and try to write notes covering the gist of what was happening. We had been very active retirees, belonging to several different organizations and doing quite a bit of volunteer work. People just did not understand what was going on. They would see my husband speak to me and I would answer, I didn't look sick. So I quit going to church. We really tried to get the word out that I couldn't hear, but most people seemed to ignore that, even the ministers in church. I have a feeling that they were only used to dealing with sick people, and I just didn't fit in that category. During this time I actually saw some people walk to the other side of the room to avoid having to talk to me, but they were very kind and made a point of asking my husband, Jim, how I was doing. Is it any wonder I became depressed and hated to walk outside the front door?

All this time Jim encouraged me and tried to keep my spirits up. He suggested maybe we should take signing classes, just to be prepared. What we didn't realize was learning to sign is like learning another language. We found it extremely difficult, but stayed in class for a semester. Actually, we retained very little of what we learned.

By this time it was nearly Christmas and I was out by myself doing some shopping. All of a sudden I noticed the steering on the car became erratic as I was pulling into a parking lot. A man close by started pointing at my tire. He came over and showed me that I had a flat on the right front. As he was starting to walk away and I was thanking him, I suddenly realized there was no way for me to get help. I ran over to him and explained that I was deaf and couldn't use a phone and asked him to call the Auto Club for me. He very nicely did that, and then when the truck driver came and changed the tire, he was also very nice and patient. It really turned out to be a good experience, but there for a minute I was terrified.

Before losing my hearing, we had been planning a six-week trip to England and Ireland and would be traveling with friends who lived in Bristol, England. Our plans went forward and we did do that trip, and

364

most of it I really enjoyed. Our friends were patient and tried to make sure I understood what was going on.

Back to the doctors. It just so happened that the HMO ear doctor I had been seeing became ill and some kind of executive doctor saw me for an appointment. Now, I haven't mentioned that several years before becoming deaf I had started to take speechreading classes. After three years of these classes, I was able to sit in a quiet situation, one on one, and have a fairly lucid conversation. This new doctor sat with my records in front of him, including my hearing tests. After about a 10-minute conversation, he announced that he would not recommend me for a cochlear implant because I was hearing everything that he said.

This was a very disturbing announcement, and I must have sat for a second with my mouth hanging open. After taking a very deep breath, I proceeded to tell him that I had been reading his lips and that I was indeed deaf, and if that became the final decision I would fight it vigorously. Thank goodness, I only saw that person one time and the matter was resolved by recommending me to House Ear Clinic for further study. I saw Dr. Luxford and had several tests, which determined my candidacy for the implant.

After returning home from our trip, and having many more tests, my date for surgery was set for May 16. After the operation, my husband brought me home wearing my white turban and I had it on the next day when we celebrated our 50th wedding anniversary.

Exactly a month later, I was hooked up and heard my first words electronically. It was a miracle. The first few days everyone sounded the same and the sound had robotic-like tones. Within weeks, Jim's voice became what it had once been, and then our children's voices were recognizable, and so on. Now, when our family is together and someone speaks behind me, I almost always recognize who is talking. The telephone can be a bit more of a problem, and I'm not always sure who is answering and sometimes have to go through all the names in the family before getting it correct, but even that is improving.

I am now 74 years of age and have had my implant for almost four years. Most people I meet do not realize that I am deaf and only hear through my appliance. When they find out they say, "But you are hearing very well." This is not a perfect device by any means. Crowd noises are extremely bothersome. Most music is not enjoyable for me, but I am still working on this and it has improved immensely. I can now enjoy a single voice when the background music is kept minimal. Restaurant music tends to drive me crazy, and I won't go back to places that have it. We have not ventured to a movie or live play yet, but we keep talking about trying.

A lady I know, older than myself, has just lost her hearing and I am recommending that she check into getting a cochlear implant. It is such a miraculous thing. I don't believe that anyone who has not gone through the loss of his or her hearing can really appreciate what a gift it is to be able to hear again. My personal theory is that any hearing person who becomes deaf should not spend one day longer than necessary without being able to hear.

One of the most frustrating things my husband and I have dealt with was looking for a person or group to talk with, so that I could have somebody say, "I understand because I went through the same thing." We found some names in the phone book, but most of the groups dealt with deaf children or hard of hearing people. Adult-onset deafness seemed to be a thing no one had ever heard about. It wasn't until we went to the House Clinic and met Darlene Fragale that we learned about a support group. We attended the first meeting we could, and still don't miss a meeting unless we have to. The group has let me know that I was not the first person that this happened to, and my husband now knows he is not the only supportive spouse. It has been very helpful because we have both been able to ask questions and gain information.

Well, if you could know me now I think you could see I have gotten over my depression. I am once again outgoing and willing to be with other people. As a result of my experiences, I have been asked several times to speak in front of groups of people in our retirement community. Last year I was given the privilege of working with some researchers at the House Clinic. This was something I really wanted to do and I hope my contribution was helpful. My reason was very personal. Jim and I have three children with normal hearing, and one son who has already suffered Sudden Hearing Loss in one ear and is gradually losing his hearing in the other. Hopefully, when he is ready for a cochlear implant it will be even better than the one I have. Modern science has figured large in our life as a couple. My husband received an artificial heart valve about eight years ago, without which he would not be alive today. So now we tell our children and grandchildren we are the bionic couple with our artificial parts making our life together longer and better.

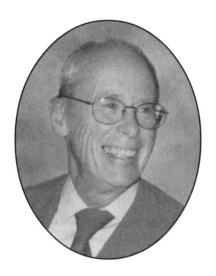

My CI...By Kenyon Riches

My first month

History: Male – born with normal hearing – (mother wore hearing aid after age 60). The first sign of my hearing loss at age 37 – during employment physical – down 15dB. Possible factor contributing to hearing loss (?) – ran a rifle firing range in Army for six months using no ear protection. At 45 years began with binaural in-the-canal hearing aids (both ears almost equal), and "graduated" to in-the-ear, then to BTE by age of 51.

3M's "Memory Mate" BTE hearing aids were my "life-saver" for seven years, but I still had to give up season tickets to the theater (even with assistive listening devices and seats in the second row center), and movies. By age 58, I could no longer hear on the telephone, radios, TV (thank goodness for captioning), sermons at church; conversations were getting more ragged. Social interactions became drastically reduced. At age 60 with hearing test results showing a loss in both ears at >199 dB. I investigated CI surgery at the suggestion of my otolaryngologist. For two years prior to receiving the CI, I was pretty much limited to one-on-one conversations – provided there were no other noises. I felt like I was living in a "BOX" that was getting smaller and smaller. Many of you have walked this road. The increased stress during those 2-3 years helped me to qualify for a "Mr. Grump" award.

I monitored the CI listserve during the year prior to my operation and throughout my HMO application and scheduling. My thanks to Joanne Syrja at Advanced Bionics for her advocacy on my behalf to my HMO and to Arlene London, Lorie Singer, and others on the Forum for helping me to know more about the CI and the "Players" in NYC than did my HMO, which wanted to send me to a doctor at Westchester Medical Center, who had no recent implant surgery experience, no active affiliation with an implant center, and no audiological support group. My HMO deferred to my research and allowed me to proceed as I requested.

I chose the Clarion CI system because of the broader choice of programming strategies and the commitment by Advanced Bionics to include them all in the BTE's, which was under development. CI surgery was on Nov 5, 1998, at the NYU Med Center by Dr. Noel Cohen. I was under anesthesia for a little over four hours for the operation and subsequent X-ray and in-the-ear testing. No complications – thank you, Dr. Cohen. Monitoring the CI Forum for a year prepared me well for what to expect. Interesting comment by one of the nurses on the CI surgical team, who said, "I love this work, because we can actually fix something!"

Device activation occurred on Nov 30 with audiologist Betsy Bromberg at NYU. The first 20-30 seconds were like 4th of July fireworks listening to an old-time radio with the volume turned up high and the dial being moved between stations – squeaking and squawking. It sounded also like someone was in the next room firing a pistol. Then all of a sudden I could understand words that Betsy was speaking. Although her voice sounded like she was from another world – electronic, reedy, and high-pitched, I could make out the words she was saying. I could hear "f", "s", and "th" sounds. After comparison of several two-syllable words, Betsy set my threshold and comfort levels, and we had a normal conversation with Betsy's lips "masked." Only the CIS program was placed in my processor (at my four-week session I was to be exposed to SAS). Needless to say, I was very satisfied with my first day (ecstatic).

Noises on NYC streets and the subway were a somewhat bewildering experience (couldn't make out too much) as I made my way uptown to stay with an old school chum. I could immediately hold a normal conversation with him and get most of what he was saying, even though he had a cold and his voice was weak and electronic. We went out for dinner and I clipped the auxiliary mike to his shirt and we continued to have a very normal quiet conversation.

I could understand 25% of what I heard from a TV newscaster. I heard sounds that I hadn't heard in years – squeaking floors, light switches, coffee being poured in a cup, paper rustling, the dog's nails walking on the tile floor, my whistling for her. My wife, Inge, called and I answered the phone. I could understand her when she said what I expected to hear, but when I asked her a question, I could not understand her response.

Day #2 – 20 hours later, Betsy reset my "levels"; threshold didn't change much, but "comfort" level increased by 25%. We moved to a testing booth for a consonant confusion test (score was 30%), and sentence recognition test (score was 50%). I was hearing (and scoring) much better than I did with my hearing aids. Used public transportation to get to LaGuardia airport and flew back to Buffalo. Inge was ecstatic when she didn't have to repeat everything two or three times. I ventured to an early Tae Kwan Do class using a headband to secure the mike, and a regular belt to hold the processor under my uniform. I couldn't hear very much during class, but Tae Kwan Do is mostly visual anyway. I could hear conversations later in the changing room. My "box" was definitely getting bigger….I woke up at 3:30 a.m. and reflected on the past two days. Then the tears flowed on my pillow…. I felt a great relief and "release" of the tensions built-up over the past few years. I gave silent thanks and prayers to God and all those who helped to make it happen.

Day #4 – I tried the telephone at work and was "moderately successful" hearing the telephone signal through a special device I used when I had hearing aids. It is a "Parametric Equalizer 242" manufactured by Professional Products in Salt Lake City (a Harmon International Company), and is used by bands and orchestras to eliminate feedback microphone noises. It allows for amplification/attenuation of three separate frequency bands with adjustable frequencies and bandwidths. I used the "suction cup" pickup on the device. I called my wife who read a grocery list to me over the phone and I understood about 80% - I couldn't understand the words "flour" and "salmon."

Day #7 – Tried the phone again with my wife – got almost all of the conversation with her speaking slowly – had to repeat a couple of words.

Day #8 – I read an article and at breakfast I indicated to my wife that I had a desire to work in that area of activity when I retired. I realized then that it was the first time in several years that I felt that I

369

could develop plans that included other people. It was an emotional moment for me…my "BOX" was getting bigger and bigger….

Two Weeks after "turn-on"

The first two weeks were wonderful. I could communicate with others, even though their voices still sounded electronic, and nowhere near what I remembered as "normal." My wife said my face showed a lot less strain. We went to a noisy restaurant, and I used the auxiliary mike clipped to my wife's blouse and had a normal quiet conversation. For the first time in years I could hear whispers. Every day I listened to the news on the car radio and could understand a little more. I understood more than 80% of the stock listing report. My comprehension was better using the auxiliary mike, and if I placed it near the speaker I could understand almost everything.

Two-Week Remap

I missed my plane from Buffalo to NYC and called my audiologist's office. Using the magnetic "suction cup" telephone pickup, I had no problem hearing the secretary and called again just before my next flight to confirm a rescheduled appointment. What a relief to casually use the phone again. At my two-week "remap," my tolerance and threshold level adjustments were considered in the "normal" range of improvement. I was still with the CIS program.

Since this was Christmas season, I sang a lot and experienced an "echo" of a simultaneous higher note that may have been a harmonic or an octave higher – I'm not sure. It was a pleasant sound and I wound up singing softly a good deal of the time. The captioning on one of the TV programs was not working. I placed my auxiliary mike near the speaker and I could understand without the captioning. We went to a neighbor's home for a Christmas party with more than 50 people. I was able to have decent conversations with no difficulty.

At my four-week remap I was introduced to the SAS program – Yuck!! It sounded like I was under water… I think the CIS program is for me.

I was a partner and CEO in a small manufacturing business, and my responsibilities included marketing and sales – rather tough when you can't use the phone – thank goodness for fax and e-mail, but they have their limitations. It was great to be able to use the phone again. To sum

370

up my first month – HALLELUJAH!! I wish I had done this 3-4 years prior, because during the years my hearing reduction went from –90 dB to–110dB, it was most frustrating. My advice to those who have a hearing loss at –90dB, and whose condition is worsening, if you are a candidate for a CI – DO IT NOW!!

Subsequent

During the next three months my hearing and my test scores improved significantly, particularly in the "noisy background environment" test. My brain was getting used to filtering out the significant from the insignificant. My social life slowly returned to almost what it was before I lost my hearing, and it was fun to again participate in discussions, debates, and arguments – whatever. I could hear birds again, and I was thrilled. After two years I still cannot make enough sense of music to enjoy it – I do miss it, although I would put it in the "nice-to-have" category, when compared to having the ability to again communicate with people on an "almost normal" basis. Although I use captioning on the TV, I can hear reasonably well if I sit close to the speaker, and I hear well on the car radio. A graphic equalizer helps "tune" the radio to my hearing limitations. My hearing is limited when I am far from a speaker in a meeting or hearing a sermon at church. My comprehension is directly related to the speaker's articulation.

I was satisfied enough with my hearing after 18 months to apply to the FAA for renewal of my third class medical certificate to allow me to exercise the privileges of my private pilot's license. The manager of the FAA Aeromedical Certification indicated that they had not granted medical certification to anyone with a cochlear implant, but I persisted and when I took my medical flight exam I also provided my audiological test scores that showed I met the applicable FAA regulation 67.305. As a result, I received my third class medical certificate and a Statement of Demonstrated Ability. I flew recently as a passenger and could hear quite well with my microprocessor plugged into the aircraft radio. I recently retired and now expect to enjoy flying on a regular basis. I feel very fortunate to live during a period of this technological innovation, and I look forward to having a lot more fun in my retirement because of it.

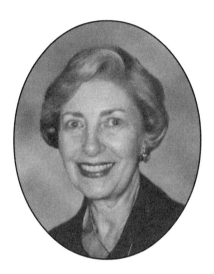

Suddenly Surrounded By Silence...By Barbara Liss Chertok

I was born into the world, like most healthy newborns, with my sense of touch, taste, smell, sight, and sound intact. For the next 21 years, I took them for granted, as most people often do. Then without warning, my precious sense of sound was taken from me — and I was suddenly surrounded by silence. For the next 41 years, I masqueraded through life as a hearing person, doing things hearing people did, only without being able to hear what was going on around me.

The sun shone brightly in my hometown of Boston on that breezy, spring day with that never-to-be-forgotten date of May 24, 1957. Although it took place more than four decades ago, it could have happened yesterday because my deafness has enveloped me every waking hour of my life since that fateful day.

It began when my balance suddenly gave out as I walked back from lunch with two co-workers. My friends helped me back to the advertising agency where we worked, and I rested on a couch waiting for the vertigo to subside. Instead it worsened, and a coworker drove me home to the apartment I shared with my aging parents in Dorchester, a suburb of Boston.

The next day, my left ear was blocked and I could not hear on that side. In a few days, my right ear began to feel the same way. I thought that it must be a temporary condition, so I did not worry, even though I was straining more to hear the television and people on the phone.

My mother called the family doctor who treated me for a cold, even though no cold symptoms were present. Over the next several days, my eyes became inflamed, first one, then the other. Light was painful and I was forced to lie in a darkened room until the condition cleared up. In the meantime, my loss of balance remained severely affected to the point where I could not walk unaided without leaning on someone or something. By now, what had merely felt like a blocking sensation in both ears had resulted in total deafness. It was two weeks before our family doctor finally summoned an ear specialist who immediately had me admitted to the hospital.

During my three-week hospital stay, I underwent a variety of tests and X-rays, but the doctors remained stumped. As the steady stream of physicians, nurses, and aides, as well as family, friends, and co-workers came through my hospital room, I became an 'instant' lipreader, communicating in this new way with people who spoke clearly and had good mouth movement. Doctors with accents, however, were another story. However, one doctor, a world-famous Harvard neurologist from England — with a stiff upper lip and a strong accent — had to resort to using pencil and paper. I have kept his notes to this day, one that reads: "You will regain all of your hearing within two to eight weeks." Those words lifted my spirits and stopped my tears from flowing. It was this same doctor who later diagnosed the cause of my deafness as herpes virus, and was wrong on both counts.

Meanwhile, my parents seemed to be having a more difficult time coping with my deafness than I was. Both were Russian immigrants who had married later in life and came from a different culture where a disabled child might be locked away somewhere. Neither my mother or father was fluent in English, and my father's speech had become slurred from a recent stroke. I struggled to read their lips and, despite my lipreading ability, communicating with them was difficult. I worried about them and put on a brave front for their benefit, which, in the end, may have helped me, as well.

After four months, an audiological test revealed a small amount of residual hearing in my right ear only and I was fitted with a powerful body hearing aid, which allowed me to re-enter a new world of very limited sound. At this time, I began six months of private, weekly lipreading lessons. The lessons brought me great pleasure for I was able to understand every word my teacher spoke, which was not always the

374

case in the real world. This wonderful experience led me to become a lip-reading teacher myself — 30 years later, a subject I taught for 10 years at a community college in Maryland and privately from my home.

But one year later, I was no longer able to hear with my hearing aid, and once again, I was suddenly surrounded by silence. This time I consulted an ear specialist who diagnosed the cause as hydrops, a build-up of fluid in the inner ear. In the year that followed, I lived in a silent world, totally dependent on lipreading. Then by chance, I met a hearing aid salesman who wanted me to try one of his powerful body hearing aids. I was both delighted and surprised that I could hear some of my own voice and a few close-range sounds with it, and purchased it immediately.

As the years passed, I never gave up hope that I might one day regain my hearing. It would take four decades and a technological miracle device to make that happen. In the meantime, armed with my expert lipreading skills and my hearing aid, I attended lectures, took classes, went to concerts and parties, and enjoyed foreign films with subtitles. Although there was much that I missed, I was determined to stay in the mainstream and experience life's pleasures.

My social life continued and despite an awkward first date with my future husband, Benson contacted me again. Telephone relay services back then, so he had to call my mother to make a second date with me, and a third, and all those that followed until our marriage one and a half years later. Fortunately, it only took a couple of dates until I could read Benson's lips perfectly. During our 20-year marriage, it was my husband's lips I read from the side at lectures, across the table at dinner parties, in the dark at movies, and facing him as he repeated phone messages to me. And it was all done silently, without using his voice.

For nearly 30 years, our family lived in Bethesda, Maryland, just over the Washington, D.C. line where the national headquarters of many major organizations for hard of hearing and deaf people are located. In the early 1970s, I began advocating for the rights of people with hearing loss by volunteering, consulting, lecturing, and serving on boards and committees. When my husband passed away in 1981 after a short bout with cancer, I began teaching lip-reading and writing articles.

Although cochlear implants were approved for adults in 1985, it was not until 1992 that I decided to undergo cochlear implant testing at Johns Hopkins Medical Center in Baltimore. It was Dr. John Niparko who correctly diagnosed the cause of my deafness as Cogan's Syndrome, an autoimmune disorder. I also learned, from a balance test, that I had no vestibular inner ear function and compensated for my loss of balance with my eyes and a hearing test confirmed I was indeed a candidate for a cochlear implant. Nonetheless, I decided to wait until the technology had advanced a bit further since I was functioning with lipreading and the few sounds my hearing aid provided.

In 1996, 15 years after my husbands death, I moved to Boca Raton, Florida, where I had a few friends and relatives. The following December, I made the big decision to be implanted. My successful cochlear implant surgery was performed by Dr. Loren J. Bartels in Tampa in December 1997, and I received a Clarion S-Series device. I had been forewarned by Dr. Bartels that the operation might leave me with a black and blue eye, which it did. The next day, as I walked from my hotel to the doctor's office to have the stitches removed, I held a newspaper in front of my face because the 'shiner' and my hair was greasy with bacterial ointment.

I returned home to Boca Raton long enough for the incision to heal and came back to Tampa six weeks later for the 'hook up' or activation of my implant device. As I entered the audiologist's office, the same question kept running through my mind: Given my long history of deafness, would I be able to hear anything with my implant? I would soon have the answer.

My son Maxwell had flown to Tampa to be with me for this exciting moment. The initial stimulation of the device began with audiologist Heather attached a cable leading from her computor to my newly aquired processor. As she set the threshold and comfort levels, she asked me to listen for some beeps. I listened intently, trying to hear something — anything. The tension in the room began to build. I concentrated very hard as I strained to hear the first beep, and amazingly enough, I HEARD the first one and all the beeps that followed. I could even distinguish the different pitches. The whole room lit up with everyone grinning broadly and I could hardly contain my emotions. When Heather announced she was going to have me listen to speech through my processor, I was tempted to ask for a drum roll, but I crossed my fingers instead. She tapped the keys on her computer and began talking to me. I sat there reading her lips, listening for all I was worth. Then, I began to talk out loud and as I spoke I realized what was happening. "Oh, that's me, I said haltingly, I'm hearing my own voice!" What I heard sounded mushy and distant, as if it was being transmitted from Mars. But, the fact that I heard anything was so thrilling that I didn't care what it sounded like. As I looked around the room, I noticed everyone's eyes glistening, particularly my son's.

For the next four days, I returned to the audiologist's office where now Donna took over the programming of my processor. With each new adjustment, speech sounds became clearer as my brain relearned how to hear again. After the fifth day in Tampa, I left and returned home to continue my programming sessions with audiologist Lynn in Juniper, one hour north of Boca.

I made steady progress with my implant for the following three years, after which time my hearing began to plateau. I have since upgraded from my original S-Series processor to a Platinum sound processor, and finaaly to a behind-the-ear processor (BTE), wireless model. With the wireless BTE, I feel like a truly liberated woman.

Almost four years have elapsed since I received my cochlear implant, and you may be wondering what I actually hear with it. Before I answer that, let me back up to the time when my daughter Victoria was two and a half years old and the phone would ring and little Vicki would run over to the phone, pick up the receiver and say into it: "Take a message for mommy?" A chore she (and the rest of the family) would repeat countless times until she left home for college. Now, after more than 40 years of not being able to hear on the phone, I'm thrilled to say "I finally can." I can once again enjoy my love of opera, jazz, and other kinds of music, I can follow the lecturers at a local university, using an infrared receiver with a patch cord plugged directly into my processor. I feel so much safer now that I can hear environmental sounds, such as fire engines and police sirens. And, how wonderful it is to hear birds and crickets and feel a part of nature! Of course, communication is the key, and I can converse more easily with anyone I choose, even with the bearded gentleman or the person with an accent.

This technological marvel has been such a blessing that in 1998 I founded the Cochlear Implant Support Group of Southeast Florida, which meets monthly at a local hospital and is open to all adults, with or without an implant, who are interested in sharing and learning about cochlear implants. My miracle has given me a new life mission, and that is to share my blessing with others.

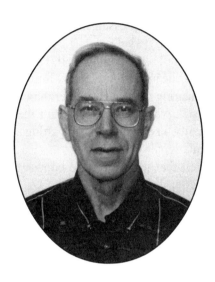

Strong Words Nearly Fell On Deaf Ears...by Bruce Berney

It's well known that childhood diseases are bad for adults. In my early forties about 25 years ago I contracted the mumps. It gave me vertigo so bad that I would have to crawl to the bathroom, and the fever deafened my right ear. Fortunately, my left ear seemed normal except for brief periods when I'd whistle and hear two notes instead of one. I was able to finish my career as the director of the Astoria Public Library.

Only a few months after I retired in 1997, I was working in the yard, and I suddenly realized that I was hearing the clicking of clippers with my bad ear and nothing with my good ear. The specialist I consulted with told me about the possibility of getting a cochlear implant but stated that one of the side effects could be dizziness. I misunderstood and thought this would be permanent, therefore I opted to face the world as a profoundly hard of hearing person. With my right ear I could hear low voices, but without consonants, understanding speech was almost impossible.

My wife, teenage son, and I took sign language classes and I also had lipreading classes; however, communication was still a struggle. My pastor gave me photocopies of his sermons, which I would read, in church. About two years ago, a church friend gave me a copy of Gordon Nystedt's newsletter that contained personal stories from cochlear implant users. I was very impressed that only one contributor complained of dizziness.

I wrote to Gordon to tell him about myself. I said that I was doing so well that I didn't think the implant was in my future. His reply was very blunt. He said that hearing is so much better than not hearing and that anyone who held back was foolish. I couldn't think of a convincing argument, so, gradually, I knew I would be getting an implant. But first I had to have a hernia repair operation.

When I finally felt that it was time to choose a surgeon, I tallied names in the newsletter. I decided to go with Dr. Sean McMenomey. Replying to my introductory letter, he said that he and his colleagues at OHSU perform about 75 implants a year. He also stated that while dizziness sometimes happens, it is usually for a very brief time.

On July 12th I received a Nucleus 24 cochlear implant. My audiologist, Alexandra Hatten, has had the joy of seeing my word recognition jump from 0% without the implant to nearly 100% within just a few weeks. How miraculous it is for me to now hear my three-year old granddaughter and to converse freely with people (when there is minimal background noise)! Although I had dreaded the operation, it turned out to be lots nicer than the hernia repair. I shudder to think how I nearly choose to be deaf for the rest of my life. I thank God for Gordon Nystedt and his newsletter and for his bluntness that opened my eyes and mind.

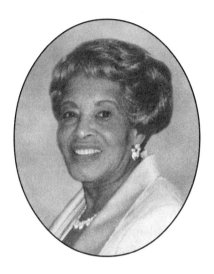

Among the Living and Hearing Again…By Thelma Beaubain

My implant story will be very similar to all who have had the cochlear implant surgery, the need to hear. But first let me preface it with what lead me to make the decision to have this procedure. The loss of three loved ones in such a shocking manner and the possibility of a hereditary factor, I believe aided in my hearing loss. The first was losing my daughter to SIDS (Sudden Infant Death Syndrome) at two months of age. Next came the loss of my husband, within two days of a stroke. This was 11 years ago and only seven weeks after we retired to South Carolina. This was a lifestyle that I was not familiar with, since I was born and raised in the suburbs of New York City. At the time we relocated, we also brought my 80-year old mother with us, which was quite a challenge for both of us. She missed all of her familiar routines, such as getting on a bus and going whereever she pleased, when she pleased, now she had to depend on me to take her where she wanted to go and the loss of that little independence was very difficult for her. Having her with me was a godsend because attending to her needs helped me through a very difficult period. Unfortunately she was only with me for four years. She took sick, in late July, and by August 1st was given a short time to live——from one to three months. We could see it was going to be very short, so my two children came down to help me the

381

last few days of her life and she left us mid-August. At this time, they realized I was having difficulty hearing and made an appointment for me to be tested while they were there, which resulted in me getting my first hearing aids. Now for the hereditary end of it, my father was profoundly deaf and has always found a reason why he couldn't adjust to wearing a hearing aid. But after I found I needed the hearing aids, in 1994, I knew I had no choice but to get use to them, since I was going to be totally alone. I had no one to tell me the doorbell or the phone was ringing. Between 1994 and the year 2000 I had five new aids, each getting stronger and stronger, until they didn't seem to be of much help. The moment of truth came when I visited with my children in New York for a month. My son and his family seemed to adjust, having to repeat things many times before I understood, but my daughter had a very hard time dealing with me. She is my eldest, by eleven years, and she wanted her mother to be the same person she always knew, which was not going to happen. At this point, I realized I was losing her. We were not able to communicate and I felt she really didn't like being around me. Maybe she felt embarrassed for me when I was around her friends or that she was so hurt at what had happened to me, that she couldn't cope. One day she said, "I thought now that you don't have to take care of Gram any longer we would be able to enjoy each other and now you can't hear." It sort of made me feel like I had done something deliberately to get this condition, to block her out of my life. I was hurt by the way she felt, and I didn't know where to turn or what to do. When I returned home I discussed my hearing loss with some-one who was about to get a new type of hearing aid. She suggested I go to her audiologist and investigate the possibility of it helping me. But I had an audiologist that had become a friend as well as a consultant, so I took the information I was given to her to see what she thought. After having spent many dollars over the past six years, I really didn't want to invest in something that was not going to be much help. She immedi-ately gave me a hearing test, since I hadn't had one in a while. The results were: there wasn't a hearing aid on the market that would do much to improve my hearing. Thus she took test results to the ENT physician in the same office for her evaluation. The physician felt I was definitely a candidate for a cochlear implant. They asked if I was interested and since I didn't know much about it I thought maybe I would look into it and then decide.

The ENT doctor made an appointment at a hospital she was affiliated with in North Carolina, and I went for evaluation and orientation in

382

early October 2000. The North Carolina team all concurred that I was a good candidate for the cochlear implant; my hearing loss was at the point where the implant would be beneficial and my health was excellent, for a lady of 71 years. So I decided then and there that I would go through with the procedure. I went through the pre-op and waited for the okay for surgery, before I told my children what I was planning to do. Their reactions were quite different. My son said, "Go for it, if you think it will help," and my daughter was afraid it might make bad matters worse and maybe I should think about it a while before I decided to have it done. I have a very close friend that I've met since coming to this town and she has stuck by me, even with my difficulty. I told her of my plans and she accompanied me back and forth to North Carolina for all of my visits and surgery. When I told her I wanted to be able to hear my grandchildren, she cried and said, "Do it." She later told me it broke her heart to hear me say that.

I had the implant surgery in early November and it was a relatively painless and quick healing operation. My children took turns and came and stayed with me for three weeks following the surgery. I went back for my first hook-up and mapping session in early December. That is when the bottom fell out for me. Based on the video I was given as to what to expect from the implant, I was totally disappointed. I couldn't hear the phone, my device would not stick to my head and most of what was said to me I didn't understand any better than before. I thought I was listening to a lot of aliens from outer space, thus I though maybe my daughter was right and I had made a mistake in doing it. I told my son about my mapping session and maybe the problems I was having were my fault. I found it very difficult to understand, "Tell me when the sound is comfortable"…what is comfortable, when you haven't really heard for years. So many choices may not have been set at the proper range for my needs. My son said, "Don't give up, it will get better." He spent a lot of time on the Internet researching this procedure and he told me the sounds I was hearing were normal for now. And my technician in North Carolina said the same thing. My North Carolina team communicated with me, via e-mail, never ceasing to show their interest in my progress in between visits. I went back in early January for a re-mapping. This was a little better and I had made up my mind that this had to work or else. So I did all I could do, in the line of self help, to get used to the new voices and sounds that were going to be with me for the rest of my life—from that day on. I would check out books on tape from the library, and I played them daily, following along with the printed book to train my ears to understand. I visited as many people as I could, who would just sit and talk with me to help me improve my hearing skills. This was a very slow process, but it was effective to some degree. When I went back for my second mapping, in early February, the results were like a rebirth. I started hearing things I couldn't remember the last time I heard them; like the phone, the microwave beep, the kettle whistle, the directional signals in the car, the birds chirping, the rain hitting my umbrella, and my grandchildren when they came to visit in mid-February. As we all know, very young children like to whisper in your ear, and whispering into mine is like whispering to the wind, so I plugged in my telephone coil and let them whisper into it and they loved it. It made them think they were talking into a mike. I went back in early March for more mapping and an evaluation test, and as far as I'm concerned the results were outstanding. The summary said I was making excellent progress with the cochlear implant and that I was able to understand speech at both the sentence level and monosyllable word level. My understanding of speech in noise is impressive. I am scheduled to return in three months for routine follow-up. I am now able to use the phone with a lot less repetition. If I ask the person I am speaking with to talk slower and not too loud, I can hold a pretty intelligent conversation. Although I know I will never hear like I heard before I started losing my hearing, I am so grateful and appreciative to the entire team that worked with me. The cochlear implant has transformed me back into the independent woman I have always been. Prior to having my hearing restored, I was not totally deaf, I could hear, but not always understand, I would have been forced to give up my home and go back to New York, where I would be near my family or to some assisted living facility. Where I live, if you can't drive, you can't function, and that would have been the first privilege I would have had to give up. What a joy it is to know that I am still my own person.

My favorite pastime is playing bridge and now that I can hear, I can appreciate how difficult I made the game for others because we have a few ladies with hearing disabilities and I can now see what I was like for those who can hear. Because of my faith in God, the prayers and support I have gotten from my family and friends, I have been able to succeed in my venture with the cochlear implant. If you are thinking about having the implant surgery and your advisors feel you will benefit from it, "do it." I will never regret my decision.

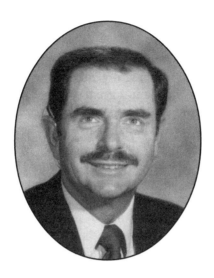

The Long Road…By Craig Carpenter

My hearing problems began at the age of 18 months, when a high fever or sulfa medication resulted in a severe hearing loss in both ears. I attended a residential deaf school, began using hearing aids at the age of seven, and experienced a gradual loss of my remaining hearing. The teachers at the school felt that I was not challenged and that I needed to be mainstreamed to the public school system. They felt that with my excellent lipreading skills I would be able to carry my own with my hearing peers.

Public school was agonizing for me because the teachers were not trained for my kind of disability. For the most part, they would lecture the class while writing notes on the blackboard, giving me little opportunity to lipread. At that time, there was no help from notetakers or interpreters. School became very difficult and making friends was very hard. High school had become a very traumatic experience for me, and my grades slipped from honor roll to just barely passing, while my social life became nil.

After graduating high school, I attended a technical college, majoring in automotive technology with a minor in electricity. I excelled once again because I had wonderful professors, who cared enough about this deaf man to help him after hours in their homes. While I did not hit the Deans List, I did manage to achieve high honors in the courses that I was interested in.

I am employed as Journeyman Electrician with the second largest suburban school district in Western New York, where I have been employed for 36 years, beginning my employment as a sweeper/cleaner and working my way up to my current position.

I began using hearing aids at the age of seven, back when they were still using vacuum tubes. The aids consisted of two major parts, a huge body aid that enclosed the tubes and volume controls and a separate, equally huge battery pack. I continued using the body aids until the age of 25 when I reached the profoundly deafened level with 110 dB loss in both ears. I used the most powerful aid I could obtain at that time but rather than help me become aware of sound, they caused severe tinnitus and I had to discontinue using the aid.

My mother was very adamant about making sure that I maintained a good vocabulary and that I used the spoken word as much as possible, as opposed to the signed or written word. Having a sense of sound at a couple of periods in my life, coupled with my hearing oriented family, gave me all the incentive I needed to seek out information on the cochlear implant. My wife and my children and now my grandchildren have no hearing loss at all, so it made sense for me to try the cochlear implant. I had nothing to lose and everything to gain.

After watching a television program about this experimental device called a cochlear implant, we began investigating the possibilities of implantation. After much testing, it was determined that I would be a good candidate and we initiated the process. I did lipreading tests, voice value recordings prior to implantation, all recorded by video. I went through tests prescribed by the manufacturer to give them some assurance that I could make use of the device. Finally, in April of 1985, at the age of 44, I was implanted with an experimental device. I recall that there was a house full of people in attendance at my first surgery, because we were making history here in Buffalo, New York. There was a full television crew as well as a large number of medical people on hand. I asked one of the people at the scene to please collect five dollars from each person in attendance, thinking I would pick up a few bucks for being the central figure in this, but as I spoke, I succumbed to sleep. The surgery was relatively painless, I felt more like I had some dental surgery and there was that dull pain for several days.

This first device (I was implanted three times in the same ear!) was a non-invasive single-channel multi-frequency device called a 3M/Vienna extracochlea device. It was similar to the early House single-channel devices with two very important differences. It did not enter the inner ear, the electrode rested on the round window and was capable of presenting sound at varying frequency levels, enabling one to distinguish not only by loudness but by pitch, something other devices were not capable of at that time.

Five weeks after the implantation there were many excited people at the long awaited initial stimulation, at which time we would find out if the device would function or not. I was hooked into a computer via my processor and we began the stimulation. When I did not respond despite the device being at full volume, the professionals called a conference of everyone in attendance. Everyone was very disappointed, and I was asked to leave the room for a few minutes while they discussed the next step. On the way out of the room, I asked if anyone had charged the battery before placing it in the processor. It turned out that the battery was not charged. A quick search turned up a battery in good condition and the stimulation began in earnest with everything functioning very well.

I once again took the lipreading tests and performed the voice value recordings. The lipreading tests showed that I had increased my ability to hear and understand substantially and my voice quality had improved dramatically. My voice has undergone a complete change; before the implant, I spoke in a monotone, rapidly with the words running together. I like to think that I speak very well now, am easily understood and speak with correct inflections. The research people at 3M had me fly up to St. Paul, Minnesota, several different times for a week at a time so they could hook me into their computer mainframe for the purpose of creating data that would lead to better speech processing. I look back with pride on those days and being able to contribute to the improvement of the cochlear implant.

Later, this device failed due to the implanted electrode breaking, causing the device to go on and off much like a hearing aid with a broken cord. We tried cord after cord until tests finally showed that the problem was internal. I had surgery again in 1987 to replace the implanted portion of the device with a newer 3M/Vienna intracochlea device whose electrode did penetrate the inner ear. This second device did not function nearly as well as the first one, and I began leaving it off for lengthy periods of time because I just was not getting anything from it. You have to understand that these devices were experimental and I was allowing myself to be used as a guinea pig. We were all disappointed with the results of this device and began looking into replacing it with the only device available at that time which had been approved by the FDA.

After a lot of hassle with health insurance, approval to go ahead with implantation of the Nucleus 22 multi-channel device was obtained. This surgery was performed in 1990 and turned out to be the easiest, at least for me! I returned to work four days after surgery, and was hooked up four weeks later. I took to the device right away and have been steadily improving ever since. I have done two external upgrades since then, turning in my old MSP processor for the Spectra that had improved capabilities for processing voice sounds. I am able to hear and understand the spoken word many times without visual stimulation. I can make use of the telephone, the car radio, and even my cell phone. I had never experienced BTE devices before; they certainly offer the user more versatility, two maps, no cords to snag, clothing selection, and longer battery life.

The implant has had a profound effect on my life. I have become much more independent, taking advantage of everything that the new world of sound has opened up to me. At work, I've gone from being a helper, to a take-charge guy with my own crew and a better position, that of lead electrician for one of the largest suburban school districts in Western New York. I take part in discussions covering a wide range of subjects that confront the schools of tomorrow. I do most everything without any thought about my deafness. Deafness which is still there, with reminders everywhere, from not being prepared with spare batteries to accidentally getting too close to metal framing and having my transmitter come off. I do encounter people who have poor diction and I require help in understanding those people.

I was very actively involved in the deaf community, serving as President, Chief Financial Office, newsletter editor and publisher for the Buffalo Club of the Deaf. President/Chief Executive Officer, Board Member, Treasurer and Home Office Director of the Cochlear Implant Club International, now known as CIAI. I was a member of the Board of Trustees of St. Mary's School for the Deaf for nine years serving as Vice-Chairman for three years; and Founder and Executive Director, Editor and Publisher for Buffalo Implant Group.

Socially, I have evolved from someone totally immersed in the deaf community, to one that is becoming involved in different issues, dealing with subjects other than deafness. I have found that some of the fundamental rights the deaf are claiming are not in step with the real world.

I am still a strong advocate for the deaf, however, I am not a member of deaf culture, nor was I ever, mostly because of my associations with the hearing world my entire life. The position that the deaf take concerning the cochlear implant was, at one time, based on fact and actual results. As time went on and implant technology improved, making those arguments invalid, the deaf chose to ignore the news coming out and kept on with their stance that there is nothing wrong with a deaf person. They say that they were born into a different culture and should be accepted for what they are, with everyone else expected to learn how to communicate with them, much as we have to learn how to communicate with anyone else who speaks a different language. The National Association of the Deaf has a new president who has taken a more liberal approach to accepting the implant, however, there are many local groups who are still completely opposed to the implant in children.

I take the position that if a person is qualified and motivated, they should take advantage of what is out there. The cochlear implant is not a sure thing, but is sure a very good aid in helping one function in the real world. I would and have recommended taking this step to anyone I thought wanted it for the right reasons. I strongly support the implantation of children at an early age, the earlier the better.

I had no way to prepare for this surgery; it had never been performed here or anywhere nearby. There was no one to consult with as to the problems that may crop up, what pain was involved surgically, how much therapy was required post hook-up and what could I realistically expect from the implant. This lead to my connecting with a group, Cochlear Implant Club of the South, in Nashville, Tennessee, led by Betty Meadows Longwith, that consisted of 16 people who had already gone through the implant process and wanted to share their experiences with others. These people were, for the most part, patients of Dr. William House from Los Angeles, using the single-channel device. In 1985 there was no such thing as a computer in every home, no such thing as personal e-mail, and it was much more difficult to get the word out. There seemed to be a real need for the ability to network with each other and to counsel prospective patients on the pros and cons of getting the implant. We all knew that the cochlear implant was the thing of the future.

In 1985, I began The Buffalo Implant Group along with Howard Tagg (deceased) because there was no one to turn to for advice and support. We began with six members and currently have a readership of 150. My implant center made me aware of the existence of CICI and we become affiliated with this group. The intent was to provide accurate information and peer support. In May 1986, CICI held its first convention at the Baptist Hospital in Nashville, Tennessee where people from all over the country who had or were planning to get an implant got together for the first time. There we realized that we needed to spread the word. In 1988, the board meeting was held in Buffalo. CICI reorganization was the primary target of the discussions. Much to my surprise, William Rogers, Chairman of the Board at that time, nominated me for the position of President and Chief Executive Officer, based on the many hours I had spent in an attempt to make CICI work in what was then our current setup, a working relationship with Baptist Hospital in Nashville. The board then proceeded to second the nomination and elect me to that position. I took over the organization as the first elected President/Chief Executive Officer. I was fortunate to have Judge Richard Brown as Vice President, Dave Emerson as Secretary and Cliff Cleary as Treasurer as well as the support of some very bright people with cochlear implants from all over the country on the board as we began the process of being completely independent from any outside influence. Determination to make this organization succeed coupled with a paid membership of 25 people gave me the drive to revive this organization. Much letter writing to people who had attended other conventions and expressed interest in CICI resulted in some very strong support from people who had otherwise decided we were not for real. The support from these contacts became the foundation upon which we grew.

We decided to publish a worthy news journal which provided much updated information on cochlear implants. With the help of Editors Connie Wild, Cliff Cleary, and Larry Orloff and a talented, capable staff, we disseminated the best information possible. We also helped provide information for chapter development and personal contact.

The home office for Cochlear Implant Club International in 1987 had been a spare bedroom in our home in Buffalo, New York, which grew and virtually took over our lives for 11 years. In the beginning, we spent about four or five hours a week on CICI matters; this had exploded to an unbelievable six hours per day or more. We were handling around 15 requests for information per day. On top of that, we were getting out a news journal printed and mailed, keeping track of membership and mail. We were also handling a lot of lengthy person-to-person phone calls, via TTY or voice, to help assist other people in making the decision to implant or not. Because of the demands of the organization,

390

the board decided it was time to take the next step and hire an executive director and open up a real office, with a paid staff in Washington, DC. The process of selecting an Executive Director was completed and the move began. We made several automobile trips to Washington, carrying with us carton after carton of CICI related records and materials and floppies containing data vital to the operation.

Needless to say, we are relieved to have our lives back after such an investment in time and energy. Of course my wife Jackie and I miss it at times because it was such a large part of our lives for so long, however, we stay busy with the Buffalo Implant Newsletter (BIG). We are very pleased with the new direction the organization has undertaken and hope that Cochlear Implant Assocation International will be a valuable resource for many years to come. As I mentioned before it is very important to have a support group to learn from each other and grow in your understanding as you journey through life with your implant. In closing I would like to say as one of the 'pioneers' of this miraculous medical technology, "You've come a long way, baby!"

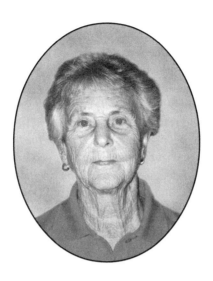

It's a New World…By Marjorie Howard

I had my Clarion cochlear implant in May 2000, and the speech processor was fitted a month later. At that time I was 74 years old. Now I wish it could have happened years earlier. I started to have hearing problems when I was a teenager, growing up in Lancashire, England, but my problem did not prevent me from being employed when I left school. I was married in 1947 to a husband who was very supportive. In 1952, I had a fenestration operation on my left ear in Edinburgh, Scotland. This was not successful and I thought at that time that my left ear was useless. In 1954, my husband and I immigrated to Canada. Shortly afterwards, I bought my first hearing aid which was a body type and used in my right ear. This worked very well, and most people were not aware that I had a hearing problem. I worked as a school secretary and dealt with teachers, students, and parents. I could use the telephone with no problems. Some years later I was fitted with a behind-the-ear model which seemed to be just as good as the body type and was more convenient.

I did not give up hope of surgical help, however, and had three more operations in Toronto on the left ear. When these operations were also unsuccessful, I believed that the left ear was dead. In spite of this, I continued to lead a fairly normal life because the hearing aid was so

393

helpful. However, my right ear continued to deteriorate, and I eventually had to go back to a body-type hearing aid. As my hearing got worse, I had to go to a more powerful hearing aid, and eventually even the most powerful aid available was not effective. Finally, in 1983 I had to give up the job I enjoyed, because I could not cope, and I now entered a dismal period in my life.

Socializing became very difficult. When we went to happy events, such as weddings and retirements, I could not tell what was being said, or what was making people laugh. This made me so miserable that we stopped going to these occasions, and we stayed home where I was the happiest. I bought a decoder for captions on the television, flashing lights for the doorbell and telephone, and a TDD. My husband and I even took sign language lessons, but as no one else in our small town understood the signs, we gave up after one course. Music had always given me great pleasure and I played the piano for my own enjoyment. Now, music was just a lot of noise, and most unpleasant. My husband always had to accompany me to appointments with the doctor, dentist, etc., and do the talking. So my pleasures were now at home. I have always loved to sew, quilt, and embroider, and these activities now filled my life, but I often wished I could attend classes to get more knowledge of these hobbies.

In 1984, my husband retired from his work, and we began to spend our winters in Florida. I have played and enjoyed golf for a long time, so I joined a ladies group at a golf club where we stay. I enjoyed playing the game, but the socializing afterwards made me feel left out. I even tried attending a few tournaments, but had to stop because not being included in conversations was just too hard to take.

During the winter of 1998-1999, I was reading a Canadian Hearing Society publication, and I read about Clarion. I already had an article by a person who had the implant, and I became very excited. I made a phone call to Advanced Bionics on the TDD, and they sent me all the information about the implant, including a list of implant clinics in Canada. I have a son who lives in Ottawa, so when I saw that the Ottawa Civic Hospital was on the list I was very happy, as I would be able to stay with him. My husband immediately called the Ottawa Civic Hospital, and that phone call was the beginning of a change in my life, and I began to feel that perhaps this time I would have some success. I was given appointments for five days of tests to find out if I was a suitable candidate for the procedure.

It was always assumed that the implant would be done on the right ear, and all the testing went well until the last one. When the surgeon, Dr. David Schramm and audiologist Chrisiane Seguin performed the last test my right ear did not respond. My husband and I at this stage were downcast, as we thought this was the end of the road. However, Dr. Schramm said he would repeat this test on the left ear, just in case there was still something there. I can't describe the elation I felt when this ear, which I thought was dead, showed a good response. Because of previous operations, however, Dr. Shramm would have to do a reconstruction operation before the implant, which would be just as invasive as the implant itself. In order to avoid two operations, Dr. Schramm offered to do a stapedectomy on the right ear, which would be a much simpler procedure. If it didn't work, I could still go ahead with the reconstruction and implant. I decided to go ahead with the stapedectomy, which was done in May 1999. Unfortunately the improvement was minimal. So in September of the same year, Dr. Schramm did the reconstruction, and when this had healed he did the implant in May 2000.

When the speech processor was fitted in June, I could hear sounds, the first sounds from that ear since 1952. From there on, my life changed. Aft first, of course, everyday sounds were all new to me. I couldn't believe my feet made so much noise when I was walking, and the traffic was louder than I could ever remember. I was able to hear speech, and I could hear the birds singing. Later, when I became used to the sound of the birds, I would sometimes say to my husband "The birds are very noisy this morning." As all the sounds were new to me, I had to learn what they meant. Working in the kitchen became easier and more enjoyable when I could recognize the sound of the kettle boiling, the tap running, the microwave pinging when it had finished. My husband doesn't hear some of the high frequencies as well as he used to do, and it is amusing when I hear the ping of the bread machine as it finishes baking, and that is a sound he has never heard. Of course I had lots of work to do to help myself. The most important was to learn to concentrate. My husband read children's storybooks to me, a sentence at a time, and I would repeat what I heard. Then I graduated to talking books with the written text. I am now also having some success with using the telephone with special people, who will speak more slowly, but I still need more practice.

The cochlear implant has really changed my life and that of my husband's as well. I am much more independent. I can do things for myself and enjoy the freedom that hearing again gives me. I will be able to take sewing courses now. I have already attended a demonstration of a new sewing machine. I could hear everything and was even able to ask questions. I have had some amusing experiences as well. Last summer I was with my son watching my 10-year-old granddaughter play soccer. It was raining, so I was standing talking to my son with my umbrella covering us. Suddenly my speech processor went silent. I was concerned, because I had replaced the battery before attending the game. As I turned to go to the car to investigate the problem, I saw that my microphone was not on my head, but had attached itself to the shaft of my umbrella. The lesson learned was not to use an umbrella with a metal shaft, or be sure to put the umbrella over the shoulder opposite the microphone.

As I had agreed to take part in a clinical trial for the high-frequency electrode, one of the things I had to do was keep a daily diary for three months, after the speech processor was fitted. Now a year later, it is very interesting to read of my early experiences. Perhaps one year from now, I will be able to look back to today and see that the improvement is continuing. I feel very fortunate to have had an implant, and I would recommend it to anyone with a profound hearing loss. I was only in the hospital overnight, and had no pain or discomfort afterwards. I am particularly fortunate to be a Canadian citizen, because the Ontario Health Insurance Plan covered all my expenses. The only thing that I had to pay for myself was the behind-the-ear processor, which was an option. It really is terrific to feel a part of the family and community once more, and I enjoy each and every day in this new world.

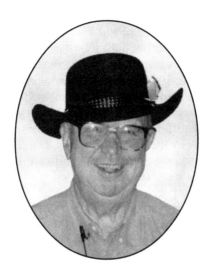

SHHH Article...By Rocky Stone

Many of you have very kindly inquired about my physical well being during the last year. In fact, your continued love and support have sustained me through a very difficult period of my life. Since I was not able to thank each of you individually, I am taking the liberty of thanking you all in this article in the *SHHH Journal.*

By April 1994, I had lost all of my central vision as a result of macular degeneration. I had been blind in my right eye since age 19. And I knew that I would be in serious trouble if something happened to my left eye, which I depended upon for hearing because I was predominantly a speechreader. As a result of that knowledge, I have followed cochlear implant research for many years, first, as a member of the Veterans Administration scientific review panel; second, as a member of the National Institute on Deafness and Other Communication Disorders advisory council.

I was aware of the recent rapid improvements in cochlear implants, and I knew that this presented at least one option to me in the event of deaf-blindness. As I had now reached that point, it became clear to me that I had to make a decision quickly. Because, as the vision disappeared and as my ability to lipread went with it, I was unable to access information or to communicate effectively with anyone including my family. I knew many people who had benefited significantly from cochlear implants and, because of my eyesight, it seemed like a logical

397

choice for me. I discussed all this with audiologists and with my chosen surgeon, Dr. Noel Cohen at New York University Medical Center. We began testing to see whether or not I would be a candidate for a cochlear implant. I went through all the normal audiological tests and assured that Medicare would take care of most of the costs.

On Tuesday, July 26, 1994, I underwent implant surgery. On August 23, 24, and 25, I was "stimulated" as they say in the professional circles and "hooked up" as many of us consumers say. I was given a program to test based on nine different programs in the computer with specifications devised for me by the audiologist after extensive testing. Within one and a half hours, I was receiving significant benefit from the implant. My responses were sufficiently good that I was permitted that first night to take the speech processor back to the hotel. The next two days consisted of more testing and further development of more programs to determine which would be most beneficial for me. We selected the program I thought as the best and headed home. En route home, my wife, Ahme, had the big band tape on and asked if I could enjoy it. I said, –"No, its just noise." She pointed out that a trumpet was playing. As soon as my mind knew what the instrument was, the irritation of noise disappeared. And over the next four hours, I began to listen for clarinets, saxophones, pianos, violins, and so forth, and identify those instruments. By the time we reached home, four hours later, I heard more music than noise. Four days after I received the speech processor, our son had a family gathering to celebrate the success of my operation. There were 16 people present, five of them were children screaming like banshees. The others were in one-on-one conversations, which created an atmosphere with considerable background noise. Previously, under these circumstances, I would simply said hello to everyone and, at the first possibility, slipped into another room and watch the TV in silence and isolation. My interaction with the family had become non-existent.

On this day, however, with all the conversations going on around me even with the children shouting and playing. I did not ask that they be silenced, I did not move into another room. I stood with my son in-law and listened for 30 minutes in a conversation and did very well. I then had conversations which each of the other adults and heard what they all said. The implant was working exceedingly well in noise.

The second major change I noticed had to do with eating outdoors. Ahme loves to eat outdoors in good weather but our house is located directly under the flight path from National Airport and I was constantly driven indoors because of the noise of the airplanes, which augmented the noise of autos passing the house. Now, I can sit on the patio with Ahme and conduct a conversation, in spite of the noise. The speech processor has a power and a volume switch, as well as a sensitivity switch. What I have learned is that increasing the volume is not the

398

way to go. With the implant, the trick is to get the sensitivity and the volume in balance with the particular situation and to remove as much noise as possible but not turn it off completely. I am getting increasingly good at finding the proper settings. This is also giving me an opportunity to expand my range of speech understanding.

The third very significant behavioral change occurred when, on the eighth day after receiving the speech processor, the phone rang and I was alone. I thought, well, I'd take a chance. So, I answered the phone and recognized the voice of Betsey Bomberg, my audiologist in New York. We had a wonderful conversation. She was astonished...happy and even joyful.

Low-frequency tones still sometimes elude me. But I find that I am getting better in each conversation. People I am talking to are more relaxed because the tension that I used to have communicated itself to others.

Let me tell you, too, about some little things that I have been enjoying, things that don't mean much to people, which now affect me in a way that I find truly significant. For example, Ahme and I went to San Diego recently since I was receiving the President's Citation from the American Academy of Otolaryngology. While we were there, we visited my two sisters. One morning, Ahme and my sisters were away, and I decided to turn on Mr.Coffee. Normally even with good sight, I would pull the coffee pot out while it was still dripping and make a mess. This time, when the coffee pot appeared to be full, I reached for it; but before I got my hand on the handle, I heard drip, drip, drip, and I knew that it wasn't finished. So, I stood there and waited for it to stop dripping, and then pulled the coffee pot out. No mess. A little thing, but it made me very happy.

Cooking in the microwave is sometimes a frustrating process because our microwave does not always respond to the pressure of my finger. I would think that I had pushed the numbers because I have numbers to tell me which is which, and when nothing happened I would be frustrated and it would waste time. Now, I push a number and if I don't hear the beep, I know I have to push it again.

These little things have tended to make me less irritable, more relaxed. Life is more enjoyable in the sense that the things I haven't heard for a long time, I am now experiencing and life is a lot more fun than it used to be. The most important thing of all, of course, is that I am back in the family with conversation and interaction, even with more than one person. That means more to me than anything else. Hearing my grandchildren's voices, not everything, but something, has been a new source of joy for me. One of the major things I have noticed about this whole experience is how relaxed I am. I no longer have that tense, tight feeling that comes with speechreading all the time. The professor who worked with me on this implant told me that I shouldn't worry about television for the time being because TV sound is of such poor quality. But, Sunday, August 28, is a day I will long remember. Just five days after hookup, I flipped through the TV channels on Sunday when many talk shows are on. I then tested 13 voices, male and female, different nationalities, and I heard at least one sentence clearly from all 13. In one case, I had a full report from a school superintendent who had major problems. Now, as I have continued listening to the TV, I have become able to hear and understand more and more. I no longer use captioning because I can't read it. But, to my delight, I am able to hear. In some cases, I can follow a plot of a program. Most importantly, however, on TV and radio is the access to information. Being cut off from reading, I know if I couldn't access information through the hearing mode, I would be in trouble, as it would take me some time to learn Braille. And, I knew that I couldn't wait that long because I'd go stir crazy without information. In October, on our last trip to the audiologist in New York, I actually listened to the radio! I understood what was being said. The commentator was saying that 300,000 illegal immigrants have received $600 million dollars of medical care from the city of New York, and I heard a long dissertation on the implications of this particular problem.

Obviously, my cochlear implant is working very well for me. Cochlear implants have proven to have a positive impact on the quality of life for thousands of individuals. Results and progress vary with each individual case and which implant you choose is up to you and depends on your situation. In my experience, I have successfully achieved all three of my goals for my cochlear implant, a short learning curve, quick access to information, and recognition of familiar voices. So, I personally am very happy with my decision. To sum it up, the cochlear implant has changed me in many ways. More importantly, it's given me an opportunity for a third career instead of spending days on how to figure out how to fill them - not being able to read or hear - I will now be able to return to the mainstream of life and continue in some productive vein for some time longer.

I would like to thank you all once more for your interest in what I am doing and how I am doing. On October 11, I went to Westhaven, Connecticut, for a 14-week blind rehabilitation program. By the time you read this article, I will have completed that course and, hopefully, be able to use my residual, peripheral sight much better than I can at this writing. Meanwhile, keep up the spirit and enthusiasm, which makes SHHH such a great organization. I love you all.

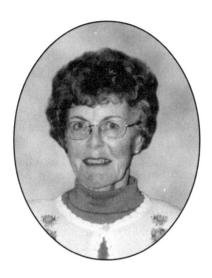

Marilyn's Miracle...By Marilyn Robillard

Praise the Lord! I am a Christian who believes in miracles. At age 65 I received my hearing miracle by way of a Clarion CII Bionic Ear. Each day has a new surprise for me! Imagine, for a moment, how profoundly different your life would be if you couldn't hear, or discriminate speech, well enough to be part of a discussion with your own family members. Imagine being around a campfire with dear friends and missing fun conversation, stories, and laughter. Being part of this world of communication and the endless new inventions for it, but still, not really "a part." When alone and the telephone rang, I didn't know if it was a family emergency or a telemarketer. "I'm sorry, I'm hearing impaired" was my obligated answer to everyone.

It hurts. Especially since I am a very ambitious, positive, intelligent, and friendly female, married 46 years to Dick, mother of four daughters and grandmother to eight precious souls. How it hurt to be an outsider in my own family discussions, always feeling stupid for not understanding the plans that were made until someone, one to one, would kindly explain them. Although I'd accepted my hearing impairment, I felt like an outsider. This acceptance was a long, hard one, as being from a small town I had no support group and had to discover my helpful technology on my own. I was thankful for the SHHH magazine that I'd subscribed to after seeing one in my audiologist's waiting room. This led to my first SHHH convention, which I attended and learned what technology offered that could possibly help me.

It's not that I didn't try. I spent a fortune periodically updating my hearing aids until even the digital ones couldn't help me discriminate speech. The TDD (telephone for deaf) helped me to be independent for making my own telephone calls, captioning on TV, and for several years my ALD (assistive listening device) helped me in seminars, various classes, and restaurant situations.

The beginning for my hearing miracle was when attending my second SHHH Convention, which was held in St. Paul. Determined to find new ways to be a better communicator, I had my schedule filled with workshops for new, or different, equipment and ways for communicating - pretty much a repeat of what I was already knowledgeable about. On the last morning, for lack of anything innovative I attended a workshop that featured six recipients of cochlear implants. Imagine my surprise when these people, sitting in front of an audience of inquisitive persons, were able to hear our questions! They were each so happy about their ability to hear after receiving their cochlear implant.

The next workshop was with two surgeons, including Dr. Samuel Levine, who explained who could be a candidate for cochlear implants and the technical aspects. At this time I was told that I could very possibly be a candidate. Although I knew Dr. Levine was at the University of Minnesota, with pages of telephone numbers, how was this hearing impaired person going to begin her quest for this newfound miracle. Only hearing impaired persons can understand how this would be an obstacle. Now, comes a third part of my miracle. My daughter, LaRita, has a friend with a cochlear implant, Cynthia Farley, who sent an e-mail to me that exploded with enthusiasm for her implant and offered her help. Eureka, I was scheduled for four appointments at the University, at which time Sharon Smith accepted me as a candidate for my surgery.

Let me explain that I had very good hearing until 1970, when my doctor told me that the best help for my arthritis was aspirin. "The sky is the limit—if your ears start ringing, slow down" was his theme. I didn't use common sense, and I did just that. My ears started ringing, and the tinnitis never stopped. From that time my hearing kept getting worse. However, the tone remained quite stable at 30 dB for high and low tones, and 70 dB for talking tones. It was my discrimination which kept getting worse until my evaluations showed only 10% to 20% comprehension. I was accepted as a candidate for my cochlear implant only because of my poor discrimination. But I was hearing many environmental sounds!! Besides, my tests had shown that I had diagnoses for possible AN (auditory neuropathy) which could be the reason for my poor discrimination. How could the cochlear implant help if my hearing nerve was not transmitting properly?

Next was research concerning my situation, although my surgery date was scheduled. This research was obtained via computer information over the Web, personal stories from persons in two e-mail groups which I'd joined, and spending my winter at our winter home in Texas with the possible surgery always on my mind.

Finally, I'd heard of no other new technology to help me, I had nothing but positive input from implantees, and my decision was made. The surgery on May 21, 2001, was successful. My hook-up was June 19th. I wondered what I'd gotten myself into. The sound was terrible. Although I'd been told that it takes time and patience, it's easier "said than done."

Our very busy summer which included several 'mappings' and my homework paid off!! Actually, I didn't have any aural rehabilitation until three months after my surgery, but it went so well that Beth Brady gave me A+ and said I'd accomplished nearly everything on her assignment sheet. After one more appointment with her, she told me there would be no reason for another. She merely recommended certain CD's for me to listen to and work on discriminating the music's lyrics.

My two-month 'mapping' with Sharon Smith on July 26th was a day of jubilation!! I could hardly contain myself!! I got 80% correct repeating sentences, 70% correct for sentences with noise, and 39% correct for single words. It has been six months since my surgery and I am so excited about my accomplishments. I am able to understand TV without captioning, listen to the radio, and even make telephone calls with both our speaker and cell phones!! I am also overhearing conversations—about ME!! A person who knew me from last year was puzzled and asked Dick why I'm hearing so much better. I answered from across the room, with a pleased smile. Life has become so much more full, and as my hearing continues to improve I will continue to add more challenges in my life. I praise the Lord for my miracle of hearing.

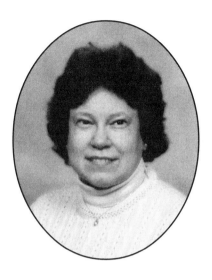

To Do Nothing Is Not an Option…By Ruth Fox

I was born with a moderate to severe hearing loss. My two sisters had hearing impairments as well. Their hearing loss was less severe than mine, but still a significant problem for them. My brother had normal hearing. Other than us three girls, there was no hearing loss in any other generations of the family. My parents were very intelligent people, but they made the only wrong decision that is possible in addressing a hearing loss. Their decision was to do nothing and pretend that the hearing loss did not exist. When I was a child, special education and hearing aids were an option. Even though the hearing aids available then were not as advanced as the hearing aids that are available today, they still helped. I went to the neighborhood public school where the only accommodation I had was to sit in the front seat, when everyone else was seated in alphabetical order. Outwardly, I became the child my parents wanted. I acted normal and looked normal. I was an average student in school, and even learned to play the violin and excel with it.

Inside, hidden from everyone, including my parents, I was frustrated, angry, lonely, and isolated. I appeared to be an exceptionally good girl in public ... too good, because I was afraid to do anything. At home I was a problem child, who was always in trouble, had a short fuse, and was excellent at having tantrums. In a family, with three children with unapprised hearing losses, communication misunderstandings ruled the emotional atmosphere of the home.

When I was 17, a teacher finally intervened and my hearing loss was addressed. I received my first hearing aid. My mother and I went to get it on a cold spring day. On the way home; I could not figure out what was making the loud sound in the car, I discovered it was slush in the wheels. Never before in my life had I heard that sound. I began speech therapy. I was an excellent violinist, playing first chair in my high school orchestra, yet I could not pronounce my own name because of the 'W'. I continued on in school, obtaining a Bachelor of Music in Performance. When a music vocation no longer seemed practical in the light of deteriorating hearing loss, I received my Masters of Science in Librarianship. I graduated with honors, having "done it right" academically.

However, as a person I was a mess, lacking in social skills and having unstable emotional health. I spent the next 10 years working to put my life back together. SHHH, doctors, counselors, teachers, ministers, and many other dedicated and caring people moved in and out of my life, helping me to put the missing pieces of my life together. Eventually, I became a functional person. Library work was not the answer for me. Therefore, after receiving certification in special education, I became a teacher of children with multi-disabilities. By the time, I was 30, I had lost all functional hearing. I continued to teach, as my students were nonverbal, a perfect match for a teacher with hearing loss.

Just before I was 40, I received a cochlear implant. That returned my hearing loss back to a functional level of hearing. I was like a person with mild to moderate loss of hearing. My whole world opened up, and the total isolation that I had felt for so many years was greatly reduced. I was able to communicate one to one with ease, and even participate to a moderate degree with groups. The telephone, which had become totally unusable, now became a functional tool again, allowing me independence.

Though my world was opening up in regards to my hearing, it had been closing down physically. In my twenties, and thirties, I had started to notice that my muscles were fatiguing with use. My muscle problem has been slowly progressive, like the loss of my hearing was. It has made it difficult for me to stand, walk, or do anything physically for any great length of time without my muscles becoming tight and hurting. I use a motorized cart for places where I would have to stand over five minutes or walk a long time. The combination of physical and hearing

406

difficulty proved to be too much for me to handle along with my job. I retired from teaching after almost 25 years. Now, using my life experiences and my ability to communicate by means of my cochlear implant and writing, I am trying to help people, both those with hearing loss and the parents of children with hearing loss, to avoid making the same mistake that my parents did. There are many ways to compensate for hearing loss, and to be functional in society in spite of it. To do nothing is not an option.

In the past year, my cochlear implant use was beginning to be less functional. I was not tolerating the stimulation of the electrodes even at very low levels. The cause is unknown, but the ear that was implanted was always extremely sensitive to sound. Last November, I was implanted in the opposite ear. My cochlear implant use has been excellent since that time, with no difficulties from any of the electrodes. To date I have used the cochlear implant for 14 years.

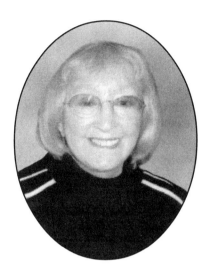

The Road to Success…By Bette Thompson-Westin

My autoimmune hearing loss started about 15 years ago, progressing gradually into total loss in one ear, and decreased comprehension in the other. Discouraged that my Tacoma doctor was doing nothing to help me, I requested a referral to the Otolaryngology Department at the University of Washington's Medical Center. The doctor I was scheduled to see was Dr. Larry Duckert, who is internationally respected for his academic contributions to the field of otology with many scientific papers and presentations and a full professor as well.

After a comprehensive examination and analysis of my hearing history, Dr. Duckert told me the news that I was hoping I would never hear, that I would eventually go deaf. I left his office in an emotional meltdown. Tears streamed onto my favorite red jacket as I was hugged and comforted by Jenny Stork, Patient Care Coordinator, a petite package of warmth, caring, and compassion.

A year's treatment with drugs stabilized what little hearing remained. I continued working full time in the travel and tourism industry. Once a month for four years I traveled to Seattle for hearing tests monitoring my steadily declining hearing. After all those months being in a soundproof room having hearing tests, I became friends with Kevin Kimele, Clinical Audiologist. Kevin always showed concern about my general health, as well as my hearing scores. We made each other laugh a lot. We both needed a good giggle in such a serious world.

At the onset of my treatment, I was accepted as a candidate for a cochlear implant, and thought, "Hey this is great!" not really knowing what it entailed. When I found out the mechanics of it, the whole idea depressed me. I complained about the prospect of a microphone draped on my ear, and wearing hardware on my body, in the form of a body-worn speech processor. Imagine being in the middle of a romantic conversation (or "situation") and having to say, "Hold that thought a minute...my batteries just went dead." My vanity was getting in the way as I thought of evolving into a bionic woman wired for sound. But that was my only option. I became determined it would work. I would be a good subject and, make the best of things, and view it as another new adventure in life. Dr. Duckert smiled and reassuringly said that he thought I would do very well.

January and February of this year were spent in the Cook Islands, and it was then my hearing took a fast nosedive. By February I couldn't carry on a decent conversation, and people were forced to write messages. That sure gets old fast! The date for my surgery was set before our trip so, I looked forward to March 9th, the BIG DAY when Dr. Duckert would implant my Nucleus 24.

I felt no apprehension as I went into surgery about 9 am. It was all over in about two hours. "Surgery went perfect and there were no complications, "reported" Dr. Duckert. After a brief stay in the Recovery Ward and two cups of coffee, we were heading for home at 11:30, and felt much better than I thought I would. Yahoo!

Twenty-four days later, when my audiologist Tina Worman finished my first mapping, she explained, "Don't expect too much the first time." Most patients don't hear as well right away. Hooked up, with processor turned on, my husband David asked, "Can you hear me?" "Yes. Yes," I cried! We all cried. It was a miracle! David moved down the halls, in and out of offices. "Can you hear me?" Yes, I could. It was incredible! Dr. Duckert arrived on the scene, followed by the rest of my support team, Kevin and Jenny, who were all smiles and happy for me. Dr. Duckert wanted to know how he sounded to me. "The way you always do, "I said, "but a little louder." What a day. Everyone was thrilled!

On the way home I could hear David in the car for the first time in over two years. We tried music, but that was going to take some time. When we got home, I plugged into the phone attachment, and called friends to surprise them. I knocked on doors in our condo build-

410

ing and surprised neighbors. "I can hear again." They were happy, since they had become tired of writing messages. I stood on my balcony and enjoyed hearing birds again. I will always remember those moments as one of the most joyful times in my life.

A few weeks after that April 2 mapping, David and I, along with my new implant, processor, and headgear, headed for Bali and Hong Kong. We packed the battery charger, converter, adapter, and a dozen spare batteries. I was curious to see how the implant worked in airports and on aircraft. I could hear airport announcements, but couldn't understand them . . . but then who does? Next I tried plugging into the armrest to see how the music and movie sounded. No go, my jack wouldn't fit in their double-plug connector. As for desk clerks, waiters, shopkeepers, and street people trying to sell us fake Rolexes ... no problem. I experienced some difficulty on tour buses, but not in private cars if the guide spoke slowly and a little louder. A great advantage was being able to switch off the processor on the plane and sleep in total silence.

Tina has since added new maps for me to try. So far, I'm trying to listen 20 minutes a day to only piano music. When I master that, I'll try the flute. Tina says the most difficult and complicated instrument to hear with an implant is the violin. I attribute my implant success to being almost completely deaf for only a short period, having an upbeat attitude, a great surgeon, and wonderful support team. When September arrives, I'll receive the new behind-the-ear processor, and then it will be off to Cambodia, Vietnam, Burma, and Thailand. Watch out, world! Here comes Bette with her new ears. And she still wears her red jacket, but now there are no tear stains.

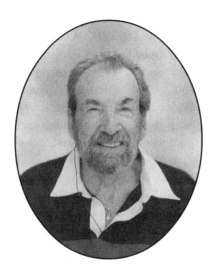

World of Words...By Don Clemons

I lived in a world of words, first as a student, as a teacher, as a college dean, and then as a president. Hearing is important to everyone, but to me it was necessary to earn a living. I stopped working because I could not hear or understand the students, faculty, board members, or the public that I needed to deal with daily. At 74 years I have had a hearing loss for 25 years, and I don't remember ever speaking to my father without raising my voice. My older brother also had a severe hearing loss and retired early. Therefore I believe my hearing loss is hereditary.

I was fitted for a hearing aid after a series of tests performed by a hearing and speech facility at the age of 50. After annual testing over the next ten years, my hearing loss became so profound that I could not continue in an educational environment. I retired, and my hearing continued to decline. At the age of 69, I was tested with two behind-the-ear aides. My level of understanding speech was 28%. I was a very active senior citizen, sailing, playing tennis and golf. I could not hear the water lapping on the hull of the sailboat or the tennis ball bounce, but most important I could not hear or understand the voice of my lovely wife or the wonderful sounds of nature.

I was a prime candidate for the cochlear implant. Four years ago I was implanted with an Advanced Bionics Clarion S-series device. I was the first adult to have the operation by a surgeon in the Fort Myers area. The first patient was an 11-year-old boy. The only negative side effect after surgery was poor balance. I did have trouble standing alone and walking for several days until my equilibrium stabilized, but the pain was negligible. I was able to play tennis after about three weeks, but allowed six weeks for all healing after the surgery.

At that point the audiologist programmed my speech processor and I was told to expect to understand closed sentences but not open ones. The first day I could understand about 80% of what was said to me. During the first six months, I found that the first time a person spoke to me it would be a little difficult to understand them, but after a few minutes of listening I could understand. It seemed as if the brain was relearning communication and when it heard a familiar voice it could understand more easily. After six months of using my "bionic ear" I was tested and my comprehension was 98%. So it seems the brain had relearned all audio input.

The hearing person receives two kinds of sounds, mechanical and natural. Mechanical is the most difficult for the cochlear implant user to understand. The telephone and the television are examples of these mechanical mediums, and it will take the implant user longer to master. The use of the telephone for a profoundly hearing impaired person can be a nightmare. For a cochlear implant user it will take time to use the telephone; the brain will have to learn new sounds and it will take time to communicate intelligent messages to the user. The days of typing on a TTY or using a third party to assist with the voice-over telephone are gone. In the beginning I used a telephone pickup cord, which has been used to tape telephone messages in the past. The short patch cord has a suction cup at one end that is attached to the telephone receiver and plugs into the speech processor. I would practice and practice listening to automated menus until my brain understood the message. Now they have invented a telephone to accommodate the cochlear implant user; one model is the Ameriphone Dialogue XL-40. This phone has an outlet for a cord with two male plugs. One plugs into the phone and the other end plugs into the speech processor. This new cochlear implant-compatible telephone makes the use of the telephone a pleasure.

During the first year it was still difficult to understand television without closed captions, so I attached the microphone, which came from Advanced Bionics, to the speaker on the television and used a patch cord. I found I could hear and understand television without closed captions.

I bought an inexpensive microphone ($24.95) from Radio Shack and a 12-foot patch cord ($2.95) to take with me on trips so I may enjoy television with or without closed captions. One of our favorite restaurants is Appleby's which has a high noise level. I attach the microphone to my wife's lapel and plug it into the speech processor. This bypasses the head microphone, and this technique allows me to almost eliminate background noise. We have found that I can hear the waitress and my wife, when the waitress cannot hear us. When I am in a noisy environment, I attach the mike to my shirt and it helps reduce the swirl of mixed sounds that you would have from the head microphone in the same environment. We have an 11-year-old Regatta convertible that we love to drive with the top down. With the microphone we can carry on a clear conversation as we drive. After you use the cochlear implant, you will find it difficult to be without it.

Another suggestion is to have your audiologist provide you with a copy of your mapping strategies on a disc in case your speech processor is lost or damaged. In my situation, my wife carries the floppy disc in her purse whenever we travel. When Clarion sends your new speech processor they can also provide the name and address of the nearest Clarion trained audiologist to re-program your speech processor. If you are a cochlear implant candidate, you may find it helpful to talk to an implant user, especially with a background similar to yours. Since I was one of the first adults in this area to receive the implant, my audiologist has referred many candidates to me and I have shared my experiences with them. In conclusion, the "bionic ear" is not the same as the natural ear, as it has some limitations. However, I am thankful that I can hear the water lapping on the side of the sailboat, the tennis ball bounce, and the birds chirping, but most of all for hearing and understanding my loved ones, especially my grandchildren.

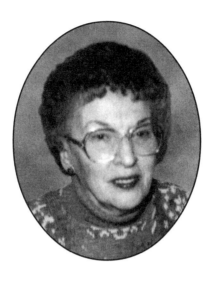

My Story…By Gerry Stewart

The year was 1953, I had just turned 21 and I was becoming aware that I couldn't hear as well on the phone when I used my right ear. When I switched to the left one, sound seemed normal. I was puzzled, but not too concerned. I married about six months later and life went on. My husband was in the Air Force and we moved to California, I had two babies. My hearing seemed less helpful, and I looked for an ear doctor. There weren't any ear doctors at the base in California, so I let it slide until we moved to Massachusetts. By this time, my lack of distinct hearing was becoming a major nuisance and I finally managed to get an appointment with the ear clinic on the base where we were stationed. After a few standard hearing tests, I was told that I had nerve deafness and that there was nothing to be done for it, therefore I would eventually be totally deaf. I was 24 years old and devastated.

This was a total blow for a young person with small children. I was having trouble hearing the babies at night when they cried for feedings, and my husband would hear them first and wake me up. (No equal opportunities here, women still got up to feed the babies!) I didn't even consider hearing aids at first as we were too broke to afford one at that time. Military pay has never been very good; a roof over our head and food for the babies seemed more important. Two more babies came

417

along and after the fourth and last child was born, I woke up one morning to realize that I was hearing almost nothing—it was the third time that my hearing had dropped drastically overnight. I was unaware that much could be done for the situation, so I just kept putting one foot ahead of the other. Taking care of four small children was exceptionally hard with so little hearing. I would have to check on them every few minutes to be certain that all was okay with each one, especially the smallest, as the older ones were so small that they were apt to treat the baby as another doll, if not watched closely. Luckily, I managed to cope and the kids thrived.

Someone my husband knew had lost a relative who wore a hearing aid, and he bought the deceased person's hearing aid for thirty dollars. This was not a lot of help. I was still not aware that one could be "fitted" with hearing aids that would cater to each hearing problem. At that time, I'm not even sure there was very much "fitting." The technological revolution in hearing aids was yet to come. I was now 30 years old.

I did go back to the ear clinic, and after more testing, the doctors recommended that I try a better hearing aid as it was apparent that I wasn't going to be able to cope if I didn't do so. We went to an audiologist, where I was evaluated and it was determined that I could benefit from a hearing aid. However, my husband had been sitting in the car for about three hours with four small children and by the time I finished my appointment and came back out and told him the price would be $500.00, he blew his stack and didn't speak to me for a month. I canceled the hearing aid purchase. I did eventually manage to find a body model, by Sonotone, for a lesser price and he did agree that I could buy that, therefore I finally had one that was tailored to my hearing loss. My hearing continued to degenerate and I kept going to audiologists and ear doctors through the years with little success. I couldn't hear in crowds and I had to listen carefully to my husband and kids to understand them.

The children were pretty good for small kids—they didn't "sass" nearly as much as might be expected, but I did realize that they "sassed" when they didn't think I was aware of it. I did manage to raise an incredibly thoughtful family of four children who have, in turn, taught the grandchildren to be thoughtful of my hearing problems. I consider myself very, very lucky in that respect.

My husband, on the other hand, didn't seem able to cope with my hearing loss and tossed out such "gems" as "Well, if you'd pay attention when I'm talking, you'd hear me." And "Well, I hope I have enough insurance to keep you going, if I die. You'll never find another man with those ears." My husband walked out when I was 41 years old. We were, by then, living in the DC area, where he had been transferred to Andrews Air Force Base. In fact, by the time he had retired, we had lived at two other bases and moved 49 times. I survived all of this with four children, a severe hearing loss, and a very good sense of humor. It kept me going, and threaded throughout this time were innumerable ear doctor and audiologist visits.

I did remarry, and needless to say, he was a man with much more compassion—my hearing never seemed to be an issue with him. My children were in high school. I was working. It was always minimum wage jobs as no one really wanted to give a deaf person much respon-sibility and I never had been to college, so I was stuck in a rut. The kids graduated, got jobs, got married, and did quite well, considering that they came from a broken home where Mom couldn't hear and didn't make much money. It made them more independent if anything. I'm very proud of my children. About this time, my mother had a stroke. I moved back to New York State to care for her, with my second hus-band, who, as always, was more concerned with others well-being than with his own. He was a very special person. Unfortunately, he died when I was 50, and my ears were still headed down and out. I decided that I really had been lucky to at least hear well enough to get my family raised, but from age 50 to 60 I worried more about the big WHEN? When might I be totally deaf? I tried to be thankful that I wasn't blind.

During these years, I had kept up with anything pertaining to ad-vances in hearing aid technology and I immediately noticed when im-plants were first mentioned. I still have two old yellowed newspaper clippings about implants—one mentioned a cost of $5,000 and the other, a cost of $10,000. Both cautioned that while sounds would be ampli-fied, understanding speech was still not good. In 1986 (I was 54) I went to an audiologist to be tested to see if I could benefit from an implant. I was told that my hearing wasn't bad enough to qualify—plus, Medicare didn't cover it. (I was by this time on disability and had no other insurance, so the operation was not for me.) I was terribly disappointed, but in retrospect it was just as well as no one really wants to hear more noise. We all want better understanding. I had tried to take sign language classes three times during the years but even though my family had gone with me, none of us had the stick-to-it-ness to sign when we were not in class and I never became proficient at it. I also tried lipreading but I have severe eye problems, so I could never see well enough to get a good grip on lipreading. I found that I did better than I thought possible, though, after I had my implant.

I met my present companion, Don, shortly before I tried for the first time to have an implant (he encouraged it) and we have been together ever since. Here is another man with infinite patience who has never treated me as though deafness was synonymous with stupidity. I am fortunate, indeed. It's amazing how cruel people can be with their remarks about deafness, and I'm sure we have all experienced more than our share of those. My mother and sister came up with such "gems" as "Well, I sure wouldn't want one of those hanging out the side of my head," (referring to my hearing aid) and "I cannot stand to repeat myself three times every time we talk." Sometimes strangers are more merciful than family.

I was 68 when I tried the new digital hearing aids and found they did no more good than my 13-year-old hearing aid. A couple months after trying the new digital hearing aids, I read an article on implants again—this time, the surgeon's name was mentioned, and included was the fact that Medicare now covered the operation. I reached for the phone and made an appointment—after all, I reasoned, they could do no more than say "No" again. Of course, this took a few more weeks and another appointment with my primary caregiver for a referral and a lot more waiting for a busy doctor and audiologist to find time for me.

This time, though, I hit the jackpot, as they assured me the hearing loss was great enough to qualify me for the cochlear implant; the machinery started whirring for Medicare approval and I carried secondary insurance to cover the rest of the costs. I was euphoric the day I discovered that something really, truly could be done and maybe I wouldn't go totally deaf as those doctors had "promised" in my younger years. The operation took place four days before Christmas; the timing didn't make me too happy, and then my sense of balance took a steep drop, making me even more worried about my decision. Then, of course, like everyone else, I had to wait out those first few weeks of no hearing before I was connected to my speech processor.

Finally, of course, the big day arrived; my processor was connected; once again I wondered if this was what all the uproar was about. I couldn't hear that well—oh, woe to me! Then, I realized that I could understand speech a bit better—we left the audiologist's office and I heard the cars driving on the street (they sounded like they were driving over crushed glass). I wondered just how much adjusting I would have to do. After 48 years of less and less hearing and understanding, I finally realized that if it takes a long time to lose one's hearing, it's obviously going to take quite a while to regain a sense of good hearing and understanding. It may never be perfect hearing, but it's so much better than what I have been capable of for the past few years. (I have had to have most people write notes to me for the past couple years because the understanding was so bad and so I was beginning to withdraw almost totally from social situations and meeting new people.)

It's been six months since my operation. I hear better, although I have a long ways to go. I still cannot understand well on the phone but I do still practice with a friend and hope to get more understanding. I still lipread to a certain extent, but I understand so much more and can sit in a room with others and actually understand most of the conversation going on around me. This is something I haven't been capable of for years, and I am ecstatic when I realize that this implant has opened up a whole New World for me. I have done it and many others have done it. If you are hesitating, you need only to talk to the people who have benefited from the implant to take your chances for a better, more fulfilling life. I look forward to my 70th birthday with a new appreciation for life and for my newfound hearing. If you are hesitating, remember.........Just do it!!!

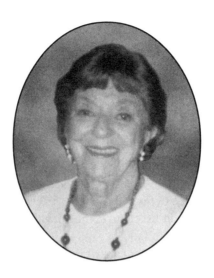

The Telephone is My Friend Again...By Beatrice Fish & Caren

For 68 years, I was blessed with perfect hearing. I worked, I had a busy social life, and enjoyed shows, concerts, TV, and the telephone. I was working in the travel business when I started to realize that the phone was becoming difficult to use. I went to an audiologist to have my hearing tested and sure enough, I needed a hearing aid in one ear. All was fine for about two years. Again, trouble with the phone, and I was fitted with a hearing aid for the second ear. Gradually my hearing became worse and in a period of eight years, after many changes in hearing aids and continued adjustments, I was told that I had a profound hearing loss. I was forced to quit the travel business and found it necessary to use the TTY. I was feeling very isolated, and one sleepless night inspired the following poem:

I have had a best friend from the time that I was a little girl.
We met when I was old enough to speak on the telephone.
We talked about school, boys, parties, and sometimes homework.
And my friend always had the right answers for me.
As I got older we talked about college, my studies and my dreams for the future.

And then we even made my wedding plans together.

Time went on, and my friend was still always there for me.

Now, I talked about my husband, about my children and about work.

I spoke to my friend about our new house, the furnishings and the decor.

When there were health problems, I was able to get all the needed answers.

My husband and I started traveling and again I shared this with my friend.

More years passed, and my children were grown and out of the house.

As I grew older, there didn't seem to be as much to talk about

But I still always spoke to my old friend.

However, my friend didn't seem to come up with the right answer. And my friend's voice began to fade.

Until one day, my friend did not answer me at all.

I knew then that my best friend, the telephone, had died.

I do miss you.

At the suggestion of my audiologist, I was tested for a cochlear implant. They informed me that I was a candidate and I decided to go for it. Next came the big decision. Which company do I choose? I was fortunate to have a daughter who researched the cochlear implant on her computer and gave me a ton of information. I then obtained names of former patients, whom I called. I discovered that those with Med-El implants seemed to handle the phone calls better.

The surgery was done two and a half years ago. Of course, for the first 30 days, I heard nothing. I admit, it was frightening, not hearing and not knowing if I ever would hear. I had been told that voices would sound like Mickey Mouse in the beginning. On my first day I was "connected', my sister and brother-in-law came to visit for two weeks. Good news. I could hold a conversation, and they did not sound like Mickey Mouse. And within a couple of months I was back on the telephone. My hearing's not perfect enough to go back to my earlier work as a travel agent. There was always the fear that I would send a client to the Caribbean, when they said Carolina.

A Daughter's Note

When you live 1,300 miles from your Mom, the phone is your lifeline. When my Mom stopped being able participate in conversations anymore because her hearing had dramatically declined, it was enormously painful. I found myself culling conversations down to the lowest common denominator. I become creative, learning how to share my daughter's illness, my son's first day of school, difficulties at work in a sentence or less. But we both felt sad and disconnected at the end of each conversation.

My two young children learned to shout one-word answers into the phone or listen to my Mom's running commentaries. It was so difficult for them to build a strong relationship with my Mom. They were so patient through my incessant prodding to speak clearly and loudly. And so often they weren't even talking about the same subject, which led to a little humor and a lot of frustration.

After a lot of thought, my Mom decided to try a cochlear implant. We chose Med-El after a conversation I had with part of the research and development team. They were articulate about the technology, patient with the explanations, and above all compassionate. The implant isn't perfect. But it is a miracle. My relationship with my Mom has been restored to the richness that was temporarily robbed by hearing loss. As I type this I can see my Mom and my three-year-old daughter in the next room. They're playing beauty parlor, exchanging the many spoken pleasantries that come with that game. My Mom is not facing my daughter and yet she's able to keep the game running at full hilt. My daughter asks "Did I cut enough, Grandma?" My Mom says "A little more off the top please." And I witness another generation now able to build a relationship with my Mom. Thanks to a little piece of heaven inserted in my Mom's head.

Resource Guide

Organizations

American Speech-Language-Hearing Assoc. (ASHA)
10801 Rockville Pike
Rockville, MD USA 20852
1-800-638-8255
www.asha.org

ASHA publishes materials for professionals in the hearing/communication field. A series of informational packets are available to the public at no charge. They can also provide referrals to audiologists and other professionals.

Alexander Graham Bell Assoc. for the Deaf
3417 Volta Place N.W.
Washington D.C. USA 20007
(202) 337-5220 (voice/tty)
www.agbell.org

AG Bell is the world's leading membership organization for pediatric hearing loss, advocating the use of technology to maximize residual hearing, and the development of written and spoken language. AG Bell addresses a broad spectrum of issues related to children with hearing loss. They can provide ongoing support and advocacy for parents and professionals. Publishes the *Volta Voice* six times a year and the *Volta Review* quarterly. They also publish informational brochures about issues related to hearing loss as well as a catalog of resources, books, and videotapes. They also host annual conferences for parents and professionals.

Auditory Verbal International (AVI)
2121 Eisenhower Ave., Suite 402
Alexandria, VA. USA 22314
(703) 739-1049 (voice)
(703) 739-0874 (tty)
www.auditory-verbal.org

AVI is dedicated to ensuring that all children with hearing impairments who have the potential to develop speech and language have the opportunity to do so. AVI certifies qualified therapists and has conferences. Publishes a newsletter the *Auricle* and *Backtalk* for parents.

Cochlear Implant Association Inc. (CIAI)
5335 Wisconsin Ave., N.W., Suite 440
Washington D.C. USA 20015-2052
(202) 895-2781
www.cici.org

CIAI is a non-profit organization dedicated to educating and supporting cochlear implant recipients and their families. They also provide information to those who have an interest in the cochlear implant technology. Publishes a quarterly magazine, *Contact* and hosts a convention every other year. Membership fees range from $25- $60 per year and include the magazine as a benefit. There are chapters of CIAI throughout the United States that offer information and support on a local basis for members and candidates.

Deafness Research Foundation
1050 17th street, N.W., Suite 701
Washington D.C. USA 20036
(202) 289-5850 (voice)
1-800-829-5934
www.drf.org
www.hearinghealth.net

Sponsors of the National Campaign for Hearing Health and the grassroots initiative "Hear Us" campaign to promote awareness of hearing loss and advocate for solutions.

John Tracy Clinic
806 West Adams Blvd.
Los Angeles, CA. USA 90007
(213) 748-5481 (voice)
1-800-522-4582
www.jtc.org

The John Tracy Clinic provides a correspondence course on hearing rehabilitation for parents and educators of hearing impaired children.

League for the Hard of Hearing
71 W. 23rd St.

430

New York, N.Y. USA 10010-4162
(917) 305-7700 (voice)
(917) 305-7999 (tty)
www.lhh.org

Founded in 1910, the League is a non-profit rehabilitation agency for children and adults who are hard of hearing, deaf, and deaf-blind. Provides hearing rehabilitation and human service programs for people who are hard of hearing or deaf. The League has a hearing museum on hearing impairment open to group tours on appointment as well as a catalog of publications, videos, and audiotapes for sale.

National Institute on Deafness and Other Communication Disorders (NIDCD)
31 Center Drive MSC 2320
Bethesda, MD. USA 20892-2320
(301) 496-7243
www.nidcd.nih.gov

Call the NIDCD for a free "Cochlear Implant Information Package" at 1-800-241-1044.

Self Help for Hard of Hearing People, Inc. (SHHH)
7910 Woodmont Ave., Suite 1200
Bethesda, MD. USA 20814
(301) 657-2248 (voice)
(301) 657-2249 (tty)
www.shhh.org

SHHH is the world's largest international organization for hard of hearing people. Publishes *Hearing Loss* magazine and organizes regional and national conventions. Has chapters throughout the United States and advocates for the hard of hearing in many areas. They also have a catalog of books and videos pertaining to hearing loss issues.

The Listening Center at John Hopkins University
PO Box 41402
Baltimore MD. USA 21203-6402
(410) 955-9397 (voice/tty)
www.listeningcenter.org

The Listening Center provides on-site rehabilitation services for children with cochlear implants through therapy sessions and computer-based training exercises. They also offer parent training and educational support in the child's school as well as professional training through seminars and videos.

Websites for Information and Research

You can do a very comprehensive search by going to one of the search engines such as google.com or yahoo.com and entering the term "cochlear implant" in the search subject box.

Cochlear Implant Manufacturers

www.bionicear.com
www.cochlear.com
www.medel.com

Other Sites Related to Hearing Loss and Cochlear Implants

www.agbell.org	Alexander Graham Bell Assoc.
www.audiology.org	American Academy of Audiology
www.asha.org	American Speech-Language and Hearing Assoc.
www.auditory-verbal.org	Auditory-Verbal International,Inc.
www.cici.org	Cochlear Implant Assoc. Inc.
www.drf.org	Deafness Research Foundation
www.esl-lab.com	Great listening practice site
www.hearthisorg.com	Facts about hearing loss and info
www.healthyhearing.com	Healthy hearing newsletter
www.jtc.org	John Tracy Clinic
www.listen-up.org	Lots of great information on hearing loss and CIs
www.lhh.org	League for the Hard of Hearing
www.ncd.gov	National Council on Disability
www.nidcd.nih.gov	NIDCD
www.oraldeaf.org	Oral Deaf Education
www.saywhatclub.org	Information about hearing loss issues

Advanced Bionics

Manufacturers of the Clarion cochlear implant. You can access their website for further information at www.bionicear.com or call 1-800-678-3575 for a free information packet for candidates.

Corporate Headquarters
Advanced Bionics Corp.
12740 San Fernando Road
Sylmar, California 91342
Telephone: 818-362-7588
Toll Free: 1-800-678-3575

European Headquarters
Advanced Bionics SARL
76 rue de Battenheim
68170 Rixheim
France
Telephone: +33 (0) 3-89-65-98-00

Pacific Rim Headquarters
Advanced Bionics
25129 Rye Canyon Loop
Valencia, California 91355
USA
Telephone: 1-661-362-1400
Toll Free: 1-800-678-3575

Latin America Office
Advanced Bionics Latin America
Carrera 16 No. 86A-53
Oficina 201
Santafe de Bogata, Columbia
South America
Telephone: (571) 610-8174

Cochlear Corporation

Manufacturers of the Nucleus cochlear implant device. You can access their website for more information at www.cochlear.com or call 1-800-523-5798 for a free information packet for candidates.

Cochlear Headquarters

14 Mars Road
PO Box 629
Lane Cove NSW 2066
Australia
Telephone: 61-2-9428-6555

America

Cochlear Corporation

400 Inverness Drive South
Suite 400
Englewood Colorado 80112
USA
Toll free: 1-800-523-5798
Telephone: 1-303-790-9010

Other Toll Free Numbers

Brazil   000-8111-004-5924
Canada   800-523-5798
Chile   1230-020-0717
Columbia   980-912-1730
Mexico   011-800-672-6126
Venezuela   800-11-120

Med-El Corporation

Manufacturers of the Med-El cochlear implant. You can access their website at www.medel.com for further information or call toll free 1-888-633-3524 for a free informational packet.

Med-El Headquarters

Furstenweg 77
A-6020 Innsbruck, Austria
Telephone: +43-512-28 88 89

America

Med-El Corporation
2222 East NC Hwy 54, Suite B-180
Durham, North Carolina 27713
Telephone: 1-919-572-2222
Toll Free: 1-888-633-3524

List of Cochlear Implant
Centers by State

ALABAMA
Alabama Institute for the Deaf and Blind
PO Box 698
Talladega, AL 35161
Phone: 256-761-3238
Birmingham Hearing and Balance Center.
2700 10th Ave S, Suite 502
Birmingham, AL 35205
Phone: 205-933-2951
Children's Hospital of Alabama
Speech/Hearing Center
1600 7th Ave
South Birmingham, AL 35233
Phone: 205-939-5815
Kirklin Clinic - University of Alabama
2000 6th Ave S
Birmingham, AL 35233
Phone: 205-801-7993
Pappas Cochlear Implant Center
2937 7th Ave South
Birmingham, AL 35233
Phone: 205-251-7169
Premier Medical ENT Group
2880 Dauphin St
Mobile, AL 36606
Phone: 251-473-1900
VA Medical Center - Birmingham
700 S 19th St
Birmingham, AL 35233
Phone: 205-558-4704
East Alabama ENT
1965 1st Ave.
Opelika, AL 36801
Phone: 334-705-0012
Steven Favrot, M.D.
840 Montclair Road, Suite 218
Birmingham, AL 35213
Phone: 205-591-6570

ARIZONA

Arizona Hearing and Balance
2550 East Guadalupe Road, Suite 106
Gilbert, AZ 85234
Phone: 480-558-5306
Arizona Otologic Association
222 W Thomas, Suite 114
Phoenix, AZ 85013-4480
Phone: 602-265-9660
Good Samaritan Health Services
1515 N 9th St, Suite B
Phoenix, AZ 85006
Phone: 602-257-4228
Good Samaritan Medical Center
Department of Audiology GSRMC
1111 E McDowell Rd.
Phoenix, AZ 85006
Phone: 602-239-4577
John Macias, M.D.
1515 N. 9th Street, Suite B
Phoenix, AZ 85006
Mayo Clinic - Scottsdale
13400 East Shea Blvd
Scottsdale, AZ 85259
Phone: 480-301-5256
Speech & Hearing Sciences
PO Box 210071
Tucson, AZ 85721-0017
Phone: 520-626-3710
University Physicians, Inc.
Department of Surgery ENT
1501 N Campbell Ave, 5th Floor Clinic
Tucson, AZ 85724
Phone: 520-694-7222

ARKANSAS
Arkansas Center of ENT and Allergy
1500 Dodson Ave
Ft Smith, AR 72901
Phone: 501-709-7405
Arkansas Childrens Hospital

800 Marshall, Mail Slot 113
Little Rock, AR 72202
Phone: 501-320-6679
Arkansas Otolargngology Center
10201 Kanis Rd
Little Rock, AR 72205
Phone: 501-227-5050

CALIFORNIA
California Ear Institute
801 Welch Road
Palo Alto, CA 94304
Phone: 650-462-3158
California Ear Institute at San Ramon
5801 Norris Canyon Rd Suite 200
San Ramon, CA 94583
Phone: 925-830-9116
CCHAT - Sacramento
9350 Keifer Blvd
Sacramento, CA 95826
Phone: 916-361-7290
Children's Hospital San Diego
Speech and Hearing Center
3020 Children's Way
M.C. 5010
San Diego, CA 92123
Phone: 858-576-5838
Children's Specialists
3030 Children's Way, Suite 402
San Diego, CA 92123
Phone: 858-966-4085
CCHAT Center - San Diego
2210 Encinitas Blvd.
Encinitas, CA 92024-4358
Phone: 760-634-7953
Children's Hospital - Oakland
Pediatric Audiology Department
747 52nd St
Oakland, CA 94609
Phone: 510-428-3344

Children's Hospital and Health Centers.
Speech, Hearing & Neurosensory Center
8010 Frost St, 2nd Floor
San Diego, CA 92123
Phone: 858-576-5838
Ear Specialty Center
9850 Genessee Avenue, Suite 650
La Jolla, CA 92037
Phone: 619-452-4327
Hearing and Balance Services
Ear and Balance Center
361 Hospital Rd, Suite #325
Newport Beach, CA 92663
Phone: 714-574-7744
House Ear Clinic
2100 W Third St, 1st Floor
Los Angeles, CA 90057
Phone: 213-483-9930
House Ear Institute
2100 W Third St.
Los Angeles, CA 90057
Phone: 213-483-4431
House Ear Institute CARE Center
2100 W Third St
Los Angeles, CA 90057
Phone: 213-353-7005
House-Shohet Hearing Associates
361 Hospital Rd, Suite 327
Newport Beach, CA 92663
Phone: 949-631-0409   .
Kaiser Permanente - Oakland
280 West MacArthur Blvd.
Oakland, CA 94611
Phone: 510-752-6398 and 510-752-6419
Kaiser Permanente - San Diego
4647 Zion Ave
c/o Audiology Dept
San Diego, CA 92120
Phone: 619-528-5006
Kaiser Permanente Medical Group

441

4900 Sunset Blvd, Suite 6B
Los Angeles, CA 90027
Phone: 323-783-4669
Jennifer Maw, M.D.
2030 Forrest Avenue, Suite 210
San Jose, CA 95128
Phone: 408-885-9500
Loma Linda University
Medical Surgical Group
11370 Anderson St, FMO 2100
Loma Linda, CA 92354
Phone: 909-558-2343
Oakland Children's Hospital
747 52nd Street
Oakland, CA 94609
Phone: 510-428-3344
Oralingua School for the Hearing Impaired
7056 S Washington Ave
Whittier, CA 90602
Phone: 562-945-8391
Pacific Neuroscience Center
2888 Long Beach Blvd, Suite 150
Long Beach, CA 90806
Phone: 562-997-1266
Pulec Ear Clinic
1245 Wilshire Blvd., Suite 503
Los Angeles, CA 90017
Phone: 213-482-4442
Sacramento ENT Surgical and Medical Group
3810 J Street
Sacramento, CA 95816
Phone: 916-736-1911
Scripps Memorial Hospital
Audiology Department
9834 Genesee Ave, Suite 224
La Jolla, CA 92037
Phone: 858-626-6394
UC Davis Medical Center-Sacramento
2521 Stockton Blvd, 7th Floor
Sacramento, CA 95817

Phone: 916-734-5398
UC Irvine Medical Center
101 The City Dr, Rte 13, Bldg 22C
Orange, CA 92868
Phone:714-456-6781
UCLA Medical Center
UCLA Medical Center Audiology Clinic
200 UCLA Medical Plaza, #540
Los Angeles, CA 90095
Phone: 310-825-5721
UCSD Medical Center
Audiology Center #8660
200 W Arbor Dr.
San Diego, CA 92103
Phone: 619-543-5683
UCSF Cochlear Implant Program
Department of Otolaryngology,
400 Parnassus Ave, Rm A-701
San Francisco, CA 94143-0340
Phone: 415-353-2464
USC University Hospital
1510 San Pablo Street, Suite 201
Los Angeles, CA 90033
Phone: 323-442-5795
VA Medical Center-Long Beach
Audiology Section (126)
5901 E 7th Street
Long Beach, CA 90822
Phone: 562-494-5698
Valley Children's Hospital
Speech/Language Pathology
6159 N Fresno St, Suite 103
Fresno, CA 93710
Phone: 559-353-6877
William F. House Hearing Association
361 Hospital Road, Suite 327
Newport Beach, CA 92663
Phone: 714-631-4327

COLORADO

Children's Hospital - Denver
1056 E 19th Ave, Box 030
Denver, CO 80218
Phone: 303-861-6814

Colorado Head and Neck
701 E Hampden Ave, #130
Englewood, CO 80110
Phone: 303-788-6632

Colorado Hearing & Balance Clinic
2125 E LaSalle St, Suite 201
Colorado Springs, CO 80909
Phone: 719-442-6984

Kaiser Permanente
2045 Franklin Street
Denver, CO 80205
Phone: 303-861-3404

Rocky Mountain Cochlear Implant Center
Medical Office Bldg III
799 E Hampden Ave, #510
Englewood, CO 80110
Phone: 303-788-7838

United States Air Force Academy
10th Medical Group/SG
4102 Pinon Dr, Suite 100
USAFA, CO 80840
Phone: 719-333-5102

University of Colorado Health Science Center
Department of Audiology
360 S Garfield St, Suite 400
Denver, CO 80209
Phone: 303-372-3190

CONNECTICUT

Connecticut Children's Medical Center
Speech Department
282 Washington St.
Hartford, CT 06106
Phone 860-545-9670

CREC Soundbridge

444

Marion Radeen
123 Progress Drive
Wethersfield, CT 06109
Phone: 860-529-4260
ENT Medical and Surgical Group
46 Prince St.
New Haven, CT 06109
Phone: 203-752-1726
New England Center for Hearing Rehabilitation
354 Hartford Turnpike
Hampton, CT 06247
Phone: 860-455-1404

DISTRICT OF COLUMBIA
Washington Hospital Center
Hearing and Speech Center
110 Irving St NW
Washington, DC 20010
Phone: 202-877-6779

DELAWARE
Christiana Care Health Service
4755 Ogletown-Stanton Rd
Newark, DE 19718
Phone: 302-733-6773

FLORIDA
All Children's Hospital
Physician's Office Bldg, Suite 170
880 6th St South
St Petersburg, FL 33701
Phone: 727-892-8989
Celebration Children's Health
Department of Audiology
400 Celebration Place
Suite A-360
Celebration, FL 34747
Phone: 407-303-4003, ext. 6518
ENT Associates of South Florida
900 N.W. 13th St., Suite 206

445

Boca Raton, FL 33486
Phone: 561-393-9150
Farrior Ear Clinic
509 W Bay St
Tampa, FL 33606
Phone: 813-253-0916
Florida ENT Associates
4340 Newberry Road, Suite 301
Gainesville, FL 32607
Phone: 352-972-9414
Florida Ear and Balance Center
400 Celebration Place, Suite A-360
Celebration, FL 32607
Phone: 407-303-4220
Florida Ear & Sinus Center
1961 Floyd St., Ste D
Sarasota, FL 34239
Phone: 941-951-0440
Fort Meyers ENT Associates
3487 Broadway
Fort Meyers, FL 33901
Phone: 941-936-0721
Jacksonville Hearing and Balance Institute
836 Prudential Dr., #1405
Jacksonville, FL 32207
Phone: 904-399-0350
Office of John Li, M.D.
210 Jupiter Lakes Blvd.
Bldg. 5000, Suite 105
Jupiter, FL 33458
Phone: 561-748-4445 and 561-748-0367
Mayo Clinic - Jacksonville
Audiology Department
4500 San Pablo Rd
Jacksonville, FL 32224
Phone: 904-953-2265
Miami Speech & Hearing
3661 S Miami Ave, Suite 410
Miami, FL 33133
Phone: 305-854-8171

Nemour's Childrens Clinic
ENT Department
807 Children's Way
Jacksonville, FL 32207
Phone: 904-390-3707

Office of June Kennedy, Ph.D.
115 W Columbia St, Suite C
Orlando, FL 32806-1055
Phone: 407-422-2200

Physician's Hearing Center
900 NW 13th St., #204
Boca Raton, FL 33486
Phone: 561-393-9150

Ress Institute
7284 Palmetto Park Road West, Suite 105
Boca Raton, FL 33433
Phone: 561-347-1611

St. Mary's Hospital of West Palm Beach
5325 Greenwood Ave, Suite 201
West Palm Beach, FL 33407
Phone: 561-659-2266

Tampa Bay Hearing and Balance Center
Harbour Side Medical Tower
4 Columbia Dr, Suite 610
Tampa, FL 33606
Phone: 813-844-4900

University of Florida
Department of Communicative Disorders
Box 100174 UFHSC
Gainesville, FL 32610-0174
Phone: 352-392-8888

University of Miami
Audiology - Box 016960 (R56)
1666 NW 10th Ave., Suite #306
Miami, FL 33136
Phone: 305-585-6747

University of Southern Florida Hearing and Balance Center
Department of Communication Sciences and Disorders
4202 E Fowler Ave, PCD 1017
Tampa, FL 33620-8150

447

Phone: 813-974-9832
VA Medical Center - Miami
Audiology Services (126)
1201 NW 16th St
Miami, FL 33125
Phone: 305-324-3148

GEORGIA
Atlanta Center of ENT
3193 Howell Mill Rd, Suite 215
Atlanta, GA 30327
Phone: 404-355-1312
Atlanta Ear Clinic
980 Johnson Ferry Road N.E., Suite 470
Atlanta, GA 30342
Phone: 404-851-9093
Atlanta Speech School
3160 Northside Pkwy NW
Atlanta, GA 30327
Phone: 404-233-5332
Auditory Education Center
1447 Peachtree St, Suite 210
Atlanta, GA 30309-3034
Phone: 404-815-4321
Children's Health Care of Atlanta
1405 Clifton Road NE
Atlanta, GA 30322
Phone: 404-315-2454
Ear Consultants of Georgia
993-C Johnson Ferry Road, N.E., Suite 240-C
Atlanta GA 30342
Phone: 404-943-0170
Emory Clinic
Department of Otolaryngology
1365 Clifton Rd NE
Atlanta, GA 30322
Phone: 404-778-4331
Georgia Ear Institute
4700 Waters Avenue
Savannah, GA 31404

448

Phone: 912-350-5000
Medical College of Georgia
Audiology
BP 4114
Augusta, GA 30912-6700
Phone: 706-721-6009
Office of Terrence Murphy, M.D.
5505 Peachtree Dunwoody Rd., Suite G51
Atlanta, GA 30342
Phone: 404-250-1216
Scottish Rite Children's Hospital
1001 Johnson Ferry Rd.
Atlanta, GA 30363
Phone: 404-256-5252, ext.3535
The ENT Center of Central Georgia
Georgia Hearing Institute
PO Box 4508
Macon, GA 31208
Phone: 478-741-1800
VA Medical Center - Decatur, GA
Audiologist Services
1670 Clairmont Rd
Decatur, GA 30033
Phone: 404-321-6111, ext.7625

HAWAII
Audiology Associates of Hawaii
Queen's Physician's Office Building
1380 Lusitana St, Suite 209
Honolulu, HI 96813
Phone: 808-524-1432
Kaiser Permanente-HI
Audiology Dept.
3288 Monanalua Blvd.
Honolulu, HI 96819
Phone: 808-533-3368
Queens Medical Center
1329 Lusitana Street
Box 407, Building 2
Honolulu, HI 96813

Phone: 808-533-3368
University of Hawaii at Manoa
1410 Lower Campus Rd
Honolulu, HI 96822
Phone: 808-956-5836

IOWA
Iowa Ear Clinic
1000 73rd St, Suite 21
Des Moines, IA 50311
Phone: 515-223-7177
University of Iowa
Department of Otolaryngology
200 Hawkins Dr, Rm 21201 PFP
Iowa City, IA 52242-1078
Phone: 319-356-7361
VA Medical Center - Iowa City
Audiology Services (126)
Highway 6 W
Iowa City, IA 52246
Phone: 319-339-7126

IDAHO
Idaho Elks Rehabilitation
Director of Audiology Services
124 W State St
Boise, ID 83702
Phone: 208-344-4843

ILLINOIS
Carle Clinic and Foundation
ECHO Program - NCW4 (Children)
602 West University Avenue
Urbana, IL 61801
Phone: 217-383-3130 and 217-383-4389
Chicago Otology Group
Division of Evanston Northwestern Healthcare
950 York Rd, Suite 102
Hinsdale, IL 60521
Phone: 630-789-3110

Children's Memorial - Chicago
Communication Disorders
2300 Children's Plaza, Box 38
Chicago, IL 60614
Phone: 773-880-4605

Evanston Northwestern Healthcare
Division of ENT
1000 Central Street, Suite 610
Evanston, IL 60201
Phone: 847-570-1360

Loyola University Medical Center
Department of Audiology
2160 S First Ave, Dock 4, Bldg 106
Chicago, IL 60153
Phone: 708-216-3821

Mercy Hospital and Medical Center - Chicago
Department of Audiology
2525 S Michigan Ave
Chicago, IL 60616
Phone: 312-567-5650

Northwestern University Medical Center
Dept. of Otolaryngology Head & Neck
675 North Clair Street, 15th floor, Suite 200
Chicago, IL 60611
Phone: 312-695-8182

Office of Dennis Moore, M.D.
1875 Dempster St, Suite 625
Park Ridge, IL 60068
Phone: 847-518-1200

Otology Group West
950 York Road, Suite 102
Hinsdale, IL 60521
Phone: 630-789-3110

Rush Presbyterian-St Lukes Medical Center
Department of Communicative Disorders
1653 W Congress Pkwy,
Chicago, IL 60612
Phone: 312-942-7068

University of Chicago
Center for Advanced Medicine

5758 S Maryland Ave., MC9020
Chicago, IL 60637
Phone: 773-834-2548
University of Illinois Eye and Ear
1855 W Taylor, Suite B46
Chicago, IL 60612
Phone: 312-996-6525

INDIANA
ENT Associates
10021 Dupont Circle Court
Fort Wayne, IN 46825
Phone: 219-426-8117
Indiana School of Medicine at Riley Hospital
702 Barnhill Dr, Suite 0860
Indianapolis, IN 46202
Phone: 317-274-6684
Jerry House & Associates
9002 North Meridan Street, Suite 204
Indianapolis, IN 46260
Phone: 317-848-9505
South Bend Clinic and Surgical Center
211 N Eddy
South Bend, IN 46617
Phone: 574-237-9200
Southlake Speech & Hearing
99 E 86th Ave, Suite A
Merrillville, IN 46410
Phone: 219-738-2528
St. Vincent Hospital
Department of Audiology
2001 West 86th Street
Indianapolis, IN 46260
Phone: 317-338-2270

KANSAS
University of Kansas Hearing and Speech Department
Child Development Unit
3901 Rainbow Blvd
Kansas City, KS 66160-7605

Phone: 913-588-5730
University of Kansas Medical Center-Clinic
Oto Head and Neck Surgery
3901 Rainbow Blvd
Kansas City, KS 66160-7380
Phone: 913-588-6707
Wichita Ear Clinic
427 N Hillside
Wichita, KS 67214
Phone: 316-686-6608

KENTUCKY
Heuser Hearing Institute
111 East Kentucky St
Louisville, KY 40203
Phone: 502-589-6314
University of Kentucky
Chandler Medical Center
Dept. of Communication Disorders
740 South Limestone
B317 Kentucky Clinic
Lexington, KY 40536-0284
Phone: 859-323-5572
University of Louisville
Myers Hall, Otolarygology
Louisville, KY 40292
Phone: 502-852-0339

LOUISIANA
Ear, Nose and Throat Specialists
17050 Medical Center Dr, Suite 315
Baton Rouge, LA 70816
Phone: 225-293-6973
LSU Medical Center
Kresge Hearing Research
Department of Otolaryngology
533 Bolivar, 5th Floor
New Orleans, LA 70112
Phone: 504-568-4785

Memorial Medical Center
Joachim Hearing & Speech Center
2820 Napolean Ave, Suite 250
New Orleans, LA 70115
Phone: 504-896-1170
Ochsner Clinic
Audiology Department, 4th Floor
1514 Jefferson Highway
New Orleans, LA 70121
Phone: 504-842-4080
Pierremont Ear, Nose and Throat
8001 Youree Dr, Suite 820
Shreveport, LA 71115
Phone: 318-798-8989

MASSACHUSETTS
Associates in Otolarynology/ Head & Neck Surgery
48 Elm Street
Worchester, MA 01609
Phone: 508-792-2924
Children's Hospital - Boston
300 Longwood Ave, Fegan 9
Boston, MA 02115
Phone: 617-355-6417
Clarke School for the Deaf
47 Round Hill Rd
Northampton, MA 01060-2199
Phone: 413-584-3450, ext. 1188
Mass. Eye & Ear Infirmary
Dept. of Otolaryngology
243 Charles Street
Boston, MA 02114
Phone: 617-573-3266
New England Medical Center
750 Washington St, Box 850
Boston, MA 02111
Phone: 617-636-9049
The Learning Center for Deaf Children
848 Central St
Framingham, MA 01701

Phone: 508-879-5110
Umass Memorial Health Care
Audiology Department
55 Lake Avenue North
Worcester, MA 01605
Phone: 508-856-4161
University of Massachusetts-Amherst
125 Arnold House
Amherst, MA 01003
Phone: 508-334-8700

MARYLAND
John Hopkins University Medical Center
Department of Oto/Head & Neck Surgery
601 N Caroline St, Suite 6009
Baltimore, MD 21287-6214
Phone: 410-955-9397
University of Maryland
16 S Eutaw St, #400
Baltimore, MD 21201-1619
Phone: 410-328-0586

MAINE
Maine ENT
210 Western Avenue
South Portland, ME 04106
Phone: 207-780-6000
Warren Center for Communication and Learning
175 Union St
Bangor, ME 04401
Phone: 207-941-2850

MICHIGAN
Audiology Professionals
224 E Fulton
Grand Rapids, Ml 49503
Phone: 616-459-7122
Central Michigan University Hearing Clinic
Department of Communication Disorders
420 Moore Hall

Mt Pleasant, MI 48859
Phone: 989-774-3726
Harper Grace Hospital
4201 St Antoine 5G UHC
Detroit, MI 48201
Phone: 313-745-4651
Henry Ford Hospital
2799 W Grand Blvd
Audiology K-8
Detroit, MI 48202
Phone: 313-916-3159
Marie Caris Ear Institute
Children's Hospital
3901 Beaubien
Detroit, MI 48201
Phone: 313-745-8903
Michigan Ear Institute
30055 Northwestern Hwy, Suite 101
Farmington Hills, Ml 48334
Phone: 248-865-2222
Shawnee Park Oral Deaf Program
2036 Chesaning SE
Grand Rapids, MI 49506
Phone: 616-771-3070
Spectrum Health - Butterworth Campus
Neurodiagnostics, Butterworth Campus
l00 Michigan St NE (A Floor)
Grand Rapids, Ml 49503
Phone: 616-391-2668
University of Michigan Medical Center
Cochlear Implant Center
1904 Taubman Center
1500 East Medical Drive
Ann Arbor, MI 48109
Phone: 734-936-8006
VA Medical Center - Ann Arbor
2215 Fuller Rd
Ann Arbor, MI 48105
Phone:734-769-7100, ext. 5902

MINNESOTA
Mayo Clinic - Rochester
Cochlear Implant Facility
RMH 2-140 El
200 First St SW
Rochester, MN 55905
Phone: 507-266-1965
Minnesota Ear Head and Neck
701 25th Ave S, Suite 200
Minneapolis, MN 55454
Phone: 612-339-2836
University of Minnesota Hospital
Fairview University Medical Center
516 Delaware St SE
MMC 396, PWB 8-240
Minneapolis, MN 55455
Phone: 612-625-1689

MISSOURI
CID Hearing Central for the Deaf
4560 Clayton Ave
St Louis, MO 63110
Phone: 314-977-0100
Jacques Herzog, M.D.
11155 Dunn Road Suite 209E
St. Louis, MO 63136
Phone: 314-741-3388
McIntire Ear Nose and Throat
1331 W 32nd St
Joplin, MO 64804
Phone: 417-623-6767
Midwest Ear Institute
4200 Pennsylvania, Suite 100
Kansas City, MO 64111
Phone: 816-932-1660
Moog Center for Deaf Education
12300 S Forty Drive
St Louis, MO 63141
Phone: 314-692-7172

Office of James Benecke, M.D.
3023 N Ballas Rd, #675
St Louis, MO 63131-2330
Phone: 314-995-9021

St. John's Regional Ear, Nose and Throat Center
1965 S Fremont, Suite 1950
Springfield, MO 65804
Phone: 417-887-9828

St. Johns Mercy Medical Center
Audiology Services
615 S New Ballas Rd
St Louis, MO 63141
Phone: 314-569-6175

St. Joseph Institute for Deaf
Otolaryngology Department
1809 Clarkson Rd.
Chesterfield, MO 63017
Phone: 636-532-3211

St. Louis Children's Hospital
One Children's Place, Suite 3S23
St Louis, MO 63110
Phone: 314-454-2201

St. Louis University
Otolaryngology Head & Neck Surgery
University Medical Group Bldg.
3635 Vista Avenue
St. Louis, MO 63110
Phone: 314-577-6110

University of Missouri Healthcare
1101 Hospital Dr
DC120.00 - Audiology
Columbia, MO 65212
Phone: 573-882-7129

Washington University School of Medicine
Cochlear Implant Program
4566 Scott Ave, Box 8115
St Louis, MO 63110
Phone: 314-362-7245

MISSISSIPPI
Jackson Ear Clinic
971 Lakeland Dr, Suite 854
St Dominic W Tower
Jackson, MS 39216-4608
Phone: 601-981-2825

MONTANA
Rocky Mountain Eye and Ear
700 W Kent St, Parkside Prof Village
Missoula, MT 59801
Phone: 406-549-3997

NORTH CAROLINA
Carolina Ear and Hearing Clinic
3100 Duraleigh Rd, Suite 300
Raleigh, NC 27612
Phone: 919-876-4327
Charlotte Eye, Ear, Nose and Throat Associates, P.A.
6035 Fairview Rd
Charlotte, NC 28210
Phone: 800-654-3368
Cochlear Implant Program of Eastern Carolina
Doctor's Park, Bldg. 8
Medical Drive
Greenville, NC 27834
Phone: 252-328-4459
Duke University Medical Center
Dept. of OHNS-DUMC 3805
Room 1559, Stead Building
Blue Zone, Duke South Hospital
Durham, NC 27710
Phone: 919-668-2350
Southeastern ENT & Sinus Center
1124 North Church Street, Suite 100
Grennsboro, NC 27401
Phone: 336-273-9932
UNC - Pediatric Cochlear Implant Program
5501 Fortunes Ridge Dr, Suite R
Durham, NC 27713

Phone: 919-419-1449
UNC Hospitals
Neurosciences Hospital, Rm G0303 Adult CI Program
Chapel Hill, NC 27514
Phone: 919-843-0425
VA Medical Center - Durham
508 Fulton St
Durham, NC 27705
Phone: 919-416-5935
Wake Forest University Medical Center
Medical Center Bldg, Hearing/Speech Department
Clinical Sciences Bldg, 4th Floor
Winston-Salem, NC 27157
Phone: 336-716-4330

NEBRASKA
Boys Town National Research Hospital
555 N 30th St
Omaha, NE 68131
Phone: 402-498-6322
Ear Specialists of Omaha
8005 Farnam Drive, Suite 206
Omaha, NE 68114
Phone: 402-933-3277
University of Nebraska Medical Center
989250 Nebraska Medical Center
Omaha, NE 68198-9250
Phone: 402-559-5208

NEW HAMPSHIRE
Dartmouth-Hitchcock Medical Center
One Medical Center Dr
Lebanon, NH 03756
Phone: 603-650-8125

NEW JERSEY
Ear Specialty Group
55 Morris Ave, Suite 304
Springfield, NJ 07081
Phone: 973-379-3330

Hackensack University Medical Center
30 Prospect Avenue
Hackensack, NJ 07601
Phone: 201-996-5151
Mountain Lakes Board of Education
Lake Drive School for the Deaf & Hard of Hearing
10 Lake Dr
Mountain Lakes, NJ 07046
Phone: 973-299-9103
Overlook Hospital
99 Beauvoir Avenue
Audiology Department PO Box 330
Summit, NJ 07901
Phone: 908-522-2283
Saint Barnabas Ambulatory Care Center
200 S Orange Ave
Livingston, NJ 07039
Phone: 973-322-7102
University of Medicine and Dentistry New Jersey Hospital
Ear, Nose and Throat Clinic, Level C
150 Bergen St
Newark, NJ 07103
Phone: 973-972-4967

NEW MEXICO
Presbyterian Ear Institute
1114 Copper NE
Albuquerque, NM 87106
Phone: 505-242-5212
University of New Mexico Hospital
Audiologist Cochlear Implant Program
7801 Academy NE
Albuquerque, NM 87109
Phone: 505-272-2725

NEVADA
ENT Consultants of Nevada
3131 La Canada Street, Suite 241
Las Vegas, NV 89109
Phone: 702-792-6700

Office of Pamela Hanson, MST
9420 Calico Garden Ave
Las Vegas, NV 89134
Phone: 702-255-1378
University of Nevada
Patient Care Center
1707 Charleston Blvd., Suite 160
Las Vegas, NV 89102
Phone: 702-671-5150

NEW YORK
Albany Medical Center Hospital
Department of Otolaryngology
43 New Scotland Ave, MC154
Albany, NY 12208
Phone: 518-262-4535
Beth Israel Medical Center
10 Union Square E, Suite 2K
New York, NY 10003
Phone: 212-844-8790
Buffalo Hearing and Speech Center
50 E North St
Buffalo, NY 14203
Phone: 716-885-8318
Buffalo Otolaryngology Group
897 Delaware Ave
Buffalo, NY 14209
Phone: 716-883-6800
Capital Regional Otolaryngology
6 Executive Park
Albany, NY 12203
Phone: 518-482-9111
Central New York Ear, Nose and Throat Consultants
1100 E Genesee St
Syracuse, NY 13210
Phone: 315-476-3124
Children's Hospital of Buffalo
Dept. of Pediatric Otolaryngology
219 Byrant Street
Buffalo, NY 14222

Phone: 716-878-7569

Columbia Presbyterian Medical
Department of Oto/Head & Neck Surgery
180 Ft Washington Ave
New York, NY 10032
Phone: 212-305-4972

League for the Hard of Hearing
71 W 23rd St.
New York, NY 10010-4162
Phone: 917-305-7700

Long Island College Hospital
339 Hicks St
Brooklyn, NY 11201
Phone: 718-780-1985

Manhattan Eye, Ear and Throat Hospital
Cochlear Implant Center, 3rd Floor
210 E 64th St
New York, NY 10021
Phone: 212-605-3793

Mercy College
Department of Communication Disorders
555 Broadway
Dobbs Ferry, NY 10522
Phone: 914-674-7746

New York Eye & Ear lnfirmary
Audiology Department
310 E 14th St
New York, NY 10003
Phone: 212-979-4340

Northeast Neurotologic Clinic
#6 Executive Park Dr, Entrance C
Albany, NY 12203
Phone: 518-482-9111

NYU Cochlear Implant Center
660 lst Ave, 7th Floor
New York, NY 10016
Phone: 212-263-7567

State University of New York at Stonybrook
Dept. of Otolaryngology
Health Sciences Center

Room T 19-020
Stonybrook, NY 11794
Phone: 631-444-4191
St. Mary's School for the Deaf
2253 Main St
Buffalo, NY 14214
Phone: 716-834-7200
Stony Brook University Hospital
Speech and Hearing
33 Research Way, Suite 4
East Setauket, NY 11727-3489
Phone: 631-444-4191
SUNY Upstate Medical University
750 E Adams St
Syracuse, NY 13210
Phone: 315-464-6591
University Hospital
175 Elizabeth Blackwell St.
Communications Disorders Unit
7th Floor-Jacobson Hall
Syracuse, NY 13210
Phone: 315-464-4806
University of Rochester Medical Center
Audiology/Speech Pathology
601 Elmwood Ave, Box 627
Rochester, NY 14642
Phone: 716-275-4852
Westchester Medical Center
Speech & Hearing Center/WIHD
Cedarwood Hall, Room 431
Valhalla, NY 10595
Phone: 914-493-8191

OHIO
Children's Hospital - Cincinnati
Center for Hearing & Deafness Research
3333 Burnet Ave
Cincinnati, OH 45229
Phone: 513-636-4236
Children's Medical Center - Audiology

464

Rehabilitation Services
One Children's Plaza
Dayton, OH 45404
Phone: 937-641-3496
Cleveland Clinic
Desk A71
9500 Euclid Ave
Cleveland, OH 44195
Phone: 216-445-5024
Columbus Children's Hospital
Audiology and Speech Pathology
555 South 18th St, AB6070
Columbus, OH 43205
Phone: 614-722-3975
Dayton Head and Neck Surgeons
369 West 1 St, Suite 400
Dayton, OH 45402-3065
Phone: 937-222-0022
Ear, Nose and Throat Associates of Dayton, Inc.
4244 Indian Ripple Rd, Suite 200
Dayton, OH 45440-3272
Phone: 937-223-1234, ext.24
Lippy Group for Ear, Nose and Throat
North Mar Center II
3893 East Market Street
Warren, OH 44484
Phone: 330-856-4000, ext. 27
Office of George Bauer, M.D.
Mercy Medical Arts Bldg
2960 Mack Rd
Fairfield, OH 45014
Phone: 513-860-4771
Ohio ENT Surgeons
500 Thomas Lane, Suite 4A
Columbus, OH 43214
Phone: 614-538-2424
The Ohio State University Medical Center; Excellent, Inc.
University Otolaryngologists, Inc.
456 W 10th Ave, Room 4018
Columbus, OH 43210

Phone: 614-293-8065
University Hospitals of Cleveland
RB&C Room B4
11100 Euclid Avenue
Cleveland, OH 44106
Phone: 216-844-8168
University of Akron
School of Speech-Language Pathology and Audiology
The Poisky Building 181
Akron, OH 44325-3001
Phone: 330-972-8187
University of Cincinnati Medical Center
ENT - Audiology, Barreff Center
234 Goodman St., ML 501
Cincinnati, OH 45219-0501
Phone: 513-475-8453

OKLAHOMA
Eastern Oklahoma Ear, Nose and Throat
5020 E 68th St
Tulsa, OK 74136
Phone: 918-492-3636
Hough Ear Institute
Cochlear Implant Program
3434 NW 56th St
Oklahoma City, OK 73112
Phone: 405-947-6030
Oklahoma Ear Institute
825 NE 10th St, Suite 4200
Oklahoma City, OK 73104
Phone: 405-271-8046

OREGON
Eugene Hearing and Speech
1500 W 12th Ave
Eugene, OR 97402
Phone: 541-485-8521
Office of F. Owen Black, M.D.
PO Box 3950
Portland, OR 97208

Phone: 503-233-6068
Oregon Health Science University
3181 SW Sam Jackson Park Rd
PV-01, Suite 250
Portland, OR 97201
Phone: 503-494-5171
Portland Ear Testing Center
921 NW 18th Ave
Portland, OR 97209
Phone: 503-227-3666
Tucker Maxon Oral School
2860 S.E. Holgate Blvd.
Portland, OR 97202
Phone: 503-235-6551

PENNSYLVANIA
Children's Hospital of Pittsburgh
Pediatric Cochlear Implant Program
3705 5th Ave
Pittsburgh, PA 15213-2583
Phone: 412-692-6680
DePaul Institute
2904 Castlegate Ave
Pittsburgh, PA 15226
Phone: 412-561-4848
Gelsinger Medical Center
Audiology Department
100 N Academy Avenue
Danville, PA 17822-1333
Phone: 800-441-6211, ext.4045
Hershey Medical Center
PO Box 850 UPC Bldg, Suite 700
500 University Dr
Hershey, PA 17033
Hospital of University of Pennsylvania Health System
Division of Audiology, 5th Floor Silverstein
3400 Spruce St
Philadelphia, PA 19104
Phone: 215-662-2784
Office of Robert T. Sataloff, M.D.

467

1721 Pine St
Philadelphia, PA 19103
Reading Hospital and Medical Center
Speech and Hearing Center
PO Box 16052
Reading, PA 19612-6052
Phone: 610-988-8694
Temple University
Kresge West Bldg, Room 302
3440 N Broad St
Philadelphia, PA 19140
Phone: 215-707-8077
The Children's Hospital of Philadelphia
Ear, Nose and Throat, 1st Floor
34th St & Civic Center Blvd, Wood Bldg.
Philadelphia, PA 19104-4399
Phone: 215- 590-7461
University of Pittsburgh Medical Center / Eye & Ear Inst.
203 Lothrop St
4th Floor, Eye & Ear Institute Bldg
Pittsburgh, PA 15213
Phone: 412-647-2030
VA Medical Center - Pittsburgh
Division of Audiology/Speech Pathology
University Dr C
Pittsburgh, PA 15240
Phone: 412-688-6157
Western Pennsylvania School for the Deaf
300 E Swissvail Ave
Pittsburgh, PA 15218
Phone: 412-244-4272

RHODE ISLAND
Atlantic Hearing and Rehabilitation, Inc.
971 Reservoir Ave
Cranston, RI 02910
Phone: 401-942-8080

SOUTH CAROLINA
Carolina Hearing Services, Inc.

1543 Ashley River Rd
Charleston, SC 29407
Phone: 843-556-4327 and 803-556-3608
Charleston ENT Assoc, LLC
1849 Savage Rd
Charleston, SC 29407
Phone: 843-766-7103
Medical University of South Carolina
Otolaryngology/Head & Neck Surgery
135 Rutlrdge Ave., Rm 216
Charleston, SC 29425
Phone: 843-876-1308
Midland ENT
3 Medical Park Road, Suite 120
Columbia, SC 29203
Phone: 803-254-2495
Piedmont Ear, Nose and Throat, P.A.
701 Arlington Avenue
Greenville, SC 29601
Phone: 864-233-6881
University of South Carolina
CI Program
3 Richland Medical Park, Suite 130
Columbia, SC 29203
Phone: 803-765-1919

SOUTH DAKOTA
Ear Nose & Throat, P.C.
2908 South Phillips Avenue
Sioux Falls, SD. 57105
Phone: 605-336-3503

TENNESSEE
Baptist Ear Center
101 Blount Avenue, Suite 500
Knoxville, TN 37920
Phone: 865-212-5279
Baptist Memphis State University
807 Jefferson
Memphis, TN 38105

Phone: 901-678-5800
Baptist Memorial Hospital
6025 Walnut Grove Rd., Suite C-1011
Memphis, TN 38120
Phone: 901-227-4554
Ear Hearing & Balance Disorders
2120 Exeter Road, Suite 230
Germantown, TN 38138
Phone: 901-257-3277
Memphis Oral School for the Deaf
711 Jefferson Ave
Memphis, TN 38105
Phone: 901-448-8492
Methodist Hearing and Balance Center
1265 Union Ave
Memphis, TN 36104
Phone: 901-726-7377
Nashville Ear, Nose and Throat
2400 Patterson St, Suite 418
Nashville, TN 37203
Phone: 615-327-2314, ext.230
Shea Clinic
6133 Poplar Pike at Ridgeway
Memphis, TN 38119
Phone: 901-761-9720
Shea-Hubbard ENT Clinic, Inc.
6027 Walnut Grove Road, Suite 411
Memphis, TN 38120
Phone: 901-767-7750
Vanderbilt Bill Wilkerson Center
1114 19th Ave S
Nashville, TN 37212
Phone: 615-936-5073

TEXAS
Austin Associates of Ear Specialists
6818 Austin Center Blvd, Suite 105
Austin, TX 78731
Phone: 512-338-9840
Austin Ear Clinic

470

Medical Oaks Pavilion
12201 Renfert Way, Suite 100
Austin, TX 78758
Phone: 512-454-0341
Callier Center for Communication Disorders
1966 Inwood Rd
Dallas, TX 75235-7298
Phone: 214-905-3042
Dallas Otolaryngology Association
7777 Forest Ln, Suite A-103
Dallas, TX 75230
Phone: 972-566-7359
Ear Medical Group
4410 Medical Dr, Suite 550
San Antonio, TX 78229
Phone: 210-614-6070
Houston Ear Research Foundation
2 Memorial SW Professional Bldg, Suite 630
7737 Southwest Freeway
Houston, TX 77074
Phone: 713-771-9966
Methodist Hospital
Audiology Services
6565 Fannin St, NA200
Houston, TX 77030
Phone: 713-441-5913
Office of Claude McLelland, M.D. F.A.C.S.
3301 S Alameda, Suite 506
Corpus Christi, TX 78411
Phone: 361-855-3000
Office of Daniel Franklin, M.D.
9034 Westheimer, Suite 103
Houston, TX 77063
Phone: 713-781-9660
Office of Mark Winter, M.D.
3805 22nd St
Lubbock, TX 7941 0
Phone: 806-793-0845
Office of Philip Anthony, M.D.
901 Hemphill

Fort Worth, TX 76104
Phone: 817-332-4060
Otology Group of Texas
9150 Huebner Rd, Suite 160
San Antonio, TX 78240
Phone: 210-697-0880
Owens Ear Center
3600 Gaston Ave., Suite #1103
Dallas, TX 75246
Phone: 214-742-2194
Scott and White, Hearing and Balance Center
Ear, Nose and Throat Department
2401 South 31st St
Temple, TX 76508
Phone: 254-724-2754
Sunshine Cottage School for Deaf Children
103 Tuieta Drive
San Antonio, TX 78212-3196
Phone: 210-824-0579
Texas Children's Hospital
Feigin Center,
6621 Fannin Street, Suite 340
Houston, TX 77030
Phone: 832-822-3243
Texas ENT Specialists
450 Medical Center Blvd., Suite 540
Webster, TX 77598
Phone: 281-338-1423
University of Texas at Austin
Communication Sciences
2504A Whitis
Austin, TX 78712-1089
Phone: 512-471-7720
University of Texas Health Science
Herman Professional Bldg
6410 Fannin, Suite 500
Houston, TX 77032
Phone: 713-704-4754
University of Texas Medical Branch at Galveston (UTMB)
301 University Blvd.

472

Galveston, TX 77555
Phone: 409-772-4688
UT Southwestern Medical School
5323 Harry Hines Blvd
Dallas, TX 75390-9035
Phone: 214-648-5475
VA Medical Center - Houston
Audiology/Speech Path (126)
2002 Holcombe Blvd
Houston, TX 77030
Phone: 713-794-7112
Wilford Hall USAF Medical Center
Audiology Clinic
2200 Berquist Dr, Suite 1
Lackland AFB, TX 78236-5300
Phone: 210-292-5421
Wilson Jones Memorial
1800 N Travis, #D
Sherman, TX 75090
Phone: 903-868-2650

UTAH
University of Utah
Primary Children's Medical Center
Audiology
100 N Medical Dr
Salt Lake City, UT 84113
Phone: 801-588-3950
University ENT - Room 3C-120
c/o 1795 E South Campus Dr -Mail Room
Salt Lake City, UT 84112-9204
Phone: 801-581-8743

VIRGINIA
Atlantic Coast Ear Specialist
933 First Colonial Road, Suite 102
Virginia Beach, VA 23454
Phone: 757-422-9300
Children's Hospital Kings Daughter
Audiology Department

601 Children's Ln
Norfolk, VA 23507
Phone: 757-668-7890
Children's National Medical Center
Speech and Hearing Department
8501 Arlington Blvd, 2nd Floor
Fairfax, VA 22031
Phone: 202-884-5600
Depaul Medical Center
Hearing and Balance
150 Kingsley Ln
Norfolk, VA 23505
Phone: 757-889-6670
Medical College of Virginia
Nelson Clinic Bldg, Room 304
Division of Audiology
403 N 11th St
PO Box 980150
Richmond, VA 23298-0150
Phone: 804-828-0431
Naval Medical Center Portsmouth
Audiology Clinic
27 Effingham, Bldg 2
Portsmouth, VA 23708-2197
Phone: 757-953-2792
University of Virginia Medical Center
Audiology Section - Dept of Communication Disorders
Primary Care Center - Ground Floor
Jefferson Park Avenue
Charlottesville, VA 22908
Phone: 804-982-0129

VERMONT
Fletcher Allen Health Care
Berlin ENT, Central VT Phys.Bidg.
RR4. Fisher Road, Box 1510
Berlin, VT 05602
Phone: 802-225-7070

WASHINGTON

474

Children's Hospital - Seattle
Research and Clinical Audiology
4800 Sand Point Way NE
Seattle, WA 98105
Phone: 206-528-2712
Mary Bridge Speech and Hearing
The Pediatric Hearing Center
1220 Division Ave
Tacoma, WA 98403
Phone: 253-403-1450
Puget 'Sound Hearing & Balance
9714 Third Avenue N.E., Suite 100
Seattle, WA 98115
Phone: 206-523-5584
Seattle Ear Clinic
600 Broadway, Suite 340
Seattle, WA 98122-5371
Phone: 206-328-4327
Spokane Ear, Nose and Throat Clinic
217 W Cataldo Ave
Spokane, WA 99201-2217
Phone: 509-624-2326
Tacoma Ear and Balance Clinic
915 6th Ave, Suite 1
Tacoma, WA 98405
Phone: 253-627-6731
University of Washington
Otolaryngology Clinic NE 306
1959 NE Pacific St, Box 356161
Seattle, WA 98195
Phone: 206-598-5633
VA Medical Center - Seattle
Audiology (126) Room 2D- 189
1660 South Columbian Way
Seattle, WA 98108
Phone: 206-764-2109
Virginia Mason Medical Center
The Listen for Life Center
1100 9th Ave, MS2-LLC
Seattle, WA 98111Phone: 206-341-0984

Washington Otology Neurotology Group
901 Boren Ave, Suite 711
Seattle, WA 98104
Phone: 206-622-6987

WISCONSIN
Marshfield Clinic
ENT/Audiology Department
1000 North Oak
Marshfield, WI 54449
Phone: 715-387-5245
Medical College of Wisconsin
Koss Cochlear Implant Program
9200 W Wisconsin Ave
Milwaukee, WI 53226
Phone: 414-805-5586
Milwaukee Otologic
Forest View Bldg
11035 W Forest Home Ave.
Hales Corner, WI 53130
Phone: 414-529-3215
University of Wisconsin Hospital and Clinics
F4/262 600 Highland Ave
Madison, WI 53792
Phone: 608-263-6197

WEST VIRGINIA
Huntington Ear Nose & Throat
1616 13th Avenue, Suite 100
Huntington, WV 25701
Phone: 304-522-8800
Tri State Otolaryngology
#3 Stonecrest Dr
Huntington, WV 25701
Phone: 304-522-6388
West Virginia University School of Medicine
Physicians Office Center
Box 782, Audiology
Morgantown, WV 26507-0782
Phone: 304-293-3457

476

Index

Dominant inheritance 46

E

Enlarged Vestibular Aqueduct Syndrome 142
enlarged vestibular aqueducts 125
epidemiology 45

F

FDA Advisory Panel 50

G

genes for deafness 44
genetic research 45

H

hair cell regeneration 47
head injury 177
hearing impairment 46
Helen Beebe Speech and Hearing Center 120, 186
hereditary hearing loss 44

J

John Tracy Clinic 430
John Tracy Clinic correspondence course 152
Journal of Otology and Neurotology 18

L

labrynthitis 153
League for the Hard of Hearing 430
Lymphatic Highdrops 352

M

macular degeneration 397
Mapping 6
Meniere's disease 179
meningitis 50
MRI 5

N

newborn hearing screening 142
NIDCD 44

noise-induced hearing loss 46
non-syndromic hearing loss 44

O

oral motor apraxia 188
oral/aural 51
ossification 323
Journal of the American Medical Association 16

P

pediatric cochlear implant studies 17
plasticity 20
Programming of cochlear implant 77
progressive hearing loss 45

R

Receiver 3

S

Self Help for Hard of Hearing People, Inc. 431
Sensioneural hearing loss 2, 155
Sign Exact English 97
Speech processor 4
Surgery 6

T

The Listening Center at John Hopkins University 431
"TORCH" syndrome 145
Total Communication 94

V

vertigo 373
vibrotactile cues 186